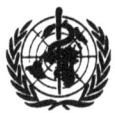

WORLD HEALTH ORGANIZATION

INTERNATIONAL AGENCY FOR RESEARCH ON CANCER

IARC MONOGRAPHS

ON THE

EVALUATION OF CARCINOGENIC RISKS TO HUMANS

Surgical Implants and Other Foreign Bodies

VOLUME 74

This publication represents the views and expert opinions
of an IARC Working Group on the
Evaluation of Carcinogenic Risks to Humans,
which met in Lyon,

23 February–2 March 1999

1999

IARC MONOGRAPHS

In 1969, the International Agency for Research on Cancer (IARC) initiated a programme on the evaluation of the carcinogenic risk of chemicals to humans involving the production of critically evaluated monographs on individual chemicals. The programme was subsequently expanded to include evaluations of carcinogenic risks associated with exposures to complex mixtures, life-style factors and biological agents, as well as those in specific occupations.

The objective of the programme is to elaborate and publish in the form of monographs critical reviews of data on carcinogenicity for agents to which humans are known to be exposed and on specific exposure situations; to evaluate these data in terms of human risk with the help of international working groups of experts in chemical carcinogenesis and related fields; and to indicate where additional research efforts are needed.

The lists of IARC evaluations are regularly updated and are available on Internet: http://www.iarc.fr/

This project was supported by Cooperative Agreement 5 UO1 CA33193 awarded by the United States National Cancer Institute, Department of Health and Human Services. Additional support has been provided since 1986 by the European Commission, since 1993 by the United States National Institute of Environmental Health Sciences and since 1995 by the United States Environmental Protection Agency through Cooperative Agreement Assistance CR 824264.

©International Agency for Research on Cancer, 1999

Distributed by IARC*Press* (Fax: +33 4 72 73 83 02; E-mail: press@iarc.fr)
and by the World Health Organization Distribution and Sales, CH-1211 Geneva 27
(Fax: +41 22 791 4857; E-mail: publications@who.int)

Publications of the World Health Organization enjoy copyright protection in accordance with the provisions of Protocol 2 of the Universal Copyright Convention.

All rights reserved. Application for rights of reproduction or translation, in part or *in toto*, should be made to the International Agency for Research on Cancer.

IARC Library Cataloguing in Publication Data

Surgical implants and other foreign bodies /
    IARC Working Group on the Evaluation of Carcinogenic Risks to Humans
    (1999 : Lyon, France)

(IARC monographs on the evaluation of carcinogenic risks to humans ; 74)

1. Foreign bodies – adverse effects 2. Foreign bodies – congresses
3. Implants, artificial – adverse effects 4. Implants, artificial – congresses
I. IARC Working Group on the Evaluation of Carcinogenic Risks to Humans
II. Series

ISBN 92 832 1274 6   (NLM Classification: W1)
ISSN 1017-1606

PRINTED IN FRANCE

CONTENTS

NOTE TO THE READER 1

LIST OF PARTICIPANTS 3

PREAMBLE 9
   Background 9
   Objective and Scope 9
   Selection of Topics for Monographs 10
   Data for Monographs 11
   The Working Group 11
   Working Procedures 11
   Exposure Data 12
   Studies of Cancer in Humans 14
   Studies of Cancer in Experimental Animals 17
   Other Data Relevant to an Evaluation of Carcinogenicity
      and its Mechanisms 20
   Summary of Data Reported 22
   Evaluation 23
   References 27

THE MONOGRAPH 33
   Introduction 35
   1. Scope of the monograph 35
   2. Host–biomaterial interactions as related to carcinogenesis 37
         2.1 Variables of the material or object 38
              2.1.1 Intrinsic chemistry 38
              2.1.2 Surface chemistry 38
              2.1.3 Chemical nature of any released soluble components 39
              2.1.4 Chemical or crystallographic nature of any released
                      particulate components 39
              2.1.5 Physical nature of any released particulate components 40
              2.1.6 Size and shape 40
              2.1.7 Surface energy and surface topography 41
              2.1.8 Hardness of the material, its elastic moduli or the
                      flexibility of the component 41
              2.1.9 Electrical or magnetic properties of the material 41

		2.1.10	Radioactivity 42
		2.1.11	Sterilization procedures 42
	2.2	Host variables 42	
		2.2.1	Species and strain 42
		2.2.2	Age, sex and size of the animal.. 42
		2.2.3	Site of implantation 43
		2.2.4	Known risk factors for human cancer 43
		2.2.5	Pharmacological status of a human host 43
		2.2.6	Indication for clinical intervention and prior or coexistent disease 43
		2.2.7	Latent period for tumour formation.................................... 43
	2.3	Host–material system 44	
3.	General mechanisms of solid-state carcinogenesis............................... 45		
	3.1	Experimental implants in rodents... 46	
4.	Pathology of sarcomas, reactive and pseudoneoplastic conditions 49		
	4.1	Introduction 49	
	4.2	Incidence and etiology 49	
	4.3	Classification 51	
	4.4	Behaviour, grading and staging 53	
	4.5	Pseudosarcomas and reactive conditions 54	
		4.5.1	Reactions to injury.. 54
		4.5.2	Reactions to foreign material.. 59
5.	General issues in epidemiological research on implants and cancer 60		
	5.1	Identification and selection of study population 61	
	5.2	Latency and length of follow-up 62	
	5.3	Statistical power 62	
	5.4	Exposure classification.. 62	
	5.5	Multiple hypothesis testing... 62	
	5.6	Control for confounding influences 63	

1.	**Exposure data** 65			
	1A.	METALLIC MEDICAL AND DENTAL MATERIALS 65		
		1A.1	Chemical and physical data 65	
			1A.1.1	Metallurgy 65
			1A.1.2	Chemical composition of metals and alloys 67
			1A.1.3	Chemical composition of dental casting alloys 75
			1A.1.4	Dental amalgam 81
			1A.1.5	Orthodontic metallic materials 81
			1A.1.6	Analytical methods... 81
		1A.2	Production 82	

1B.	NON-METALLIC MEDICAL AND DENTAL MATERIALS		84
	1B.1	Chemical and physical data	84
		1B.1.1 Polymer chemistry	84
		1B.1.2 Synthesis and composition of polymers	85
		1B.1.3 Ceramics	98
		1B.1.4 Composite materials	99
	1B.2	Production and use	99
		1B.2.1 Production	99
		1B.2.2 Use	101
1C.	COMPOSITE MEDICAL AND DENTAL IMPLANTS		102
	1C.1	Description of devices	102
		1C.1.1 Generic orthopaedic joint replacements	102
		1C.1.2 Orthopaedic fracture fixation devices	103
		1C.1.3 Cardiovascular devices	104
		1C.1.4 Dental materials	104
	1C.2	Numbers of implants used	105
	1C.3	Regulations and guidelines	107
1D.	OTHER FOREIGN BODIES		109
	1D.1	Introduction	109
	1D.2	Bullets and pellets	109
	1D.3	Shell fragments	110

2. **Studies of cancer in humans** 113
- 2A. METALLIC MEDICAL AND DENTAL MATERIALS 113
  - 2A.1 Case reports 113
  - 2A.2 Analytical studies..113
- 2B. NON-METALLIC MEDICAL AND DENTAL MATERIALS 118
  - 2B.1 Case reports 118
    - 2B.1.1 Cancer following silicone implants for the breast ..118
    - 2B.1.2 Sarcomas at the site of vascular grafts 118
  - 2B.2 Analytical studies..118
    - 2B.2.1 Cohort studies...118
    - 2B.2.2 Case–control studies..130
- 2C. COMPOSITE MEDICAL AND DENTAL IMPLANTS 132
  - 2C.1 Case reports 132
    - 2C.1.1 Orthopaedic implants 132
    - 2C.1.2 Cardiac pacemakers 132
  - 2C.2 Analytical studies..146
    - 2C.2.1 Orthopaedic implants 146
      - (a) Cohort studies..146
      - (b) Case–control studies...161

2D. OTHER FOREIGN BODIES 162
    2D.1 Metallic foreign bodies 162
    2D.2 Non-metallic foreign bodies 162

3. **Studies of cancer in animals seen in veterinary practice** 173
   3.1 Dogs 173
      3.1.1 Case reports 173
      3.1.2 Analytical studies...173
   3.2 Cats 173
      3.2.1 Case reports 173
      3.2.2 Case series 176
      3.2.3 Analytical studies...177

4. **Studies of cancer in experimental animals** 179
   4A. METALLIC MEDICAL AND DENTAL MATERIALS 179
      4A.1 Metallic chromium..179
          4A.1.1 Intrapleural administration 179
          4A.1.2 Intramuscular administration 179
          4A.1.3 Intraperitoneal administration 179
          4A.1.4 Intravenous administration...180
          4A.1.5 Intrarenal administration 180
          4A.1.6 Intraosseous administration 181
      4A.2 Metallic cobalt 181
          4A.2.1 Intramuscular administration 181
          4A.2.2 Intrarenal administration 182
          4A.2.3 Intrathoracic administration 182
          4A.2.4 Intraosseous administration 183
      4A.3 Metallic nickel 183
          4A.3.1 Inhalation exposure 183
          4A.3.2 Intratracheal administration 184
          4A.3.3 Intrapleural administration 184
          4A.3.4 Subcutaneous administration 184
          4A.3.5 Intramuscular administration 185
          4A.3.6 Intraperitoneal administration 185
          4A.3.7 Intraosseous administration 186
          4A.3.8 Intrarenal administration 186
          4A.3.9 Intravenous administration...186
      4A.4 Metallic titanium 186
          4A.4.1 Intramuscular administration 186
          4A.4.2 Intraosseous administration 187
      4A.5 Metallic foils 187
          4A.5.1 Subcutaneous administration 187

		4A.5.2	Intraperitoneal administration 187
	4A.6	Metal alloys 188
		4A.6.1	Intratracheal administration 188
		4A.6.2	Intrabronchial administration 194
		4A.6.3	Subcutaneous administration 194
		4A.6.4	Intramuscular administration 194
		4A.6.5	Intraperitoneal administration 196
		4A.6.6	Intrarenal administration 196
		4A.6.7	Intraosseous administration 197
		4A.6.8	Intra-articular administration 197
		4A.6.9	Implantation of ear tags 198
4B.	NON-METALLIC MEDICAL AND DENTAL MATERIALS 198
	4B.1	Polydimethylsiloxanes (silicones) 198
		4B.1.1	Subcutaneous administration 198
		4B.1.2	Intraperitoneal administration 199
		4B.1.3	Intraosseous implantation 200
	4B.2	Polyurethane 200
		4B.2.1	Subcutaneous and/or intraperitoneal administration 200
		4B.2.2	Inhalation and/or intratracheal or intrabronchial administration 204
	4B.3	Poly(methyl methacrylate) 205
		4B.3.1	Subcutaneous and/or intramuscular administration 205
		4B.3.2	Intraperitoneal administration 207
		4B.3.3	Other experimental systems 207
	4B.4	Poly(2-hydroxyethyl methacrylate) 208
		4B.4.1	Subcutaneous administration 208
	4B.5	Poly(ethylene terephthalate) 208
		4B.5.1	Subcutaneous administration 208
	4B.6	Polyethylene 209
		4B.6.1	Subcutaneous administration 209
		4B.6.2	Intraperitoneal administration 211
		4B.6.3	Other experimental systems 212
	4B.7	Polypropylene 212
		4B.7.1	Subcutaneous administration 212
	4B.8	Polytetrafluoroethylene 213
		4B.8.1	Subcutaneous administration 213
		4B.8.2	Intraperitoneal administration 215
	4B.9	Polyamide (nylon) 215
		4B.9.1	Subcutaneous administration 215
		4B.9.2	Intraperitoneal administration 215

		4B.10	Poly(glycolic acid)	216
			4B.10.1 Subcutaneous administration	216
		4B.11	Polylactide	216
			4B.11.1 Subcutaneous administration	216
		4B.12	ε-Caprolactone-L-lactide copolymer	216
			4B.12.1 Subcutaneous administration	216
		4B.13	Polystyrene and related polymers	217
			4B.13.1 Subcutaneous administration	217
		4B.14	Poly(vinyl alcohol)	218
			4B.14.1 Subcutaneous administration	218
		4B.15	Poly(vinyl chloride)	219
			4B.15.1 Subcutaneous administration	219
			4B.15.2 Other routes of administration	220
		4B.16	Vinyl chloride–vinyl acetate copolymer	220
			4B.16.1 Subcutaneous administration	220
		4B.17	Cellophane	221
			4B.17.1 Subcutaneous administration	221
			4B.17.2 Other experimental systems	222
		4B.18	Millipore filters	223
			4B.18.1 Subcutaneous administration	223
			4B.18.2 Intraperitoneal administration	224
		4B.19	Epoxy resins	224
			4B.19.1 Subcutaneous administration	224
		4B.20	Aluminium oxide ceramics	224
			4B.20.1 Subcutaneous administration	224
		4B.21	Glass sheet	224
			4B.21.1 Subcutaneous administration	224
		4B.22	Major factors that affect tumour incidence	225
			4B.22.1 Physical factors	225
			4B.22.2 Chemical factors	227
	4C.	COMPOSITE MEDICAL AND DENTAL IMPLANTS		228
	4D.	OTHER FOREIGN BODIES		229
5.	Other data relevant to an evaluation of carcinogenicity and its mechanisms			231
	5A.	METALLIC MEDICAL AND DENTAL MATERIALS		231
		5A.1	Degradation of metallic implants in biological systems	231
			5A.1.1 Mechanisms of degradation	231
			5A.1.2 In-vitro corrosion of dental alloys	232
		5A.2	Absorption, distribution and excretion	233
			5A.2.1 Humans	234
			5A.2.2 Experimental systems	235

		5A.3	Tissue responses and other expressions of toxicity 237

- 5A.3 Tissue responses and other expressions of toxicity 237
  - 5A.3.1 Humans..237
    - (a) Inflammatory and immunological responses ..237
    - (b) Oral contact lichenoid reactions......................238
    - (c) Allergic reactions 239
  - 5A.3.2 Experimental systems..240
    - (a) Animal studies 240
    - (b) Cytotoxicity of metal ions 241
    - (c) Cytotoxicity of metallic materials 242
    - (d) Effects of metal ions and metallic materials on cytokine levels and histamine release 242
- 5A.4 Genetic and related effects..242
  - 5A.4.1 Humans..242
  - 5A.4.2 Experimental systems..243
- 5A.5 Mechanisms of carcinogenic action..245

5B. NON-METALLIC MEDICAL AND DENTAL MATERIALS 245
- 5B.1 Degradation, distribution, metabolism and excretion 245
  - 5B.1.1 Humans..245
    - (a) Degradation of polyurethane foam..................245
    - (b) Wear of dental composites 248
  - 5B.1.2 Experimental systems..249
    - (a) Polyurethane-coated breast implants 249
    - (b) Other polyurethane implants 250
    - (c) Polydimethylsiloxanes (silicones) 251
    - (d) Degradable polymers 252
    - (e) Substances released from dental composites ..253
- 5B.2 Tissue responses and other expressions of toxicity 255
  - 5B.2.1. Humans..255
    - (a) Polydimethylsiloxanes (silicones) 255
    - (b) Polyurethane-coated breast implants 257
    - (c) Polytetrafluoroethylene implants 257
    - (d) Joint replacements, polyethylene and bone cement 257
    - (e) Dental materials 258
  - 5B.2.2 Experimental systems..263
    - (a) Inflammatory, hyperplastic and metaplastic responses..263
      - (i) Polydimethylsiloxanes (silicones) 263
      - (ii) Polyurethanes 264
      - (iii) Polyethylene..265
      - (iv) Polytetrafluoroethylene 266
      - (v) Acrylic substances 266

		(vi)	Ceramics, hydroxylapatite 267
		(vii)	Dental composites 268
		(viii)	Components of dental composites 270
		(ix)	Other materials 275
	(b)	Immunological effects 275
		(i)	Polydimethylsiloxanes (silicones) 275
		(ii)	Other materials 276
5B.3	Genetic and related effects 277
	5B.3.1	Humans 277
	5B.3.2	Experimental systems 277
		(a) In-vitro genotoxicity assays 277
		(b) Cell transformation test 280
		(c) In-vivo genotoxicity assays 281
		(d) Cytogenetic effects in tumour cells 282
5B.4	Mechanistic considerations of implantation-site sarcomagenesis in rodents 282
	5B.4.1	Major features that affect tumour incidence in solid-state carcinogenesis 282
	5B.4.2	Biological factors 282
		(a) Fibrous tissue capsule formation and continued presence of implant 282
		(b) The role of perforation in the reduction of tumorigenicity 283
		(c) Species and strain differences 283
	5B.4.3	Timing and location of preneoplastic events 284
	5B.4.4	Origin of preneoplastic parent cells 286
	5B.4.5	Stages in foreign-body tumorigenesis 287
	5B.4.6	Other data on the role of capsule and implant on tumour promotion/progression 288
		(a) Different roles of an implant during early and late stages of carcinogenesis 288
		(b) Promotion by an implant of subcutaneous carcinogenesis initiated by irradiation or a chemical carcinogen 289
	5B.4.7	Effect of different implant materials on inhibition of gap-junctional intercellular communication as an index of tumour promotion 290
	5B.4.8	What initiates the formation of preneoplastic parent cells? 293
	5B.4.9	Possible genotoxic mechanisms underlying solid-state carcinogenesis 294

5C.	OTHER FOREIGN BODIES		297
	5C.1	Degradation in biological systems	297
	5C.2	Distribution and excretion	297
		5C.2.1 Lead	297
		(a) Humans	297
		(b) Experimental systems	298
		5C.2.2 Depleted uranium	298
		(a) Humans	298
		(b) Experimental systems	299
	5.C.3	Tissue responses and other expressions of toxicity	300
		5C.3.1 Lead	300
		5C.3.2 Depleted uranium	300
	5C.4	Genetic and related effects	301
		5C.4.1 Lead	301
		5C.4.2 Depleted uranium	301

6. Summary of data reported and evaluation 303
    6.1 Exposure data 303
    6.2 Human carcinogenicity data 304
    6.3 Veterinary studies 305
    6.4 Animal carcinogenicity data 306
    6.5 Other relevant data 308
    6.6 Evaluation 309

Appendix 313
    Asbestos fibres 313
    Crystalline silica 317
    Poorly soluble particulates (PSPs) or low-toxicity dusts 319
    Relevance of these mechanisms for evaluation of the carcinogenicity
        of surgical implants and prosthetic devices 320

References 323

CUMULATIVE INDEX TO THE MONOGRAPHS SERIES 377

NOTE TO THE READER

The term 'carcinogenic risk' in the *IARC Monographs* series is taken to mean the probability that exposure to an agent will lead to cancer in humans.

Inclusion of an agent in the *Monographs* does not imply that it is a carcinogen, only that the published data have been examined. Equally, the fact that an agent has not yet been evaluated in a monograph does not mean that it is not carcinogenic.

The evaluations of carcinogenic risk are made by international working groups of independent scientists and are qualitative in nature. No recommendation is given for regulation or legislation.

Anyone who is aware of published data that may alter the evaluation of the carcinogenic risk of an agent to humans is encouraged to make this information available to the Unit of Carcinogen Identification and Evaluation, International Agency for Research on Cancer, 150 cours Albert Thomas, 69372 Lyon Cedex 08, France, in order that the agent may be considered for re-evaluation by a future Working Group.

Although every effort is made to prepare the monographs as accurately as possible, mistakes may occur. Readers are requested to communicate any errors to the Unit of Carcinogen Identification and Evaluation, so that corrections can be reported in future volumes.

IARC WORKING GROUP ON THE EVALUATION OF CARCINOGENIC RISKS TO HUMANS: SURGICAL IMPLANTS AND OTHER FOREIGN BODIES

Lyon, 23 February–2 March 1999

LIST OF PARTICIPANTS

Members

J. Boice, International Epidemiology Institute, Ltd, 1550 Research Boulevard, Suite 200, Rockville, MD 20850, United States

S.A. Brown, Division of Mechanics and Materials Science, Office of Science and Technology, Center for Devices and Radiological Health, Food and Drug Administration, 9200 Corporate Boulevard, HFZ-150, Rockville, MD 20852, United States

J.A. Centeno, Biophysical Toxicology Branch, Department of Environmental and Toxicologic Pathology, Armed Forces Institute of Pathology, Building 54, Room M099A, 14th Street and Alaska Avenue, N.W., Washington, DC 20306-6000, United States

J.E. Dahl, Scandinavian Institute of Dental Materials, Kirkeveien 71B, PO Box 70, 1305 Haslum, Norway

C. Fisher, Department of Histopathology, The Royal Marsden National Health Service Trust, 203 Fulham Road, London SW3 6JJ, United Kingdom

J.E. Garcia, Biomaterials and Engineering Section, Therapeutic Goods Administration Laboratories, PO Box 100, Woden ACT 2606, Australia

W.J. Gillespie, Dunedin School of Medicine, University of Otago, PO Box 913, Dunedin, New Zealand (*Chairman*)

D. Gott, Implants and Materials Section, Medical Devices Agency, Department of Health, Hannibal House, London SE1 6TQ, United Kingdom

T. Hanawa, Biomaterials Research Team, National Research Institute for Metals, 1-2-1 Sengen, Tsukuba 305-0047, Japan

A. Hensten-Pettersen, Scandinavian Institute of Dental Materials, Kirkeveien 71B, PO Box 70, 1305 Haslum, Norway

A.B. Kane, Brown University, Division of Biology and Medicine, Department of Pathology and Laboratory Medicine, Box G-B511, Providence, RI 02912, United States

H. Kappert, Laboratory for Experimental Dentistry and Dental Material, University of Freiburg, Hugstetter Strasse 55, 79106 Freiburg i. Breisgau, Germany

D. Macy, Comparative Oncology, Colorado State University, Veterinary Teaching Hospital, Fort Collins, CO 80523, United States

D. Marzin, Laboratory of Toxicology, Institut Pasteur de Lille, 1 rue du Professeur Calmette, BP 245, 59019 Lille Cedex, France

J. McLaughlin, International Epidemiology Institute, Ltd, 1550 Research Boulevard, Suite 200, Rockville, MD 20850, United States

A. Nakamura, Division of Medical Devices, National Institute of Health Sciences, 1-18-1 Kamiyoga, Setagaya-ku, Tokyo 158, Japan

O. Nyrén, Department of Medical Epidemiology, Karolinska Institute, PO Box 281, 17177 Stockholm, Sweden

S. Olin, International Life Sciences Institute, Risk Science Institute, 1126 Sixteenth Street NW, Washington, DC 20036, United States

F.W. Sunderman, Jr, 270 Barnes Road, Whiting, VT 05778-4411, United States

J. Tinkler, Implants and Materials Section, Medical Devices Agency, Department of Health, Hannibal House, London SE1 6TQ, United Kingdom

P. Toniolo, Department of Obstetrics and Gynecology, New York University School of Medicine, Room NB9E2, 550 First Avenue, New York, NY 10016, United States

T. Tsuchiya, Division of Medical Devices, National Institute of Health Sciences, 1-18-1 Kamiyoga, Setagaya-ku, Tokyo 158, Japan

T. Visuri, Central Military Hospital, PO Box 50, 00301 Helsinki, Finland

D.F. Williams, Department of Clinical Engineering, Duncan Building, Royal Liverpool University Hospital, Liverpool L69 3GA, United Kingdom

Observer

School of Dentistry, University of Vienna

A. Schedle, School of Dentistry, University of Vienna, Währingerstrasse 25a, 1090 Vienna, Austria

IARC Secretariat

R. Baan, Unit of Carcinogen Identification and Evaluation
M. Blettner[1], Unit of Carcinogen Identification and Evaluation
P. Boffetta, Unit of Environmental Cancer Epidemiology
J. Cheney (*Editor*)
M. Friesen, Unit of Gene–Environment Interactions
C. Genevois-Charmeau, Unit of Carcinogen Identification and Evaluation
Y. Grosse, Unit of Carcinogen Identification and Evaluation
C. Malaveille, Unit of Endogenous Cancer Risk Factors

---

[1] Present address: Department of Epidemiology and Medical Statistics, School of Public Health, Postfach 100131, 33501 Bielefeld, Germany

PARTICIPANTS

D. McGregor, Unit of Carcinogen Identification and Evaluation (*Responsible Officer*)
M. Mesnil, Unit of Multistage Carcinogenesis
A.B. Miller[1], Unit of Chemoprevention
C. Partensky, Unit of Carcinogen Identification and Evaluation
J. Rice, Unit of Carcinogen Identification and Evaluation (*Head of Programme*)
R. Saracci, IARC, Emeritus
J. Wilbourn, Unit of Carcinogen Identification and Evaluation

Technical assistance
M. Lézère
A. Meneghel
D. Mietton
J. Mitchell
S. Reynaud
S. Ruiz

---

[1] Present address: Department of Epidemiology, German Cancer Research Center, Im Neuenheimer Feld 280, 69120 Heidelberg, Germany

PREAMBLE

IARC MONOGRAPHS PROGRAMME ON THE EVALUATION OF CARCINOGENIC RISKS TO HUMANS

PREAMBLE

1. BACKGROUND

In 1969, the International Agency for Research on Cancer (IARC) initiated a programme to evaluate the carcinogenic risk of chemicals to humans and to produce monographs on individual chemicals. The *Monographs* programme has since been expanded to include consideration of exposures to complex mixtures of chemicals (which occur, for example, in some occupations and as a result of human habits) and of exposures to other agents, such as radiation and viruses. With Supplement 6 (IARC, 1987a), the title of the series was modified from *IARC Monographs on the Evaluation of the Carcinogenic Risk of Chemicals to Humans* to *IARC Monographs on the Evaluation of Carcinogenic Risks to Humans*, in order to reflect the widened scope of the programme.

The criteria established in 1971 to evaluate carcinogenic risk to humans were adopted by the working groups whose deliberations resulted in the first 16 volumes of the *IARC Monographs series*. Those criteria were subsequently updated by further ad-hoc working groups (IARC, 1977, 1978, 1979, 1982, 1983, 1987b, 1988, 1991a; Vainio *et al.*, 1992).

2. OBJECTIVE AND SCOPE

The objective of the programme is to prepare, with the help of international working groups of experts, and to publish in the form of monographs, critical reviews and evaluations of evidence on the carcinogenicity of a wide range of human exposures. The *Monographs* may also indicate where additional research efforts are needed.

The *Monographs* represent the first step in carcinogenic risk assessment, which involves examination of all relevant information in order to assess the strength of the available evidence that certain exposures could alter the incidence of cancer in humans. The second step is quantitative risk estimation. Detailed, quantitative evaluations of epidemiological data may be made in the *Monographs*, but without extrapolation beyond the range of the data available. Quantitative extrapolation from experimental data to the human situation is not undertaken.

The term 'carcinogen' is used in these monographs to denote an exposure that is capable of increasing the incidence of malignant neoplasms; the induction of benign neoplasms may in some circumstances (see p. 19) contribute to the judgement that the exposure is carcinogenic. The terms 'neoplasm' and 'tumour' are used interchangeably.

Some epidemiological and experimental studies indicate that different agents may act at different stages in the carcinogenic process, and several mechanisms may be involved. The aim of the *Monographs* has been, from their inception, to evaluate evidence of carcinogenicity at any stage in the carcinogenesis process, independently of the underlying mechanisms. Information on mechanisms may, however, be used in making the overall evaluation (IARC, 1991a; Vainio *et al.*, 1992; see also pp. 25–27).

The *Monographs* may assist national and international authorities in making risk assessments and in formulating decisions concerning any necessary preventive measures. The evaluations of IARC working groups are scientific, qualitative judgements about the evidence for or against carcinogenicity provided by the available data. These evaluations represent only one part of the body of information on which regulatory measures may be based. Other components of regulatory decisions vary from one situation to another and from country to country, responding to different socioeconomic and national priorities. **Therefore, no recommendation is given with regard to regulation or legislation, which are the responsibility of individual governments and/or other international organizations.**

The *IARC Monographs* are recognized as an authoritative source of information on the carcinogenicity of a wide range of human exposures. A survey of users in 1988 indicated that the *Monographs* are consulted by various agencies in 57 countries. About 3000 copies of each volume are printed, for distribution to governments, regulatory bodies and interested scientists. The Monographs are also available from IARC*Press* in Lyon and via the Distribution and Sales Service of the World Health Organization in Geneva.

3. SELECTION OF TOPICS FOR MONOGRAPHS

Topics are selected on the basis of two main criteria: (a) there is evidence of human exposure, and (b) there is some evidence or suspicion of carcinogenicity. The term 'agent' is used to include individual chemical compounds, groups of related chemical compounds, physical agents (such as radiation) and biological factors (such as viruses). Exposures to mixtures of agents may occur in occupational exposures and as a result of personal and cultural habits (like smoking and dietary practices). Chemical analogues and compounds with biological or physical characteristics similar to those of suspected carcinogens may also be considered, even in the absence of data on a possible carcinogenic effect in humans or experimental animals.

The scientific literature is surveyed for published data relevant to an assessment of carcinogenicity. The IARC information bulletins on agents being tested for carcinogenicity (IARC, 1973–1996) and directories of on-going research in cancer epidemiology (IARC, 1976–1996) often indicate exposures that may be scheduled for future meetings. Ad-hoc working groups convened by IARC in 1984, 1989, 1991, 1993 and 1998 gave recommendations as to which agents should be evaluated in the IARC Monographs series (IARC, 1984, 1989, 1991b, 1993, 1998a,b).

As significant new data on subjects on which monographs have already been prepared become available, re-evaluations are made at subsequent meetings, and revised monographs are published.

4. DATA FOR MONOGRAPHS

The *Monographs* do not necessarily cite all the literature concerning the subject of an evaluation. Only those data considered by the Working Group to be relevant to making the evaluation are included.

With regard to biological and epidemiological data, only reports that have been published or accepted for publication in the openly available scientific literature are reviewed by the working groups. In certain instances, government agency reports that have undergone peer review and are widely available are considered. Exceptions may be made on an ad-hoc basis to include unpublished reports that are in their final form and publicly available, if their inclusion is considered pertinent to making a final evaluation (see pp. 25–27). In the sections on chemical and physical properties, on analysis, on production and use and on occurrence, unpublished sources of information may be used.

5. THE WORKING GROUP

Reviews and evaluations are formulated by a working group of experts. The tasks of the group are: (i) to ascertain that all appropriate data have been collected; (ii) to select the data relevant for the evaluation on the basis of scientific merit; (iii) to prepare accurate summaries of the data to enable the reader to follow the reasoning of the Working Group; (iv) to evaluate the results of epidemiological and experimental studies on cancer; (v) to evaluate data relevant to the understanding of mechanism of action; and (vi) to make an overall evaluation of the carcinogenicity of the exposure to humans.

Working Group participants who contributed to the considerations and evaluations within a particular volume are listed, with their addresses, at the beginning of each publication. Each participant who is a member of a working group serves as an individual scientist and not as a representative of any organization, government or industry. In addition, nominees of national and international agencies and industrial associations may be invited as observers.

6. WORKING PROCEDURES

Approximately one year in advance of a meeting of a working group, the topics of the monographs are announced and participants are selected by IARC staff in consultation with other experts. Subsequently, relevant biological and epidemiological data are collected by the Carcinogen Identification and Evaluation Unit of IARC from recognized sources of information on carcinogenesis, including data storage and retrieval systems such as MEDLINE and TOXLINE.

For chemicals and some complex mixtures, the major collection of data and the preparation of first drafts of the sections on chemical and physical properties, on analysis, on production and use and on occurrence are carried out under a separate contract funded by the United States National Cancer Institute. Representatives from industrial associations may assist in the preparation of sections on production and use. Information on production and trade is obtained from governmental and trade publications and, in some cases, by direct contact with industries. Separate production data on some agents may not be available because their publication could disclose confidential information. Information on uses may be obtained from published sources but is often complemented by direct contact with manufacturers. Efforts are made to supplement this information with data from other national and international sources.

Six months before the meeting, the material obtained is sent to meeting participants, or is used by IARC staff, to prepare sections for the first drafts of monographs. The first drafts are compiled by IARC staff and sent before the meeting to all participants of the Working Group for review.

The Working Group meets in Lyon for seven to eight days to discuss and finalize the texts of the monographs and to formulate the evaluations. After the meeting, the master copy of each monograph is verified by consulting the original literature, edited and prepared for publication. The aim is to publish monographs within six months of the Working Group meeting.

The available studies are summarized by the Working Group, with particular regard to the qualitative aspects discussed below. In general, numerical findings are indicated as they appear in the original report; units are converted when necessary for easier comparison. The Working Group may conduct additional analyses of the published data and use them in their assessment of the evidence; the results of such supplementary analyses are given in square brackets. When an important aspect of a study, directly impinging on its interpretation, should be brought to the attention of the reader, a comment is given in square brackets.

7. EXPOSURE DATA

Sections that indicate the extent of past and present human exposure, the sources of exposure, the people most likely to be exposed and the factors that contribute to the exposure are included at the beginning of each monograph.

Most monographs on individual chemicals, groups of chemicals or complex mixtures include sections on chemical and physical data, on analysis, on production and use and on occurrence. In monographs on, for example, physical agents, occupational exposures and cultural habits, other sections may be included, such as: historical perspectives, description of an industry or habit, chemistry of the complex mixture or taxonomy. Monographs on biological agents have sections on structure and biology, methods of detection, epidemiology of infection and clinical disease other than cancer.

For chemical exposures, the Chemical Abstracts Services Registry Number, the latest Chemical Abstracts Primary Name and the IUPAC Systematic Name are recorded; other synonyms are given, but the list is not necessarily comprehensive. For biological agents, taxonomy and structure are described, and the degree of variability is given, when applicable.

Information on chemical and physical properties and, in particular, data relevant to identification, occurrence and biological activity are included. For biological agents, mode of replication, life cycle, target cells, persistence and latency and host response are given. A description of technical products of chemicals includes trade names, relevant specifications and available information on composition and impurities. Some of the trade names given may be those of mixtures in which the agent being evaluated is only one of the ingredients.

The purpose of the section on analysis or detection is to give the reader an overview of current methods, with emphasis on those widely used for regulatory purposes. Methods for monitoring human exposure are also given, when available. No critical evaluation or recommendation of any of the methods is meant or implied. The IARC published a series of volumes, *Environmental Carcinogens: Methods of Analysis and Exposure Measurement* (IARC, 1978–93), that describe validated methods for analysing a wide variety of chemicals and mixtures. For biological agents, methods of detection and exposure assessment are described, including their sensitivity, specificity and reproducibility.

The dates of first synthesis and of first commercial production of a chemical or mixture are provided; for agents which do not occur naturally, this information may allow a reasonable estimate to be made of the date before which no human exposure to the agent could have occurred. The dates of first reported occurrence of an exposure are also provided. In addition, methods of synthesis used in past and present commercial production and different methods of production which may give rise to different impurities are described.

Data on production, international trade and uses are obtained for representative regions, which usually include Europe, Japan and the United States of America. It should not, however, be inferred that those areas or nations are necessarily the sole or major sources or users of the agent. Some identified uses may not be current or major applications, and the coverage is not necessarily comprehensive. In the case of drugs, mention of their therapeutic uses does not necessarily represent current practice, nor does it imply judgement as to their therapeutic efficacy.

Information on the occurrence of an agent or mixture in the environment is obtained from data derived from the monitoring and surveillance of levels in occupational environments, air, water, soil, foods and animal and human tissues. When available, data on the generation, persistence and bioaccumulation of the agent are also included. In the case of mixtures, industries, occupations or processes, information is given about all agents present. For processes, industries and occupations, a historical description is also given, noting variations in chemical composition, physical properties and levels of occupational exposure with time and place. For biological agents, the epidemiology of infection is described.

Statements concerning regulations and guidelines (e.g., pesticide registrations, maximal levels permitted in foods, occupational exposure limits) are included for some countries as indications of potential exposures, but they may not reflect the most recent situation, since such limits are continuously reviewed and modified. The absence of information on regulatory status for a country should not be taken to imply that that country does not have regulations with regard to the exposure. For biological agents, legislation and control, including vaccines and therapy, are described.

8. STUDIES OF CANCER IN HUMANS

(a) Types of studies considered

Three types of epidemiological studies of cancer contribute to the assessment of carcinogenicity in humans—cohort studies, case–control studies and correlation (or ecological) studies. Rarely, results from randomized trials may be available. Case series and case reports of cancer in humans may also be reviewed.

Cohort and case–control studies relate the exposures under study to the occurrence of cancer in individuals and provide an estimate of relative risk (ratio of incidence or mortality in those exposed to incidence or mortality in those not exposed) as the main measure of association.

In correlation studies, the units of investigation are usually whole populations (e.g. in particular geographical areas or at particular times), and cancer frequency is related to a summary measure of the exposure of the population to the agent, mixture or exposure circumstance under study. Because individual exposure is not documented, however, a causal relationship is less easy to infer from correlation studies than from cohort and case–control studies. Case reports generally arise from a suspicion, based on clinical experience, that the concurrence of two events—that is, a particular exposure and occurrence of a cancer—has happened rather more frequently than would be expected by chance. Case reports usually lack complete ascertainment of cases in any population, definition or enumeration of the population at risk and estimation of the expected number of cases in the absence of exposure. The uncertainties surrounding interpretation of case reports and correlation studies make them inadequate, except in rare instances, to form the sole basis for inferring a causal relationship. When taken together with case–control and cohort studies, however, relevant case reports or correlation studies may add materially to the judgement that a causal relationship is present.

Epidemiological studies of benign neoplasms, presumed preneoplastic lesions and other end-points thought to be relevant to cancer are also reviewed by working groups. They may, in some instances, strengthen inferences drawn from studies of cancer itself.

(b) Quality of studies considered

The Monographs are not intended to summarize all published studies. Those that are judged to be inadequate or irrelevant to the evaluation are generally omitted. They may be mentioned briefly, particularly when the information is considered to be a useful supplement to that in other reports or when they provide the only data available. Their inclusion does not imply acceptance of the adequacy of the study design or of the analysis and interpretation of the results, and limitations are clearly outlined in square brackets at the end of the study description.

It is necessary to take into account the possible roles of bias, confounding and chance in the interpretation of epidemiological studies. By 'bias' is meant the operation of factors in study design or execution that lead erroneously to a stronger or weaker association than in fact exists between disease and an agent, mixture or exposure circumstance. By 'confounding' is meant a situation in which the relationship with disease is made to appear stronger or weaker than it truly is as a result of an association between the apparent causal factor and another factor that is associated with either an increase or decrease in the incidence of the disease. In evaluating the extent to which these factors have been minimized in an individual study, working groups consider a number of aspects of design and analysis as described in the report of the study. Most of these considerations apply equally to case–control, cohort and correlation studies. Lack of clarity of any of these aspects in the reporting of a study can decrease its credibility and the weight given to it in the final evaluation of the exposure.

Firstly, the study population, disease (or diseases) and exposure should have been well defined by the authors. Cases of disease in the study population should have been identified in a way that was independent of the exposure of interest, and exposure should have been assessed in a way that was not related to disease status.

Secondly, the authors should have taken account in the study design and analysis of other variables that can influence the risk of disease and may have been related to the exposure of interest. Potential confounding by such variables should have been dealt with either in the design of the study, such as by matching, or in the analysis, by statistical adjustment. In cohort studies, comparisons with local rates of disease may be more appropriate than those with national rates. Internal comparisons of disease frequency among individuals at different levels of exposure should also have been made in the study.

Thirdly, the authors should have reported the basic data on which the conclusions are founded, even if sophisticated statistical analyses were employed. At the very least, they should have given the numbers of exposed and unexposed cases and controls in a case–control study and the numbers of cases observed and expected in a cohort study. Further tabulations by time since exposure began and other temporal factors are also important. In a cohort study, data on all cancer sites and all causes of death should have been given, to reveal the possibility of reporting bias. In a case–control study, the effects of investigated factors other than the exposure of interest should have been reported.

Finally, the statistical methods used to obtain estimates of relative risk, absolute rates of cancer, confidence intervals and significance tests, and to adjust for confounding should have been clearly stated by the authors. The methods used should preferably have been the generally accepted techniques that have been refined since the mid-1970s. These methods have been reviewed for case–control studies (Breslow & Day, 1980) and for cohort studies (Breslow & Day, 1987).

(c) *Inferences about mechanism of action*

Detailed analyses of both relative and absolute risks in relation to temporal variables, such as age at first exposure, time since first exposure, duration of exposure, cumulative exposure and time since exposure ceased, are reviewed and summarized when available. The analysis of temporal relationships can be useful in formulating models of carcinogenesis. In particular, such analyses may suggest whether a carcinogen acts early or late in the process of carcinogenesis, although at best they allow only indirect inferences about the mechanism of action. Special attention is given to measurements of biological markers of carcinogen exposure or action, such as DNA or protein adducts, as well as markers of early steps in the carcinogenic process, such as proto-oncogene mutation, when these are incorporated into epidemiological studies focused on cancer incidence or mortality. Such measurements may allow inferences to be made about putative mechanisms of action (IARC, 1991a; Vainio *et al.*, 1992).

(d) *Criteria for causality*

After the individual epidemiological studies of cancer have been summarized and the quality assessed, a judgement is made concerning the strength of evidence that the agent, mixture or exposure circumstance in question is carcinogenic for humans. In making its judgement, the Working Group considers several criteria for causality. A strong association (a large relative risk) is more likely to indicate causality than a weak association, although it is recognized that relative risks of small magnitude do not imply lack of causality and may be important if the disease is common. Associations that are replicated in several studies of the same design or using different epidemiological approaches or under different circumstances of exposure are more likely to represent a causal relationship than isolated observations from single studies. If there are inconsistent results among investigations, possible reasons are sought (such as differences in amount of exposure), and results of studies judged to be of high quality are given more weight than those of studies judged to be methodologically less sound. When suspicion of carcinogenicity arises largely from a single study, these data are not combined with those from later studies in any subsequent reassessment of the strength of the evidence.

If the risk of the disease in question increases with the amount of exposure, this is considered to be a strong indication of causality, although absence of a graded response is not necessarily evidence against a causal relationship. Demonstration of a decline in risk after cessation of or reduction in exposure in individuals or in whole populations also supports a causal interpretation of the findings.

Although a carcinogen may act upon more than one target, the specificity of an association (an increased occurrence of cancer at one anatomical site or of one morphological type) adds plausibility to a causal relationship, particularly when excess cancer occurrence is limited to one morphological type within the same organ.

Although rarely available, results from randomized trials showing different rates among exposed and unexposed individuals provide particularly strong evidence for causality.

When several epidemiological studies show little or no indication of an association between an exposure and cancer, the judgement may be made that, in the aggregate, they show evidence of lack of carcinogenicity. Such a judgement requires first of all that the studies giving rise to it meet, to a sufficient degree, the standards of design and analysis described above. Specifically, the possibility that bias, confounding or misclassification of exposure or outcome could explain the observed results should be considered and excluded with reasonable certainty. In addition, all studies that are judged to be methodologically sound should be consistent with a relative risk of unity for any observed level of exposure and, when considered together, should provide a pooled estimate of relative risk which is at or near unity and has a narrow confidence interval, due to sufficient population size. Moreover, no individual study nor the pooled results of all the studies should show any consistent tendency for the relative risk of cancer to increase with increasing level of exposure. It is important to note that evidence of lack of carcinogenicity obtained in this way from several epidemiological studies can apply only to the type(s) of cancer studied and to dose levels and intervals between first exposure and observation of disease that are the same as or less than those observed in all the studies. Experience with human cancer indicates that, in some cases, the period from first exposure to the development of clinical cancer is seldom less than 20 years; latent periods substantially shorter than 30 years cannot provide evidence for lack of carcinogenicity.

9. STUDIES OF CANCER IN EXPERIMENTAL ANIMALS

All known human carcinogens that have been studied adequately in experimental animals have produced positive results in one or more animal species (Wilbourn *et al.*, 1986; Tomatis *et al.*, 1989). For several agents (aflatoxins, 4-aminobiphenyl, azathioprine, betel quid with tobacco, bischloromethyl ether and chloromethyl methyl ether (technical grade), chlorambucil, chlornaphazine, ciclosporin, coal-tar pitches, coal-tars, combined oral contraceptives, cyclophosphamide, diethylstilboestrol, melphalan, 8-methoxypsoralen plus ultraviolet A radiation, mustard gas, myleran, 2-naphthylamine, nonsteroidal oestrogens, oestrogen replacement therapy/steroidal oestrogens, solar radiation, thiotepa and vinyl chloride), carcinogenicity in experimental animals was established or highly suspected before epidemiological studies confirmed their carcinogenicity in humans (Vainio *et al.*, 1995). Although this association cannot establish that all agents and mixtures that cause cancer in experimental animals also cause cancer in humans, nevertheless, **in the absence of adequate data on humans, it is biologically plausible and prudent to regard agents and mixtures for which there is *sufficient evidence* (see p. 24) of carcinogenicity in experimental animals as if they presented a carcinogenic risk to humans**. The possibility that a given agent may cause cancer through a species-specific mechanism which does not operate in humans (see p. 27) should also be taken into consideration.

The nature and extent of impurities or contaminants present in the chemical or mixture being evaluated are given when available. Animal strain, sex, numbers per group, age at start of treatment and survival are reported.

Other types of studies summarized include: experiments in which the agent or mixture was administered in conjunction with known carcinogens or factors that modify carcinogenic effects; studies in which the end-point was not cancer but a defined precancerous lesion; and experiments on the carcinogenicity of known metabolites and derivatives.

For experimental studies of mixtures, consideration is given to the possibility of changes in the physicochemical properties of the test substance during collection, storage, extraction, concentration and delivery. Chemical and toxicological interactions of the components of mixtures may result in nonlinear dose–response relationships.

An assessment is made as to the relevance to human exposure of samples tested in experimental animals, which may involve consideration of: (i) physical and chemical characteristics, (ii) constituent substances that indicate the presence of a class of substances, (iii) the results of tests for genetic and related effects, including studies on DNA adduct formation, proto-oncogene mutation and expression and suppressor gene inactivation. The relevance of results obtained, for example, with animal viruses analogous to the virus being evaluated in the monograph must also be considered. They may provide biological and mechanistic information relevant to the understanding of the process of carcinogenesis in humans and may strengthen the plausibility of a conclusion that the biological agent under evaluation is carcinogenic in humans.

(a) *Qualitative aspects*

An assessment of carcinogenicity involves several considerations of qualitative importance, including (i) the experimental conditions under which the test was performed, including route and schedule of exposure, species, strain, sex, age, duration of follow-up; (ii) the consistency of the results, for example, across species and target organ(s); (iii) the spectrum of neoplastic response, from preneoplastic lesions and benign tumours to malignant neoplasms; and (iv) the possible role of modifying factors.

As mentioned earlier (p. 11), the *Monographs* are not intended to summarize all published studies. Those studies in experimental animals that are inadequate (e.g., too short a duration, too few animals, poor survival; see below) or are judged irrelevant to the evaluation are generally omitted. Guidelines for conducting adequate long-term carcinogenicity experiments have been outlined (e.g. Montesano *et al.*, 1986).

Considerations of importance to the Working Group in the interpretation and evaluation of a particular study include: (i) how clearly the agent was defined and, in the case of mixtures, how adequately the sample characterization was reported; (ii) whether the dose was adequately monitored, particularly in inhalation experiments; (iii) whether the doses and duration of treatment were appropriate and whether the survival of treated animals was similar to that of controls; (iv) whether there were adequate numbers of animals per group; (v) whether animals of each sex were used; (vi) whether animals were allocated randomly to groups; (vii) whether the duration of observation was adequate; and (viii) whether the data were adequately reported. If available, recent data on the incidence of specific tumours in historical controls, as well as in concurrent controls, should be taken into account in the evaluation of tumour response.

When benign tumours occur together with and originate from the same cell type in an organ or tissue as malignant tumours in a particular study and appear to represent a stage in the progression to malignancy, it may be valid to combine them in assessing tumour incidence (Huff *et al.*, 1989). The occurrence of lesions presumed to be pre-neoplastic may in certain instances aid in assessing the biological plausibility of any neoplastic response observed. If an agent or mixture induces only benign neoplasms that appear to be end-points that do not readily progress to malignancy, it should nevertheless be suspected of being a carcinogen and requires further investigation.

(*b*)   *Quantitative aspects*

The probability that tumours will occur may depend on the species, sex, strain and age of the animal, the dose of the carcinogen and the route and length of exposure. Evidence of an increased incidence of neoplasms with increased level of exposure strengthens the inference of a causal association between the exposure and the development of neoplasms.

The form of the dose–response relationship can vary widely, depending on the particular agent under study and the target organ. Both DNA damage and increased cell division are important aspects of carcinogenesis, and cell proliferation is a strong determinant of dose–response relationships for some carcinogens (Cohen & Ellwein, 1990). Since many chemicals require metabolic activation before being converted into their reactive intermediates, both metabolic and pharmacokinetic aspects are important in determining the dose–response pattern. Saturation of steps such as absorption, activation, inactivation and elimination may produce nonlinearity in the dose–response relationship, as could saturation of processes such as DNA repair (Hoel *et al.*, 1983; Gart *et al.*, 1986).

(*c*)   *Statistical analysis of long-term experiments in animals*

Factors considered by the Working Group include the adequacy of the information given for each treatment group: (i) the number of animals studied and the number examined histologically, (ii) the number of animals with a given tumour type and (iii) length of survival. The statistical methods used should be clearly stated and should be the generally accepted techniques refined for this purpose (Peto *et al.*, 1980; Gart *et al.*, 1986). When there is no difference in survival between control and treatment groups, the Working Group usually compares the proportions of animals developing each tumour type in each of the groups. Otherwise, consideration is given as to whether or not appropriate adjustments have been made for differences in survival. These adjustments can include: comparisons of the proportions of tumour-bearing animals among the effective number of animals (alive at the time the first tumour is discovered), in the case where most differences in survival occur before tumours appear; life-table methods, when tumours are visible or when they may be considered 'fatal' because mortality rapidly follows tumour development; and the Mantel-Haenszel test or logistic regression, when occult tumours do not affect the animals' risk of dying but are 'incidental' findings at autopsy.

In practice, classifying tumours as fatal or incidental may be difficult. Several survival-adjusted methods have been developed that do not require this distinction (Gart et al., 1986), although they have not been fully evaluated.

10. OTHER DATA RELEVANT TO AN EVALUATION OF CARCINOGENICITY AND ITS MECHANISMS

In coming to an overall evaluation of carcinogenicity in humans (see pp. 25–27), the Working Group also considers related data. The nature of the information selected for the summary depends on the agent being considered.

For chemicals and complex mixtures of chemicals such as those in some occupational situations or involving cultural habits (e.g. tobacco smoking), the other data considered to be relevant are divided into those on absorption, distribution, metabolism and excretion; toxic effects; reproductive and developmental effects; and genetic and related effects.

Concise information is given on absorption, distribution (including placental transfer) and excretion in both humans and experimental animals. Kinetic factors that may affect the dose–response relationship, such as saturation of uptake, protein binding, metabolic activation, detoxification and DNA repair processes, are mentioned. Studies that indicate the metabolic fate of the agent in humans and in experimental animals are summarized briefly, and comparisons of data on humans and on animals are made when possible. Comparative information on the relationship between exposure and the dose that reaches the target site may be of particular importance for extrapolation between species. Data are given on acute and chronic toxic effects (other than cancer), such as organ toxicity, increased cell proliferation, immunotoxicity and endocrine effects. The presence and toxicological significance of cellular receptors is described. Effects on reproduction, teratogenicity, fetotoxicity and embryotoxicity are also summarized briefly.

Tests of genetic and related effects are described in view of the relevance of gene mutation and chromosomal damage to carcinogenesis (Vainio et al., 1992; McGregor et al., 1999). The adequacy of the reporting of sample characterization is considered and, where necessary, commented upon; with regard to complex mixtures, such comments are similar to those described for animal carcinogenicity tests on p. 18. The available data are interpreted critically by phylogenetic group according to the end-points detected, which may include DNA damage, gene mutation, sister chromatid exchange, micronucleus formation, chromosomal aberrations, aneuploidy and cell transformation. The concentrations employed are given, and mention is made of whether use of an exogenous metabolic system in vitro affected the test result. These data are given as listings of test systems, data and references. The Genetic and Related Effects data presented in the Monographs are also available in the form of Graphic Activity Profiles (GAP) prepared in collaboration with the United States Environmental Protection Agency (EPA) (see also

Waters *et al.*, 1987) using software for personal computers that are Microsoft Windows® compatible. The EPA/IARC GAP software and database may be downloaded free of charge from *www.epa.gov/gapdb*.

Positive results in tests using prokaryotes, lower eukaryotes, plants, insects and cultured mammalian cells suggest that genetic and related effects could occur in mammals. Results from such tests may also give information about the types of genetic effect produced and about the involvement of metabolic activation. Some end-points described are clearly genetic in nature (e.g., gene mutations and chromosomal aberrations), while others are to a greater or lesser degree associated with genetic effects (e.g. unscheduled DNA synthesis). In-vitro tests for tumour-promoting activity and for cell transformation may be sensitive to changes that are not necessarily the result of genetic alterations but that may have specific relevance to the process of carcinogenesis. A critical appraisal of these tests has been published (Montesano *et al.*, 1986).

Genetic or other activity manifest in experimental mammals and humans is regarded as being of greater relevance than that in other organisms. The demonstration that an agent or mixture can induce gene and chromosomal mutations in whole mammals indicates that it may have carcinogenic activity, although this activity may not be detectably expressed in any or all species. Relative potency in tests for mutagenicity and related effects is not a reliable indicator of carcinogenic potency. Negative results in tests for mutagenicity in selected tissues from animals treated *in vivo* provide less weight, partly because they do not exclude the possibility of an effect in tissues other than those examined. Moreover, negative results in short-term tests with genetic end-points cannot be considered to provide evidence to rule out carcinogenicity of agents or mixtures that act through other mechanisms (e.g. receptor-mediated effects, cellular toxicity with regenerative proliferation, peroxisome proliferation) (Vainio *et al.*, 1992). Factors that may lead to misleading results in short-term tests have been discussed in detail elsewhere (Montesano *et al.*, 1986).

When available, data relevant to mechanisms of carcinogenesis that do not involve structural changes at the level of the gene are also described.

The adequacy of epidemiological studies of reproductive outcome and genetic and related effects in humans is evaluated by the same criteria as are applied to epidemiological studies of cancer.

Structure–activity relationships that may be relevant to an evaluation of the carcinogenicity of an agent are also described.

For biological agents—viruses, bacteria and parasites—other data relevant to carcinogenicity include descriptions of the pathology of infection, molecular biology (integration and expression of viruses, and any genetic alterations seen in human tumours) and other observations, which might include cellular and tissue responses to infection, immune response and the presence of tumour markers.

11. SUMMARY OF DATA REPORTED

In this section, the relevant epidemiological and experimental data are summarized. Only reports, other than in abstract form, that meet the criteria outlined on p. 11 are considered for evaluating carcinogenicity. Inadequate studies are generally not summarized: such studies are usually identified by a square-bracketed comment in the preceding text.

(a) Exposure

Human exposure to chemicals and complex mixtures is summarized on the basis of elements such as production, use, occurrence in the environment and determinations in human tissues and body fluids. Quantitative data are given when available. Exposure to biological agents is described in terms of transmission and prevalence of infection.

(b) Carcinogenicity in humans

Results of epidemiological studies that are considered to be pertinent to an assessment of human carcinogenicity are summarized. When relevant, case reports and correlation studies are also summarized.

(c) Carcinogenicity in experimental animals

Data relevant to an evaluation of carcinogenicity in animals are summarized. For each animal species and route of administration, it is stated whether an increased incidence of neoplasms or preneoplastic lesions was observed, and the tumour sites are indicated. If the agent or mixture produced tumours after prenatal exposure or in single-dose experiments, this is also indicated. Negative findings are also summarized. Dose–response and other quantitative data may be given when available.

(d) Other data relevant to an evaluation of carcinogenicity and its mechanisms

Data on biological effects in humans that are of particular relevance are summarized. These may include toxicological, kinetic and metabolic considerations and evidence of DNA binding, persistence of DNA lesions or genetic damage in exposed humans. Toxicological information, such as that on cytotoxicity and regeneration, receptor binding and hormonal and immunological effects, and data on kinetics and metabolism in experimental animals are given when considered relevant to the possible mechanism of the carcinogenic action of the agent. The results of tests for genetic and related effects are summarized for whole mammals, cultured mammalian cells and nonmammalian systems.

When available, comparisons of such data for humans and for animals, and particularly animals that have developed cancer, are described.

Structure–activity relationships are mentioned when relevant.

For the agent, mixture or exposure circumstance being evaluated, the available data on end-points or other phenomena relevant to mechanisms of carcinogenesis from studies in humans, experimental animals and tissue and cell test systems are summarized within one or more of the following descriptive dimensions:

(i) Evidence of genotoxicity (structural changes at the level of the gene): for example, structure–activity considerations, adduct formation, mutagenicity (effect on specific genes), chromosomal mutation/aneuploidy

(ii) Evidence of effects on the expression of relevant genes (functional changes at the intracellular level): for example, alterations to the structure or quantity of the product of a proto-oncogene or tumour-suppressor gene, alterations to metabolic activation/inactivation/DNA repair

(iii) Evidence of relevant effects on cell behaviour (morphological or behavioural changes at the cellular or tissue level): for example, induction of mitogenesis, compensatory cell proliferation, preoplasia and hyperplasia, survival of premalignant or malignant cells (immortalization, immunosuppression), effects on metastatic potential

(iv) Evidence from dose and time relationships of carcinogenic effects and interactions between agents: for example, early/late stage, as inferred from epidemiological studies; initiation/promotion/progression/malignant conversion, as defined in animal carcinogenicity experiments; toxicokinetics

These dimensions are not mutually exclusive, and an agent may fall within more than one of them. Thus, for example, the action of an agent on the expression of relevant genes could be summarized under both the first and second dimensions, even if it were known with reasonable certainty that those effects resulted from genotoxicity.

12. EVALUATION

Evaluations of the strength of the evidence for carcinogenicity arising from human and experimental animal data are made, using standard terms.

It is recognized that the criteria for these evaluations, described below, cannot encompass all of the factors that may be relevant to an evaluation of carcinogenicity. In considering all of the relevant scientific data, the Working Group may assign the agent, mixture or exposure circumstance to a higher or lower category than a strict interpretation of these criteria would indicate.

(a) *Degrees of evidence for carcinogenicity in humans and in experimental animals and supporting evidence*

These categories refer only to the strength of the evidence that an exposure is carcinogenic and not to the extent of its carcinogenic activity (potency) nor to the mechanisms involved. A classification may change as new information becomes available.

An evaluation of degree of evidence, whether for a single agent or a mixture, is limited to the materials tested, as defined physically, chemically or biologically. When the agents evaluated are considered by the Working Group to be sufficiently closely related, they may be grouped together for the purpose of a single evaluation of degree of evidence.

(i) *Carcinogenicity in humans*

The applicability of an evaluation of the carcinogenicity of a mixture, process, occupation or industry on the basis of evidence from epidemiological studies depends on the variability over time and place of the mixtures, processes, occupations and industries. The Working Group seeks to identify the specific exposure, process or activity which is considered most likely to be responsible for any excess risk. The evaluation is focused as narrowly as the available data on exposure and other aspects permit.

The evidence relevant to carcinogenicity from studies in humans is classified into one of the following categories:

Sufficient evidence of carcinogenicity: The Working Group considers that a causal relationship has been established between exposure to the agent, mixture or exposure circumstance and human cancer. That is, a positive relationship has been observed between the exposure and cancer in studies in which chance, bias and confounding could be ruled out with reasonable confidence.

Limited evidence of carcinogenicity: A positive association has been observed between exposure to the agent, mixture or exposure circumstance and cancer for which a causal interpretation is considered by the Working Group to be credible, but chance, bias or confounding could not be ruled out with reasonable confidence.

Inadequate evidence of carcinogenicity: The available studies are of insufficient quality, consistency or statistical power to permit a conclusion regarding the presence or absence of a causal association between exposure and cancer, or no data on cancer in humans are available.

Evidence suggesting lack of carcinogenicity: There are several adequate studies covering the full range of levels of exposure that human beings are known to encounter, which are mutually consistent in not showing a positive association between exposure to the agent, mixture or exposure circumstance and any studied cancer at any observed level of exposure. A conclusion of 'evidence suggesting lack of carcinogenicity' is inevitably limited to the cancer sites, conditions and levels of exposure and length of observation covered by the available studies. In addition, the possibility of a very small risk at the levels of exposure studied can never be excluded.

In some instances, the above categories may be used to classify the degree of evidence related to carcinogenicity in specific organs or tissues.

(ii) *Carcinogenicity in experimental animals*

The evidence relevant to carcinogenicity in experimental animals is classified into one of the following categories:

Sufficient evidence of carcinogenicity: The Working Group considers that a causal relationship has been established between the agent or mixture and an increased incidence of malignant neoplasms or of an appropriate combination of benign and malignant neoplasms in (a) two or more species of animals or (b) in two or more independent studies in one species carried out at different times or in different laboratories or under different protocols.

Exceptionally, a single study in one species might be considered to provide sufficient evidence of carcinogenicity when malignant neoplasms occur to an unusual degree with regard to incidence, site, type of tumour or age at onset.

Limited evidence of carcinogenicity: The data suggest a carcinogenic effect but are limited for making a definitive evaluation because, e.g. (a) the evidence of carcinogenicity is restricted to a single experiment; or (b) there are unresolved questions regarding the adequacy of the design, conduct or interpretation of the study; or (c) the agent or mixture increases the incidence only of benign neoplasms or lesions of uncertain neoplastic potential, or of certain neoplasms which may occur spontaneously in high incidences in certain strains.

Inadequate evidence of carcinogenicity: The studies cannot be interpreted as showing either the presence or absence of a carcinogenic effect because of major qualitative or quantitative limitations, or no data on cancer in experimental animals are available.

Evidence suggesting lack of carcinogenicity: Adequate studies involving at least two species are available which show that, within the limits of the tests used, the agent or mixture is not carcinogenic. A conclusion of evidence suggesting lack of carcinogenicity is inevitably limited to the species, tumour sites and levels of exposure studied.

    (b)   Other data relevant to the evaluation of carcinogenicity and its mechanisms

Other evidence judged to be relevant to an evaluation of carcinogenicity and of sufficient importance to affect the overall evaluation is then described. This may include data on preneoplastic lesions, tumour pathology, genetic and related effects, structure–activity relationships, metabolism and pharmacokinetics, physicochemical parameters and analogous biological agents.

Data relevant to mechanisms of the carcinogenic action are also evaluated. The strength of the evidence that any carcinogenic effect observed is due to a particular mechanism is assessed, using terms such as weak, moderate or strong. Then, the Working Group assesses if that particular mechanism is likely to be operative in humans. The strongest indications that a particular mechanism operates in humans come from data on humans or biological specimens obtained from exposed humans. The data may be considered to be especially relevant if they show that the agent in question has caused changes in exposed humans that are on the causal pathway to carcinogenesis. Such data may, however, never become available, because it is at least conceivable that certain compounds may be kept from human use solely on the basis of evidence of their toxicity and/or carcinogenicity in experimental systems.

For complex exposures, including occupational and industrial exposures, the chemical composition and the potential contribution of carcinogens known to be present are considered by the Working Group in its overall evaluation of human carcinogenicity. The Working Group also determines the extent to which the materials tested in experimental systems are related to those to which humans are exposed.

    (c)   Overall evaluation

Finally, the body of evidence is considered as a whole, in order to reach an overall evaluation of the carcinogenicity to humans of an agent, mixture or circumstance of exposure.

An evaluation may be made for a group of chemical compounds that have been evaluated by the Working Group. In addition, when supporting data indicate that other, related compounds for which there is no direct evidence of capacity to induce cancer in humans or in animals may also be carcinogenic, a statement describing the rationale for this conclusion is added to the evaluation narrative; an additional evaluation may be made for this broader group of compounds if the strength of the evidence warrants it.

The agent, mixture or exposure circumstance is described according to the wording of one of the following categories, and the designated group is given. The categorization of an agent, mixture or exposure circumstance is a matter of scientific judgement, reflecting the strength of the evidence derived from studies in humans and in experimental animals and from other relevant data.

Group 1 —The agent (mixture) is carcinogenic to humans.
The exposure circumstance entails exposures that are carcinogenic to humans.

This category is used when there is *sufficient evidence* of carcinogenicity in humans. Exceptionally, an agent (mixture) may be placed in this category when evidence of carcinogenicity in humans is less than sufficient but there is *sufficient evidence* of carcinogenicity in experimental animals and strong evidence in exposed humans that the agent (mixture) acts through a relevant mechanism of carcinogenicity.

Group 2

This category includes agents, mixtures and exposure circumstances for which, at one extreme, the degree of evidence of carcinogenicity in humans is almost sufficient, as well as those for which, at the other extreme, there are no human data but for which there is evidence of carcinogenicity in experimental animals. Agents, mixtures and exposure circumstances are assigned to either group 2A (probably carcinogenic to humans) or group 2B (possibly carcinogenic to humans) on the basis of epidemiological and experimental evidence of carcinogenicity and other relevant data.

Group 2A—The agent (mixture) is probably carcinogenic to humans.
The exposure circumstance entails exposures that are probably carcinogenic to humans.

This category is used when there is *limited evidence* of carcinogenicity in humans and *sufficient evidence* of carcinogenicity in experimental animals. In some cases, an agent (mixture) may be classified in this category when there is *inadequate evidence* of carcinogenicity in humans, *sufficient evidence* of carcinogenicity in experimental animals and strong evidence that the carcinogenesis is mediated by a mechanism that also operates in humans. Exceptionally, an agent, mixture or exposure circumstance may be classified in this category solely on the basis of *limited evidence* of carcinogenicity in humans.

Group 2B—The agent (mixture) is possibly carcinogenic to humans.
The exposure circumstance entails exposures that are possibly carcinogenic to humans.

This category is used for agents, mixtures and exposure circumstances for which there is *limited evidence* of carcinogenicity in humans and less than *sufficient evidence* of carcinogenicity in experimental animals. It may also be used when there is *inadequate evidence* of carcinogenicity in humans but there is *sufficient evidence* of carcinogenicity in experimental animals. In some instances, an agent, mixture or exposure circumstance for which there is *inadequate evidence* of carcinogenicity in humans but *limited evidence* of carcinogenicity in experimental animals together with supporting evidence from other relevant data may be placed in this group.

Group 3—The agent (mixture or exposure circumstance) is not classifiable as to its carcinogenicity to humans.

This category is used most commonly for agents, mixtures and exposure circumstances for which the *evidence of carcinogenicity* is *inadequate* in humans and *inadequate* or *limited* in experimental animals.

Exceptionally, agents (mixtures) for which the *evidence of carcinogenicity* is *inadequate* in humans but *sufficient* in experimental animals may be placed in this category when there is strong evidence that the mechanism of carcinogenicity in experimental animals does not operate in humans.

Agents, mixtures and exposure circumstances that do not fall into any other group are also placed in this category.

Group 4—The agent (mixture) is probably not carcinogenic to humans.

This category is used for agents or mixtures for which there is *evidence suggesting lack of carcinogenicity* in humans and in experimental animals. In some instances, agents or mixtures for which there is *inadequate evidence* of carcinogenicity in humans but *evidence suggesting lack of carcinogenicity* in experimental animals, consistently and strongly supported by a broad range of other relevant data, may be classified in this group.

References

Breslow, N.E. & Day, N.E. (1980) *Statistical Methods in Cancer Research*, Vol. 1, *The Analysis of Case–Control Studies* (IARC Scientific Publications No. 32), Lyon, IARC

Breslow, N.E. & Day, N.E. (1987) *Statistical Methods in Cancer Research*, Vol. 2, *The Design and Analysis of Cohort Studies* (IARC Scientific Publications No. 82), Lyon, IARC

Cohen, S.M. & Ellwein, L.B. (1990) Cell proliferation in carcinogenesis. *Science*, **249**, 1007–1011

Gart, J.J., Krewski, D., Lee, P.N., Tarone, R.E. & Wahrendorf, J. (1986) *Statistical Methods in Cancer Research*, Vol. 3, *The Design and Analysis of Long-term Animal Experiments* (IARC Scientific Publications No. 79), Lyon, IARC

Hoel, D.G., Kaplan, N.L. & Anderson, M.W. (1983) Implication of nonlinear kinetics on risk estimation in carcinogenesis. *Science*, **219**, 1032–1037

Huff, J.E., Eustis, S.L. & Haseman, J.K. (1989) Occurrence and relevance of chemically induced benign neoplasms in long-term carcinogenicity studies. *Cancer Metastasis Rev.*, **8**, 1–21

IARC (1973–1996) *Information Bulletin on the Survey of Chemicals Being Tested for Carcinogenicity/Directory of Agents Being Tested for Carcinogenicity*, Numbers 1–17, Lyon

IARC (1976–1996)

    Directory of On-going Research in Cancer Epidemiology 1976. Edited by C.S. Muir & G. Wagner, Lyon

    Directory of On-going Research in Cancer Epidemiology 1977 (IARC Scientific Publications No. 17). Edited by C.S. Muir & G. Wagner, Lyon

    Directory of On-going Research in Cancer Epidemiology 1978 (IARC Scientific Publications No. 26). Edited by C.S. Muir & G. Wagner, Lyon

    Directory of On-going Research in Cancer Epidemiology 1979 (IARC Scientific Publications No. 28). Edited by C.S. Muir & G. Wagner, Lyon

    Directory of On-going Research in Cancer Epidemiology 1980 (IARC Scientific Publications No. 35). Edited by C.S. Muir & G. Wagner, Lyon

    Directory of On-going Research in Cancer Epidemiology 1981 (IARC Scientific Publications No. 38). Edited by C.S. Muir & G. Wagner, Lyon

    Directory of On-going Research in Cancer Epidemiology 1982 (IARC Scientific Publications No. 46). Edited by C.S. Muir & G. Wagner, Lyon

    Directory of On-going Research in Cancer Epidemiology 1983 (IARC Scientific Publications No. 50). Edited by C.S. Muir & G. Wagner, Lyon

    Directory of On-going Research in Cancer Epidemiology 1984 (IARC Scientific Publications No. 62). Edited by C.S. Muir & G. Wagner, Lyon

    Directory of On-going Research in Cancer Epidemiology 1985 (IARC Scientific Publications No. 69). Edited by C.S. Muir & G. Wagner, Lyon

    Directory of On-going Research in Cancer Epidemiology 1986 (IARC Scientific Publications No. 80). Edited by C.S. Muir & G. Wagner, Lyon

    Directory of On-going Research in Cancer Epidemiology 1987 (IARC Scientific Publications No. 86). Edited by D.M. Parkin & J. Wahrendorf, Lyon

    Directory of On-going Research in Cancer Epidemiology 1988 (IARC Scientific Publications No. 93). Edited by M. Coleman & J. Wahrendorf, Lyon

    Directory of On-going Research in Cancer Epidemiology 1989/90 (IARC Scientific Publications No. 101). Edited by M. Coleman & J. Wahrendorf, Lyon

    Directory of On-going Research in Cancer Epidemiology 1991 (IARC Scientific Publications No.110). Edited by M. Coleman & J. Wahrendorf, Lyon

    Directory of On-going Research in Cancer Epidemiology 1992 (IARC Scientific Publications No. 117). Edited by M. Coleman, J. Wahrendorf & E. Démaret, Lyon

    Directory of On-going Research in Cancer Epidemiology 1994 (IARC Scientific Publications No. 130). Edited by R. Sankaranarayanan, J. Wahrendorf & E. Démaret, Lyon

Directory of On-going Research in Cancer Epidemiology 1996 (IARC Scientific Publications No. 137). Edited by R. Sankaranarayanan, J. Wahrendorf & E. Démaret, Lyon

IARC (1977) *IARC Monographs Programme on the Evaluation of the Carcinogenic Risk of Chemicals to Humans*. Preamble (IARC intern. tech. Rep. No. 77/002), Lyon

IARC (1978) *Chemicals with Sufficient Evidence of Carcinogenicity in Experimental Animals—IARC Monographs Volumes 1–17* (IARC intern. tech. Rep. No. 78/003), Lyon

IARC (1978–1993) *Environmental Carcinogens. Methods of Analysis and Exposure Measurement*:

Vol. 1. Analysis of Volatile Nitrosamines in Food (IARC Scientific Publications No. 18). Edited by R. Preussmann, M. Castegnaro, E.A. Walker & A.E. Wasserman (1978)

Vol. 2. Methods for the Measurement of Vinyl Chloride in Poly(vinyl chloride), Air, Water and Foodstuffs (IARC Scientific Publications No. 22). Edited by D.C.M. Squirrell & W. Thain (1978)

Vol. 3. Analysis of Polycyclic Aromatic Hydrocarbons in Environmental Samples (IARC Scientific Publications No. 29). Edited by M. Castegnaro, P. Bogovski, H. Kunte & E.A. Walker (1979)

Vol. 4. Some Aromatic Amines and Azo Dyes in the General and Industrial Environment (IARC Scientific Publications No. 40). Edited by L. Fishbein, M. Castegnaro, I.K. O'Neill & H. Bartsch (1981)

Vol. 5. Some Mycotoxins (IARC Scientific Publications No. 44). Edited by L. Stoloff, M. Castegnaro, P. Scott, I.K. O'Neill & H. Bartsch (1983)

Vol. 6. N-Nitroso Compounds (IARC Scientific Publications No. 45). Edited by R. Preussmann, I.K. O'Neill, G. Eisenbrand, B. Spiegelhalder & H. Bartsch (1983)

Vol. 7. Some Volatile Halogenated Hydrocarbons (IARC Scientific Publications No. 68). Edited by L. Fishbein & I.K. O'Neill (1985)

Vol. 8. Some Metals: As, Be, Cd, Cr, Ni, Pb, Se, Zn (IARC Scientific Publications No. 71). Edited by I.K. O'Neill, P. Schuller & L. Fishbein (1986)

Vol. 9. Passive Smoking (IARC Scientific Publications No. 81). Edited by I.K. O'Neill, K.D. Brunnemann, B. Dodet & D. Hoffmann (1987)

*Vol. 10. Benzene and Alkylated Benzenes (*IARC Scientific Publications No. 85). Edited by L. Fishbein & I.K. O'Neill (1988)

Vol. 11. Polychlorinated Dioxins and Dibenzofurans (IARC Scientific Publications No. 108). Edited by C. Rappe, H.R. Buser, B. Dodet & I.K. O'Neill (1991)

Vol. 12. Indoor Air (IARC Scientific Publications No. 109). Edited by B. Seifert, H. van de Wiel, B. Dodet & I.K. O'Neill (1993)

IARC (1979) *Criteria to Select Chemicals for* IARC Monographs (IARC intern. tech. Rep. No. 79/003), Lyon

IARC (1982) *IARC Monographs on the Evaluation of the Carcinogenic Risk of Chemicals to Humans*, Supplement 4, *Chemicals, Industrial Processes and Industries Associated with Cancer in Humans* (IARC Monographs, Volumes 1 to 29), Lyon

IARC (1983) *Approaches to Classifying Chemical Carcinogens According to Mechanism of Action* (IARC intern. tech. Rep. No. 83/001), Lyon

IARC (1984) *Chemicals and Exposures to Complex Mixtures Recommended for Evaluation in IARC Monographs and Chemicals and Complex Mixtures Recommended for Long-term Carcinogenicity Testing* (IARC intern. tech. Rep. No. 84/002), Lyon

IARC (1987a) *IARC Monographs on the Evaluation of Carcinogenic Risks to Humans*, Supplement 6, *Genetic and Related Effects: An Updating of Selected* IARC Monographs *from Volumes 1 to 42*, Lyon

IARC (1987b) *IARC Monographs on the Evaluation of Carcinogenic Risks to Humans*, Supplement 7, *Overall Evaluations of Carcinogenicity: An Updating of* IARC Monographs *Volumes 1 to 42*, Lyon

IARC (1988) *Report of an IARC Working Group to Review the Approaches and Processes Used to Evaluate the Carcinogenicity of Mixtures and Groups of Chemicals* (IARC intern. tech. Rep. No. 88/002), Lyon

IARC (1989) *Chemicals, Groups of Chemicals, Mixtures and Exposure Circumstances to be Evaluated in Future IARC Monographs, Report of an ad hoc Working Group* (IARC intern. tech. Rep. No. 89/004), Lyon

IARC (1991a) *A Consensus Report of an IARC Monographs Working Group on the Use of Mechanisms of Carcinogenesis in Risk Identification* (IARC intern. tech. Rep. No. 91/002), Lyon

IARC (1991b) *Report of an ad-hoc* IARC Monographs *Advisory Group on Viruses and Other Biological Agents Such as Parasites* (IARC intern. tech. Rep. No. 91/001), Lyon

IARC (1993) *Chemicals, Groups of Chemicals, Complex Mixtures, Physical and Biological Agents and Exposure Circumstances to be Evaluated in Future* IARC Monographs, *Report of an ad-hoc Working Group* (IARC intern. Rep. No. 93/005), Lyon

IARC (1998a) *Report of an ad-hoc* IARC Monographs *Advisory Group on Physical Agents* (IARC Internal Report No. 98/002), Lyon

IARC (1998b) *Report of an ad-hoc* IARC Monographs *Advisory Group on Priorities for Future Evaluations* (IARC Internal Report No. 98/004), Lyon

McGregor, D.B., Rice, J.M. & Venitt, S., eds (1999) *The Use of Short and Medium-term Tests for Carcinogens and Data on Genetic Effects in Carcinogenic Hazard Evaluation* (IARC Scientific Publications No. 146), Lyon, IARC

Montesano, R., Bartsch, H., Vainio, H., Wilbourn, J. & Yamasaki, H., eds (1986) *Long-term and Short-term Assays for Carcinogenesis—A Critical Appraisal* (IARC Scientific Publications No. 83), Lyon, IARC

Peto, R., Pike, M.C., Day, N.E., Gray, R.G., Lee, P.N., Parish, S., Peto, J., Richards, S. & Wahrendorf, J. (1980) Guidelines for simple, sensitive significance tests for carcinogenic effects in long-term animal experiments. In: *IARC Monographs on the Evaluation of the Carcinogenic Risk of Chemicals to Humans*, Supplement 2, *Long-term and Short-term Screening Assays for Carcinogens: A Critical Appraisal*, Lyon, pp. 311–426

Tomatis, L., Aitio, A., Wilbourn, J. & Shuker, L. (1989) Human carcinogens so far identified. *Jpn. J. Cancer Res.*, **80**, 795–807

Vainio, H., Magee, P.N., McGregor, D.B. & McMichael, A.J., eds (1992) *Mechanisms of Carcinogenesis in Risk Identification* (IARC Scientific Publications No. 116), Lyon, IARC

Vainio, H., Wilbourn, J.D., Sasco, A.J., Partensky, C., Gaudin, N., Heseltine, E. & Eragne, I. (1995) *Identification of human carcinogenic risk in* IARC Monographs. *Bull. Cancer,* **82**, 339–348 (in French)

Waters, M.D., Stack, H.F., Brady, A.L., Lohman, P.H.M., Haroun, L. & Vainio, H. (1987) Appendix 1. Activity profiles for genetic and related tests. In: *IARC Monographs on the Evaluation of Carcinogenic Risks to Humans*, Suppl. 6, *Genetic and Related Effects: An Updating of Selected IARC Monographs from Volumes 1 to 42*, Lyon, IARC, pp. 687–696

Wilbourn, J., Haroun, L., Heseltine, E., Kaldor, J., Partensky, C. & Vainio, H. (1986) Response of experimental animals to human carcinogens: an analysis based upon the IARC Monographs Programme. *Carcinogenesis*, **7**, 1853–1863

THE MONOGRAPH

INTRODUCTION

Foreign bodies are defined as any exogenous object that has been introduced into the tissues or cavities of the body and is not rapidly absorbed. Solid materials may enter the body as a result of the implantation of medical devices, as a result of accidents (recreational, automobile, occupational and hunting) or as a result of wartime or crime-related injuries (bullets and shrapnel fragments). A biomaterial may be defined in this context as any material used in a medical device that is intended to interact with living systems. Foreign bodies may induce a wide range of local tissue reactions, in particular inflammation, giant cell formation and fibrosis.

1. Scope of the monograph

The exposure of interest in this monograph is the presence within the body of a solid metallic or non-metallic object as a result either of surgery or of involuntary penetration (as, for example, through a war wound).

Excluded from evaluation are exposures to:
- occupational handling of materials designed for implantation
- radiation emitted by any implanted object
- any device designed to lie on the surface of the body, either on the skin or within a cavity lined by endothelium (for, example, contact lenses and intra-uterine contraceptive devices)
- intra-ocular implants
- cochlear implants
- certain materials, including suture materials derived from animal tissues, foreign bodies of vegetable origin, and glasses
- allografts and xenografts of bone or other connective tissue

In this general introduction, some key concepts in our current understanding of host–material interactions are presented. These include consideration of the degradation of materials within the body, general mechanisms of chemical and solid state carcinogenesis, and a discussion of the pathology of sarcomas. This is followed by a short description of some characteristics of epidemiology as they relate to the study of cancers associated with implanted devices.

Subsequent chapters describe human exposure data, evidence from case reports and analytical studies for carcinogenicity in humans and in companion animals, evidence of carcinogenicity of implanted materials from animal experiments, and further background material on mechanisms of degradation and carcinogenicity. Finally, a summary of evidence and an overall evaluation of current evidence are provided.

Some of the substances that constitute, or may be released from, foreign bodies have been evaluated previously within the *IARC Monographs*. These are listed in Table 1.

Table 1. Substances found in (or potentially originating from) foreign bodies that have been evaluated for carcinogenicity previously in the *IARC Monographs* programme

Material	Use	Evaluation of evidence		Classification	Year/Volume
		Human	Animal		
para-Aramid fibrils	D	I	I	3	1997/68
Beryllium	D	S	S	1	1993/58
Beryllium oxide	D	S	S	1	1993/58
Beryllium salts	D	S	S	1	1993/58
Chromium	M + D	I	I	3	1990/49
Chromium trioxide	M + D	S	L	1	1990/49
Chromium[VI] salts	M + D	S	S	1	1990/49
Cobalt	M + D	I	S	2B	1991/52
Cobalt-chromium-molybdenum alloy	M + D	I	L	2B	1991/52
Cobalt(II) oxide	M + D	I	S	2B	1991/52
Cobalt salts	M + D	I	L	2B	1991/52
2,4-Diaminotoluene	M	ND	S	2B	1987/S7
Ethylene oxide	M	L	S	1	1994/60
Lead and inorganic lead compounds	Bullets	I	S[a]	2B[a]	1987/S7
Mercury	D	I	I	3	1993/58
Nickel (metallic)	M + D	I	S	2B	1990/49
Nickel compounds	M + D	S	S + L + I	1	1990/49
Nylon 6	M	ND	I	3	1987/S7
Polyethylene	M	ND	I	3	1987/S7
Poly(methyl methacrylate)	M + D	ND	I	3	1987/S7
Polypropylene	M	ND	I	3	1987/S7
Polytetrafluoroethylene	M + D	ND	I	3	1987/S7
Polyvinylpyrrolidone	M	ND	L	3	1999/71
Silica, amorphous	M + D	I	I	3	1997/68
Silica, crystalline[b]	M + D		S		1997/68
Titanium dioxide	M + D	I	L	3	1989/47
Toluene diisocyanates	M	I	S	2B	1999/71

M, medical; D, dental

[a] Lead compounds; elemental lead has not been tested adequately.

[b] Crystalline silica inhaled in the form of quartz or cristobalite from occupational sources is *carcinogenic to humans (Group 1)*. This evaluation is not relevant to implants and other foreign bodies.

Elsewhere in this introduction, statements regarding the carcinogenicity of other specific chemicals and materials should not be construed as evaluations by this Working Group and are included only to illustrate mechanistic concepts.

The approach adopted in this volume is to consider sequentially metallic, non-metallic and mixed materials, which have different profiles of biological activity. This introduction brings together a number of diverse, multidisciplinary issues that are important in evaluating the carcinogenic risks associated with implanted biomaterials and other foreign bodies. These issues are:
- Host–biomaterial interactions
- General mechanisms of solid-state carcinogenesis
- Pathology of sarcomas, reactive and pseudoneoplastic conditions
- General issues in human epidemiological research on implants and cancer

2. Host–biomaterial interactions as related to carcinogenesis

There is no doubt that the implantation of biomaterials or products related to biomaterials into tissues can be associated with the formation of tumours under certain conditions. In considering the significance, relevance and mechanistic implications of this phenomenon, a wide variety of factors must be taken into account. These factors relate to the nature of the materials themselves, to the nature of the host and to the relationship between the material and the host.

With respect to the materials themselves, disregarding host variations, the following variables are known or might be considered to have some influence on the process of carcinogenicity related to a biomaterial or foreign body: (a) intrinsic chemistry; (b) surface chemistry; (c) chemical nature of any released soluble components; (d) chemical or crystallographic nature of any released particulate components; (e) physical nature of any released particulate components; (f) size; (g) shape; (h) hardness of the surface; (i) surface energy; (j) surface topography; (k) elastic moduli of the material or the flexibility of the component; (l) electrical or magnetic properties; (m) radioactivity; and (n) sterilization procedures.

With respect to the host and disregarding material variations, general factors that should be taken into account are the site of implantation and the latent period for tumour formation. In animals, some factors that may influence the carcinogenic outcome are the species under study, the strain or breed, age, sex and size. When evaluating the possible human carcinogenic responses to implanted materials, consideration must be given to host factors such as known risk factors for cancer, such as age, sex, occupation, lifestyle and genetic factors, as well as pharmacological status, prior or coexistent disease and the indication for clinical intervention.

With regard to interactions within the host–material system, factors which should be considered include the extent and technique of surgery, subsequent complications and the duration of contact between the biomaterial and the host.

A review of the published data concerning solid-state carcinogenicity in animals and humans allows an assessment of the relative importance of each of these factors.

2.1 Variables of the material or object

2.1.1 *Intrinsic chemistry*

There is some difficulty over the identification of variations in susceptibility to solid-state carcinogenicity on the basis of intrinsic material chemistry (chemical composition), since many publications fail to identify accurately the precise materials that were used in an experimental study or were the subject of clinical observations. There are published reports in which tumours in experimental animals have been associated with the following materials, among many others:

- Aluminium oxide ceramic subcutaneously implanted in rats (Griss *et al.*, 1977)
- Stainless steel implanted intramuscularly in rats (Stinson, 1964; Gaechter *et al.*, 1977; Memoli *et al.*, 1986)
- Tantalum metal implanted subcutaneously in rats (Oppenheimer *et al.*, 1956)
- Silver and platinum metal implanted in rats (Nothdurft, 1955, 1956)
- Polyethylene implanted subcutaneously in rats and Syrian hamsters (e.g., Oppenheimer *et al.*, 1952, 1955, 1961; Bering & Handler, 1957; Bates & Klein, 1966)
- Poly(methyl methacrylate) implanted intraperitoneally in mice and rats (e.g., Laskin *et al.*, 1954; Stinson, 1964)
- Polydimethylsiloxanes implanted subcutaneously in rats (e.g., Oppenheimer *et al.*, 1955; Maekawa *et al.*, 1984)
- Glass fragments implanted subcutaneously in mice (Tomatis, 1963).

This list is not exhaustive, a longer compilation being available in Section 4 of this Monograph, but it is clear that all types of material, including pure noble metals, base metal alloys, ceramics and ceramic compounds, glasses, thermoplastics, thermosetting resins and elastomers, have been implicated. It has to be argued, therefore, that solid-state carcinogenicity is not primarily a function of inherent material chemistry. Although there is variation in carcinogenic response from one material to another, there is no evidence that the material chemistry *per se* is the key determinant.

2.1.2 *Surface chemistry*

All considerations of the biocompatibility of materials should address the basic question of whether the surface chemistry is any different from the bulk chemistry and whether the composition and properties of the outermost layer of atoms or molecules are more relevant to carcinogenesis than those of the interior of the sample. For example, it is known that different surface molecular structures on methacrylate polymers can cause differences in cell shape and proliferation of normal and malignant human cells in culture in the absence of toxicity (Kulesh & Greene, 1986). Such findings confirm that surface chemistry can modulate cell behaviour in this respect. However, even though it would seem that different surface chemistries may have different biological effects, the fact that material surfaces involving all three primary valence bonds (ionic, metallic and covalent) are tumorigenic suggests that surface chemistry is not the key determinant.

2.1.3 *Chemical nature of any released soluble components*

Chemical carcinogenesis is far better understood than solid-state carcinogenesis and some of the components of implantable biomaterials are known or suspected human or animal carcinogens. It is also clear that with virtually all biomaterials in current clinical use, there is some degree of interaction with the host tissue such that some reaction product (possibly a corrosion product, a product of polymer biodegradation or an additive released from a plastic formulation) will gain access to the tissues. It is therefore possible that solid-state carcinogenesis associated with biomaterials is related to the release of some soluble carcinogenic products, perhaps at infinitesimally low rates but over a protracted period of time.

Chromium and nickel, toluene diisocyanates and toluene diamines, that are known or suspected carcinogens, can be released from one or more biomaterials.

However, the evidence again suggests that mobilization of chemical carcinogens cannot be the cause of many cases of solid-state carcinogenesis and cannot, therefore, be a key determinant. For example, aluminium oxide ceramic is one of the most inert of all materials, being an oxide ceramic that is highly resistant to reduction to any soluble form. Polytetrafluoroethylene is the most stable of all polymers and cannot release any components under physiological conditions. Similarly, poly(methyl methacrylate) appears incapable of biodegradation under physiological conditions, although it may release residual monomers. Nevertheless, all three have been shown to produce tumours in rodents (e.g., Oppenheimer *et al.*, 1955; Stinson, 1960).

2.1.4 *Chemical or crystallographic nature of any released particulate components*

The same arguments could be made with respect to the chemistry or crystallography of solid particles released from any biomaterial. Microscopically visible corrosion products that are released from some metallic biomaterials induce chronic inflammatory reactions that are seen around them. For example, the chromium-rich deposits seen around some grossly corroded stainless steel products induce chronic inflammation, with the presence of macrophages, giant cells and even plasma cells. The crystalline form of particulate matter is important; for example, inhalation of crystalline silica is associated with lung cancer in certain occupational exposures, while inhalation of amorphous silica is not (IARC, 1997a). Both forms of silica are used as fillers in biomaterials. Nevertheless, there does not appear to be any consistent relationship between solid-state carcinogenicity and any known chemical or crystallographic feature of particulates released from materials.

2.1.5 *Physical nature of any released particulate components*

A major clinical concern is the possibility of the release of particulate matter arising from surface abrasion of biomaterials, this being especially important with the generation of particulate wear debris in orthopaedic joint prostheses. Differences in physico-chemical characteristics of wear debris influence degradation and the identity and rate of release of chemical species from the material. Once again, it might be assumed that the presence of very large numbers of particles, whose release from devices has been estimated to be in the order of hundreds of thousands per day (Doorne *et al.*, 1998), could contribute to solid-state carcinogenesis. It is very difficult to determine from the experimental evidence whether this is, in fact, the case, since it is not possible to reproduce exactly the clinical conditions in an experimental model. However, small particles of polymer are in general less likely to induce tumours than large particles (see e.g., Oppenheimer *et al.*, 1961).

2.1.6 *Size and shape*

Certain physical features of implants can influence the characteristics of the host response to them. In experimental animals, the shape of the implant influences the development of the fibrous capsule that forms around the implant. Established physical parameters that influence solid-state tumorigenicity in rats and mice are listed in Table 2. Recent studies with a silicone elastomer and cellulose acetate samples with different degrees of permeability and porosity, subcutaneously implanted in rats (James *et al.*, 1997), showed variations in acute inflammatory and chronic fibrotic responses, cellularity, proliferation and apoptotic cell death within the fibrous capsules. These differences were correlated with differences in carcinogenicity. Thus, physical attributes of

Table 2. Some physical properties of non-metallic foreign bodies that affect tumour incidence in rats and mice

Increase in tumorigenicity	Decrease in tumorigenicity
Large size	Small size
Geometry	Geometry
Discs	Fine shreds
Concave buttons	Perforated sheets
Continuous sheets	
Smooth surface	Rough surface
Pore size (filters)	Pore size (filters)
< 0.02 μm (cells do not invade)	> 0.65 μm (cells invade)

Modified from Oppenheimer *et al.* (1955), Goldhaber (1962), Bischoff & Bryson (1964), Paulini *et al.* (1975) and Moizhess & Vasiliev (1989)

the material samples are clearly important with respect to the development of tumours in rats.

2.1.7 Surface energy and surface topography

Both surface energy and the topography are able to influence cell behaviour, in the former case by virtue of the energetics of cell attachment and spreading and in the latter case by control of cell shape through direct physical interaction between cell membranes and surface features. With respect to surface energy, the fact that high-energy surfaces of metals and the low-energy surfaces of some polymers (including highly hydrophilic surfaces of polyvinylpyrrolidone and cellulosic polymers) can be tumorigenic suggests that this is not an important factor in solid-state carcinogenicity. With respect to surface topography, although macroporosity has some effect, there does not appear to be any evidence that general topographical features of solid surfaces play any part in this process.

2.1.8 Hardness of the material, its elastic moduli or the flexibility of the component

The fact that a medical device might be carcinogenic after implantation suggests that it is causing some unnatural process to take place in the adjacent tissue. One of the more obvious stimuli to a tissue associated with the presence of a foreign material is the physical or mechanical disturbance to the physiological system. If a hard, rigid, synthetic material is placed in an intramuscular site, the immediate consequence will be perturbation of the stress fields within the tissue. This could result in an increased stimulus to fibrosis through the mechanical stimulation of fibroblasts. The presence of an elastomer such as silicone within a muscle invokes less chronic inflammatory response than the presence of a rigid material, such as an aluminium oxide ceramic. There is no evidence, however, that these differences in rigidity and hardness are reflected at all in tumour formation.

2.1.9 Electrical or magnetic properties of the material

It has been speculated that some physical parameters such as the electrical or magnetic characteristics of materials are important variables that control the host response. Since some of these properties differ significantly from one material to another, and since physiological processes are known to be influenced by bioelectrical phenomena, such suggestions are quite plausible. Specific suggestions have, for example, been concerned with the possible influence of dielectric constants on biocompatibility. It does not appear that any systematic study has been performed on the relationship, if any, between carcinogenesis and these properties. Nevertheless, materials which are excellent conductors of electricity and materials which are insulators produce similar tumours under otherwise similar conditions, as do ferromagnetic and paramagnetic materials, and materials with high and with low dielectric constants.

2.1.10 *Radioactivity*

Some medical devices involve components that are radioactive. In some cases, the radioactivity is intentional as the implant is intended to deliver localized radiotherapy. In other cases, the radioactivity is associated with the presence of small amounts of impurities or additives, as with yttria-stabilized zirconia used in some joint replacement prostheses. Concern has been expressed about the possibility that these implanted sources of radioactivity could be carcinogenic, but there is no evidence of this.

2.1.11 *Sterilization procedures*

All implanted devices used in human patients have to be sterilized. Most experimental procedures with animals are performed under sterile conditions and it is assumed that most studies of the biocompatibility, including carcinogenicity, of materials involve sterilized samples. There is a theoretical possibility, therefore, that sterilization processes themselves are risk factors. One problem in examining this possibility is that not all studies specify the sterilization conditions. Additionally, there are widely different techniques for sterilization, including dry heat, steam, γ-radiation (see IARC, 2000), electron beam radiation and exposure to ethylene oxide (see IARC, 1994a). If all samples producing tumours had been sterilized by ethylene oxide, carcinogenesis initiated by residues of this gas or any product derived from it would certainly be a logical explanation. However, since tumours have clearly arisen from implants sterilized by several other techniques, it is very difficult to believe that this sterilization method could be a significant factor.

2.2 Host variables

2.2.1 *Species and strain*

Tumours have been associated with implanted devices or materials in the following species: humans, dogs, cats, rabbits, guinea-pigs, rats, Syrian hamsters and mice. There is no reason to suppose that this list represents all the species in which tumours could occur; humans, and to a much lesser extent dogs and cats, receive medical devices therapeutically and the other animals are the main experimental species in which materials are implanted for study. By far the largest incidence of solid-state tumours has been associated with rats, with a large number also seen with mice. This may reflect the fact that these rodents are most usually used for carcinogenicity studies, but also it could reflect significant species specificity. It is also possible that there is strain specificity, but this is even harder to define. Tumours have been seen in at least ten different strains of rats, but this factor has not been systematically investigated.

2.2.2 *Age, sex and size of the animal*

Carcinogenicity studies of implanted materials always involve long-term exposure and usually extend for the lifetime of the animal. There is some evidence that the latent period of solid-state tumour formation in rats decreases with the age of implantation.

Paulini *et al.* (1975) found that rats which developed sarcomas after implantation of polyester-polyurethane sponge did so at an average age of 20.6 months (range 12.5–24.5 months), irrespective of whether the material was implanted in the first or the fifteenth month of life. In most cases, however, the incidence of tumour formation as a function of age cannot be assessed from the experimental evidence. Tumours associated with biomaterials have been reported in both male and female animals, and no consistent sex bias has been determined.

With respect to size, differences within a particular rodent species are not sufficient to allow any conclusions to be reached. Large dogs, however, may be more susceptible than small dogs to sarcoma development following implantation (Stevenson, 1991).

2.2.3 *Site of implantation*

Tumours have been found at the site of materials implanted via a number of different routes. The published literature suggests that experimental animals are susceptible to implantation site tumorigenesis following subcutaneous, intramuscular, intraperitoneal, intrapulmonary, intra-articular, intravascular and possibly other routes of administration of foreign bodies.

The vast majority of experiments have been performed with subcutaneous and intramuscular implantation. There have been no controlled studies to determine whether either of these types of site is more at risk than the other or whether the incidence of tumours at such sites represents anything other than the fact that they are more commonly employed.

2.2.4 *Known risk factors for human cancer*

Any variable in the host that can be responsible for differences in inflammatory and regenerative processes may affect susceptibility to solid-state carcinogenesis. However, the very low number of confirmed cases of implant-related tumours in humans makes analysis very difficult.

2.2.5 *Pharmacological status of a human host*

Similarly, it might be expected that any drug regimen, especially one that is prolonged or repeated, and or that involves anti-inflammatory or immunosuppressive components, could have some influence on susceptibility to tumours, but again the very small patient population precludes such analysis.

2.2.6 *Indication for clinical intervention and prior or coexistent disease*

Again, due to the paucity of data, no analysis of these factors can be made.

2.2.7 *Latent period for tumour formation*

The latency of tumours arising as a result of carcinogenic exposures is, in part, a function of the longevity of the species. It is therefore logical to assume that the latent period will vary from host species to host species, so that differences in incidence at any one time period could be due to these variations. In rats the latent period is typically 15–30 weeks. Observations of tumours in clinical patients would suggest that the latent period is quite long (see Tables 33–36, Section 2D), although there are significant variations. The latent period for osteosarcomas associated with orthopaedic devices in dogs is in the range of six years (see Table 37, Section 3.1.1), which would be consistent with the period quoted above for rats and the 20 or so years in humans, on the basis of life expectancy.

2.3 Host–material system

Joint replacements in humans frequently entail lengthy and complex surgery that may be complicated by subsequent infection, or loosening or other failure of the prosthesis. These complications may predispose these patients to the development of subsequent tumours; however, the small number of patients that have developed joint replacement-associated tumours precludes analysis of these factors.

Immediately after biomaterials and foreign bodies are implanted, host proteins are adsorbed onto the surface. As described earlier, the physicochemical properties of the material surface influence the extent of adsorption. Host cells subsequently adhere to the modified material surface. The interaction between host cells and the implant varies depending on the anatomical site and the target cell. For example, albumin and fibrinogen are adsorbed from blood while fibronectin and vitronectin are adsorbed from the extracellular matrix. In general, host cell–material interactions may cause haemolysis, cytotoxicity, apoptosis, proliferation, altered gene expression, release of inflammatory mediators and cytokines, encapsulation by fibrosis and mutagenicity and carcinogenicity (Fubini *et al.*, 1998). The mechanisms leading to mutagenicity and carcinogenicity will be discussed in more detail.

In contrast to exogenous chemicals, the dose of solid material implanted into the host that produces any cellular response is difficult to quantify. This difficulty arises because metal ions and other chemical species may be mobilized from the surface of the implant, but the composition of these mobilized constituents may not reflect the composition of the bulk material. Medical implants are often complex in structure and composition. The biologically active compounds that can be or are released from a medical device depend on the original composition of the device. These compounds may arise from modification of the biomaterial by the biological environment.

For an evaluation of the biological response to a biomaterial, especially in relation to mutagenicity and carcinogenicity, it is necessary to know: the exact composition of the biomaterial or extract(s); the composition and rates of release of leachable materials into the biological environment; the potential for degradation, which may lead to the formation of compounds with different mutagenic properties or leachability; the influence of the physical environment of the biomaterial; and the surface properties. Much of the information available for assessment is inadequate in these respects, and the methods used are often not validated. It is not possible to predict whether a biomaterial is mutagenic solely on the basis of its original composition.

INTRODUCTION

Since foreign bodies and metal implants usually persist in the host for long periods of time, there is the potential for prolonged mobilization and release of metal ions and soluble chemical species from solid materials. Of particular concern is the mobilization of ions such as iron, both from the implant and from endogenous stores, because these transition elements can catalyse the generation of free radicals by Fenton reactions. Local generation of reactive oxygen and nitrogen species can be amplified by a persistent or chronic host inflammatory response (Fubini *et al.*, 1998).

Mobilized metal ions and chemical species and particulate wear debris may produce local and or systemic effects. Soluble metal ions and chemical breakdown or degradation products from polymers may be transported in plasma or blood cells and distributed to distant sites. These mobilized components may bind directly to distant target cells or host macromolecules (including proteins or DNA) or be metabolized to more toxic, reactive intermediates. Alternatively, these solubilized materials may be converted to more polar metabolites and excreted in the bile or urine. Binding of soluble ions and chemical species mobilized from the surface of solid materials to cellular molecules, especially DNA, may be involved in initiation of cancer. Binding to host proteins may also initiate local or systemic immune responses.

Particulate materials and wear debris released from the surface of biomaterials are usually phagocytosed by macrophages. Macrophages may store poorly soluble, non-degradable particulates within phagolysosomes for long periods of time. In response to large particulates or fibrous materials, macrophages may fuse to form multinucleated, foreign body giant cells. Macrophages are motile cells and may transport particulates to the lymphatics where they are subsequently stored in local lymph nodes. Systemic transport and storage of particulates within macrophages residing at distant sites such as the liver, spleen and bone-marrow have also been reported, e.g., in silicosis (Silicosis and Silicate Disease Committee, 1988).

3. General mechanisms of solid-state carcinogenesis

All carcinogens, regardless of their physical or chemical state, can be classified according to their mechanism of action (Table 3). In general, carcinogens are classified as genotoxic (positive in bacterial mutagenesis assays and mammalian assays for the induction of micronuclei or cytogenetic alterations) or non-genotoxic agents which usually induce cell proliferation (mitogenic or cytotoxic agents and hormones). Some carcinogens induce molecular alterations by epigenetic mechanisms (binding to heterochromatin or altered patterns of DNA methylation) or by interference with DNA repair mechanisms (Butterworth *et al.*, 1992). DNA damage in target cell populations may also be induced indirectly by reactive oxygen or nitrogen species released from neutrophils or macrophages at sites of persistent or chronic inflammation. Cytokines and growth factors released from activated macrophages can contribute to target cell proliferation.

Table 3. Classification of carcinogens by mechanism of action[a]

Carcinogen	Biological activity
Genotoxic	DNA adducts leading to gene mutation Clastogenic Aneuploidogenic
Nongenotoxic	
Mitogenic	Stimulation of cell proliferation
Cytotoxic	Causes necrosis or apoptosis Compensatory or regenerative hyperplasia

[a] Modified from Butterworth *et al.* (1992)

Although the mechanisms of solid-state carcinogenesis induced by implanted materials remain little studied and poorly understood, there is a considerable literature on the mechanisms which operate following the inhalation of asbestos, crystalline silica and poorly soluble particulates (reviewed in the Appendix). Asbestos and asbestiform fibres (IARC, 1977, 1987a) and crystalline silica (IARC, 1997a) have been classified as carcinogenic to humans. The relevance of these observations to solid-state carcinogenesis in implants of other materials remains uncertain, but a self-amplification mechanism of persistent inflammation, generation of oxidants and release of chemokines and cytokines, as has been proposed in relation to fibre carcinogenesis (Fubini, 1996) offers a unifying hypothesis for solid-state carcinogenesis in general.

3.1 Experimental implants in rodents

Isolated cases of sarcomas and carcinomas arising in association with metallic or plastic nondegradable foreign bodies and implants (Radio & McManus, 1996) have been reported at many anatomical sites (Table 4). An experimental model of foreign-body or solid-state carcinogenesis is implantation of smooth, nondegradable films subcutaneously in rats or mice (reviewed in Brand, 1982, 1987). Several physical factors are correlated with tumorigenicity, including surface area, surface continuity, size and shape, surface smoothness and erosion resistance (Moizhess & Vasiliev, 1989). Generally, powdered non-metallic materials are not tumorigenic. In various strains of mice, there are genetically determined differences in tumour latency (6–30 months) and frequency. These foreign-body tumours were classified as sarcomas and had a variety of histopathological appearances: fibromyxosarcoma, rhabdomyosarcoma, haemangiosarcoma, reticulosarcoma and osteogenic sarcoma. [The Working Group noted that, as with human sarcomas, these pathological diagnoses might be revised based on modern criteria.] The cell of origin has been postulated to be a pluripotential mesenchymal stem cell originating in the microvasculature (Johnson *et al.*, 1973a,b, 1977, 1980). The sarcomas have been shown to be of clonal origin and transplantable. They usually grow

Table 4. Foreign bodies and cancer

Agent	Anatomical site	Cancer
Shrapnel, bullets[a] (humans)	Soft tissues	Fibrosarcoma
	Bone	Chondrosarcoma
	Brain	Meningioma
	Lung	Bronchogenic carcinoma
Bone splinters[a] (humans)	Larynx	Laryngeal carcinoma
Experimental implants[a] (rats, mice)	Subcutaneous	Sarcomas
Asbestos fibres[b] (humans, rodents)	Lung	Bronchogenic carcinoma
	Mesothelium	Malignant mesothelioma
Crystalline silica[c] (humans, rats)	Lung	Bronchogenic carcinoma
Poorly-soluble particulates[d] (rats)	Lung	Bronchogenic carcinoma

[a] Reviewed in Brand (1982, 1987)
[b] Reviewed in IARC (1977, 1987a)
[c] Reviewed in IARC (1997a)
[d] Reviewed in Oberdörster (1997)

rapidly and spread by local invasion; metastases are rare (Brand, 1982). The term 'pluripotential cell' is no longer used and it is currently the view that the cells of origin of mesenchymal tumours cannot be identified. Instead, the tumours are classified according to their direction of differentiation (i.e., where they are going) rather than their histogenesis (i.e., where they came from) (Gould, 1986).

The morphological sequence of tissue reactions to subcutaneous foreign bodies has been described (Brand et al., 1975a). There is an initial acute inflammatory reaction with infiltration of neutrophils and monocytes at the site. Proliferating macrophages and multinucleated giant cells accumulate focally and adhere to the surface. Elongated spindle cells and collagen fibres surround the implant and new capillaries grow in. Fibroblast proliferation and collagen deposition are active until the cells become dormant at about three months. At this time, a collagenous capsule of variable density encases the implant. During this dormant phase, preneoplastic cells have been recovered from the fibrous capsule. Several months later, preneoplastic cells can also be recovered from the implant surface (Buoen et al., 1975). Neoplastic cells have been hypothesized to arise from these adherent preneoplastic cells. Since these sarcomas are presumably derived from primitive vascular cells associated with capillary ingrowth, there is no direct physical interaction between the preneoplastic cells and the surface of the implant during the initial stages of tumour development. Sarcomas are also induced by intraperitoneal implants which have become surrounded by a fibrous capsule (Brand, 1982).

It is proposed that foreign bodies are nongenotoxic carcinogens that act as mitogens by stimulating proliferation of mesenchymal cells that surround the implant. Initiated cells have been postulated to arise spontaneously from microvascular precursors within this proliferating cell population (Johnson et al., 1973a,b, 1977, 1980). Promotion or maturation of these initiated cells was assumed to occur during the dormant phase of encapsulation by dense fibrous tissue (Brand, 1982). Some biochemical and molecular mechanisms that might be responsible for these initiation and promotion stages are discussed in Section 5 of this monograph.

Since the initial observation that cellophane films implanted subcutaneously in rats induced sarcomas (Oppenheimer et al., 1948), numerous plastics and polymers developed for use as medical and dental prosthetic devices have been tested for toxicity and carcinogenicity in animals (reviewed in Rigdon, 1975). In contrast to smooth nondegradable films, similar materials implanted subcutaneously or intraperitoneally in particulate or fibrous form do not induce the types of sarcoma that are typical of foreign-body tumours. Even high doses of particulates injected intraperitoneally in rats generally do not induce sarcomas or malignant mesotheliomas, although diffuse malignant mesotheliomas are readily induced by natural and man-made fibrous materials in rats (Pott et al., 1987). An important exception is the induction of both mesotheliomas and sarcomas in rats following intraperitoneal injection of nickel and nickel alloys containing more than 50% nickel (Pott et al., 1989, 1992). Direct intraperitoneal injection of particulates such as titanium dioxide induces a mild, transient inflammatory response followed by clearance of particles to mesenteric lymph nodes with no subsequent fibrotic or carcinogenic response, even after repeated weekly intraperitoneal injections in mice (Branchaud et al., 1993). The initial inflammatory reaction and subsequent fibrosis induced by implanted biomaterials in animals depend on the species and the anatomical site (Brand, 1982).

An acute inflammatory response of variable intensity occurs that involves oedema, leukocytes and erythrocytes, as in any inflammatory reaction. The involvement of specific cell types and the extent of fibrous encapsulation depend on the kind and physical form of material implanted (Rigdon, 1975). Implanted biomaterials become rapidly coated with host plasma proteins including albumin, immunoglobulin type G (IgG) and fibrinogen. Coating with albumin appears to down-regulate the inflammatory response, while adsorption of fibrinogen appears to trigger both coagulation and acute inflammation (Tang et al., 1993, 1996). Persistent inflammation at the surface of biomaterials with localized generation of oxidants not only accelerates autoxidation (Radio & McManus, 1996), but may also induce mutations indirectly in proliferating mesenchymal cells surrounding the implant. Deposition of haemosiderin following haemolysis of extravasated erythrocytes may provide a local source of iron that catalyses generation of hydroxyl radicals from oxidants released by inflammatory cells. So far, there is no evidence for or against this mechanism in rodents or humans, although there is not a good correlation between the intensity or persistence of the acute inflammatory response and the subsequent development of foreign-body tumours (Rigdon, 1975).

The rare cases of human sarcomas arising in association with metallic foreign bodies embedded in soft tissues or bone or in association with prosthetic devices could arise by a mechanism similar to that described for foreign-body tumorigenesis in mice and rats; however, using the same techniques developed in the mouse model, no pre-neoplastic cells were identified in 50 patients who had received a variety of surgical implants (Brand, 1982). Carcinomas may develop in response to exogenous foreign bodies such as fragments of bullets or splinters of bone. In these cases, prolonged physical damage to epithelial surfaces followed by regeneration of epithelial cells may provide the stimulus for persistent cell proliferation.

4. Pathology of sarcomas, reactive and pseudoneoplastic conditions

4.1 Introduction

Both epithelial and connective tissue can undergo reactive and pseudoneoplastic proliferation in response to a variety of stimuli. The majority of reactions to foreign materials, and most diagnostic difficulties, concern the connective tissues.

The connective tissues comprise the mesodermally derived connective tissues of the trunk and extremities, i.e., bone, cartilage, muscle, fat, fibrous tissue and blood vessels, and include, by convention, peripheral nerves which are of neuroectodermal origin. Tumours of soft tissue and bone can be benign, malignant (sarcomas which metastasize) or of intermediate type (liable to recur locally but only rarely to metastasize). The commonest anatomical locations of soft-tissue sarcomas are the limbs and limb girdles, the retroperitoneum, the chest and abdominal walls and the mediastinum. Sarcomas of the head and neck form a further clinically significant subgroup, and similar tumours can occasionally arise in connective tissue elements of solid or hollow viscera. Osteo-sarcomas and chondrosarcomas, although most frequently of skeletal origin, also arise in extra-skeletal tissues.

4.2 Incidence and etiology

Benign mesenchymal tumours outnumber malignant tumours in hospital series (Enzinger & Weiss, 1995). Malignant tumours of the connective and soft tissues arise at all ages, some 5–10% of cases occurring before the age of 15 years. Age-standardized incidence rates range from 1–3 per 100 000 population per year in most areas covered by cancer registration (Parkin et al., 1997).

The cause or causes are in most cases unknown, although some of the underlying molecular events in the genesis of sarcomas are being elucidated. Associations have been reported with hereditary conditions, therapeutic or accidental irradiation, exposure to certain chemicals and immunological defects. Trauma can draw clinical attention to a pre-existing malignancy, but more commonly causes pseudoneoplastic reactions. However, sarcomas have been reported to arise in burn scars and in relation to metallic and plastic surgical implants.

Soft-tissue tumours can arise in a variety of genetic diseases or hereditary syndromes. Peripheral neurofibromatosis (NF1; also known as Von Recklinghausen's neurofibromatosis), an autosomal dominant condition with variable penetrance, is complicated by malignant peripheral nerve sheath tumours and occasionally other sarcomas. Central neurofibromatosis (NF2) is associated with bilateral acoustic neuromas. In some benign nerve sheath tumours, there is loss of part of chromosome 22 (Emory et al., 1995), and a possible mechanism of neoplasia is loss of the tumour-suppressor gene *NF2* which is localized to 22q11.2-q12. Some malignant peripheral nerve sheath tumours are associated with loss of 17p, including the locus of the tumour-suppressor gene *p53* (Menon et al., 1990).

Fibromatosis or desmoid tumour (a non-metastasizing but locally aggressive lesion) is found in about 10% of patients with the autosomal dominant condition of familial adenomatous polyposis (FAP), in whom it often arises in the mesentery. Gardner's syndrome additionally includes other benign soft-tissue, cutaneous and bone tumours (Enzinger & Weiss, 1995). The FAP locus at 5q21-22 contains the *APC* gene, mutations of which are implicated in FAP and in the genesis of colon cancer. In fibromatoses, a variety of abnormalities have been described including trisomy 7, 8 and 20 (in deep fibromatoses) and, in those associated with FAP, loss of heterozygosity due to deletion of 5q (Dei Tos & Dal Cin, 1997).

Li–Fraumeni syndrome is an autosomal dominant trait in which patients with germline *p53* mutations have a familial predisposition to cancers (Strong et al., 1992). These include childhood soft-tissue sarcomas, breast and other malignancies.

Among patients who survive familial retinoblastoma, 10–20% develop sarcomas including osteosarcoma in the first decade, then other types later in life. This is related to loss of the *Rb* tumour-suppressor gene which is located at 13q14 (Stratton et al., 1989).

Therapeutic irradiation (see IARC, 2000) (for example, in treatment of lymphomas, Hodgkin's disease or breast or gynaecological cancers) is followed, in a very small proportion (0.1%) of cases, by development within the irradiated field of sarcomas in soft tissue or bone (Laskin et al., 1988; Wiklund et al., 1991; Mark et al., 1994; Pitcher et al., 1994). Such sarcomas, which arise after a long interval (exceeding three years and frequently much longer), are, with rare exceptions, of high-grade malignancy. Reported subtypes include malignant fibrous histiocytoma, osteosarcoma, chondrosarcoma, leiomyosarcoma, angiosarcoma (which is sometimes low-grade, notably in the breast (Parham & Fisher, 1997)) and synovial sarcoma (van de Rijn et al., 1997).

Exposure to herbicides containing 2,3,7,8-tetrachlorodibenzo-*para*-dioxin has been associated with human sarcomas (IARC, 1997b), and occupational exposure to vinyl chloride has been implicated in the etiology of angiosarcoma of the liver as well as other neoplasms (IARC, 1979a; Evans et al., 1983; IARC, 1987b).

INTRODUCTION

Sarcomas can develop in immunosuppressed hosts. These include Kaposi's sarcoma linked to human immunodeficiency virus (HIV) infection (IARC, 1996) and acquired immune deficiency syndrome (AIDS), which is associated with infection with Kaposi's sarcoma herpesvirus (KSHV), a recently discovered herpesvirus previously designated HHV8 (Cesarman & Knowles, 1997; IARC, 1997c). Recently, smooth muscle tumours have been reported in immune-disordered children and adults (including transplant recipients and AIDS patients). In some of these, the Epstein–Barr virus (EBV) (IARC, 1997c) genome was demonstrated (Lee et al., 1995; McClain et al., 1995).

4.3 Classification

In contrast to carcinomas, it is not clear from which cells sarcomas arise since they have no in-situ phase. With a few exceptions, soft-tissue malignancies arise *de novo* and only rarely from pre-existing benign soft-tissue tumours, although the latter are numerically much more frequent. The most familiar example of this phenomenon is the malignant peripheral nerve sheath tumour arising in a neurofibroma, particularly in the setting of NF1.

Sarcomas are, therefore, classified by their apparent direction of differentiation, i.e., according to the cell or tissue type which they most resemble (Table 5). Thus, liposarcomas display fatty differentiation, leiomyosarcomas form smooth muscle, rhabdomyosarcomas form skeletal muscle and so on. Most sarcomas display one line of differentiation, although this sometimes changes when the tumour recurs. Because neoplasms can resemble embryonic tissues at different developmental stages, as well as adult tissues, and because of the wide variety of cell types and tissues derived from mesenchyme, there is a large number of sarcoma subtypes. The second edition of the

Table 5. Classification of sarcomas according to type of differentiation

Mesenchymal differentiation (adult or embryonic)	Other differentiation (consistent pattern)	No specific differentiation (variable pattern)
Liposarcoma (adipose tissue)	Synovial sarcoma (epithelial)	MFH (fibroblastic)
Leiomyosarcoma (smooth muscle)	Epithelioid sarcoma (epithelial)	Storiform-pleomorphic
Rhabdomyosarcoma (striated muscle)	Clear-cell sarcoma (melanocytic/neural)	Myxoid
Angiosarcoma (endothelial cell)	Ewing's sarcoma/pPNET (neural)	Giant cell
MPNST (Schwann cell)	Alveolar soft part sarcoma (nature uncertain)	Xanthomatous
Osteosarcoma (bone)		Sarcoma (NOS)
Chondrosarcoma (cartilage)		
Fibrosarcoma (fibroblastic)		

MFH, malignant fibrous histiocytoma; MPNST, malignant peripheral nerve sheath tumour; pPNET, peripheral primitive neuroectodermal tumour; NOS, not otherwise specified
The terminology used for soft-tissue sarcomas is that of WHO (Weiss, 1994)

WHO classification of soft-tissue tumours (Weiss, 1994) lists nearly 100 intermediate or malignant entities.

Cellular differentiation is apparent at a variety of levels. Morphologically, an initial assessment will include cell shape, and the presence of any obvious tissue type—for example, formation of neoplastic fat, muscle, bone, cartilage or blood vessels. In many cases, precise categorization requires further investigation by immunohistochemistry, electron microscopy or genetic techniques. Immunohistochemistry is of particular use in differential diagnosis of spindle- and round-cell sarcomas, and electron microscopy in the diagnosis of tumours with no or multiple immunohistochemical markers (Erlandson, 1994). Cytogenetic and molecular genetic techniques can reveal aberrations in a number of sarcomas and are valuable for diagnosing childhood-type small round-cell tumours and some myxoid tumours. Of special interest is the consistent presence in some sarcoma subtypes of specific chromosomal translocations, for many of which the relevant fusion genes have been identified (Cooper, 1996; Fisher, 1999) (Table 6). It is not known how these events arise, but they allow more precise classification and diagnosis and clarify the interrelationship of morphological subtypes. For example, it has been shown that round-cell liposarcoma is the poorly differentiated variant of myxoid liposarcoma (Weiss, 1996); that Ewing's sarcoma of both soft tissue

Table 6. Chromosomal translocations in malignant soft-tissue tumours

Tumour type	Usual and variant translocations	Fusion genes
Synovial sarcoma	t(x;18)(p11.2;q11.2)	*SSX1* or *SSX2*, *SYT*
MRC liposarcoma	t(12;16)(q13;p11)	*CHOP*, *TLS*
	t(12;22)(q13;q11-q12)	*CHOP*, *EWS*
Ewing's sarcoma/pPNET	t(11;22)(q24;q12)	*FLI1*, *EWS*
	t(21;22)(q22;q12)	*ERG*, *EWS*
	t(7;22)(p22;q12)	*ETV1*, *EWS*
	t(2;22)(q33;q12)	*FEV*, *EWS*
	t(17;22)(q12;q12)	*E1AF*, *EWS*
Desmoplastic SRCT	t(11;22)(p13;q12)	*WT1*, *EWS*
Alveolar rhabdomyosarcoma	t(2;13)(q35;q14)	*PAX3*, *FKHR*
	t(1;13)(q36;q14)	*PAX7*, *FKHR*
Myxoid chondrosarcoma (extra-osseous)	t(9;22)(q21-31;q12.2)	*CHN*, *EWS*
Clear-cell sarcoma	t(12;22)(q13;q12)	*ATF1*, *EWS*
DFSP/GCF	t(17;22)(q22;q13)	*COL1A*, *PDGFB1*
CIFS	t(12;15)(p13;q25)	*ETV6*, *NTRK3*

MRC, myxoid/round cell; pPNET, peripheral primitive neuroectodermal tumour; SRCT, small round-cell tumour; DFSP, dermatofibrosarcoma protuberans; GCF, giant-cell fibroblastoma; CIFS, congenital-infantile fibrosarcoma
From Fisher (1999)

INTRODUCTION

and bone, peripheral primitive neuroectodermal tumours (pPNET) and thoraco-pulmonary small round-cell tumours (Askin tumour) all have the same underlying genetic abnormality; and that clear-cell sarcoma of soft parts and malignant melanoma are separate conditions, as are soft-tissue and osseous variants of myxoid chondrosarcoma (Brody et al., 1997a).

A number of soft-tissue sarcomas do not resemble any normal mesenchymal element and many of these have been found to display non-mesenchymal differentiation (see Table 5). Thus synovial sarcoma (Fisher, 1986) and epithelioid sarcoma (Fisher, 1988) show epithelial differentiation, Ewing's sarcoma and pPNETs are primitive neural tumours and clear-cell sarcomas of tendons and aponeuroses have melanocytic features (Chung & Enzinger, 1983).

Malignant tumours composed of neoplastic fibroblasts have a particularly wide variety of manifestations. The lower grades include fibrosarcomas classified according to the accompanying stromal changes—myxoid (Angervall et al., 1977), fibromyxoid (Evans, 1993) or inflammatory (Meis & Enzinger, 1991). The higher-grade or pleomorphic sarcomas have been classified as malignant fibrous histiocytomas (Weiss & Enzinger, 1978), and until recently the commonest adult soft-tissue sarcoma was malignant fibrous histiocytoma of the storiform pleomorphic type (Fisher et al., 1992). The application of modern pathological techniques has, however, enabled many of these to be identified as poorly differentiated examples of various specific types of sarcoma (Fletcher, 1992; Fisher, 1996). It is also clear that some carcinomas, melanomas and even lymphomas can assume malignant fibrous histiocytoma-like patterns in solid organs and in soft tissues (Fletcher, 1992). The residual group of pleomorphic sarcomas, in which no differentiation is detected, show fibroblastic features, and should perhaps be called pleomorphic fibrosarcoma but the term malignant fibrous histiocytoma is well established and useful in diagnostic and clinical practice.

In contrast to the sarcoma types listed in Table 5, malignant fibrous histiocytomas do not show consistent genetic abnormalities, although they display a number of non-specific aberrations.

4.4 Behaviour, grading and staging

Sarcomas grow and infiltrate locally, and many eventually metastasize. They spread commonly to the lungs and bone, and in some cases to lymph nodes. Their behaviour can be predicted to some extent by histological subtypes; some types are known to metastasize early, while others are indolent.

For the remainder, which form the majority of soft-tissue sarcomas, the behaviour is variable. One of the principal factors in assessing prognosis and determining management is the histological grade. Grading is an attempt to predict behaviour from microscopic features and usually relates to the degree of differentiation or resemblance to normal tissue. For carcinomas, where the degree of differentiation is readily assessed, grading is relatively straightforward, but the task is more difficult for sarcomas, which include many different types of tumour. Some resemble adult tissue, e.g., smooth muscle or fatty tumours, yet may have a poor prognosis even when well differentiated. Others recapitulate normal embryonic tissue but can have either a good or bad prognosis: although rhabdomyosarcoma is high-grade, myxoid liposarcoma is not. Additionally, many soft-tissue sarcomas do not resemble any normal tissue, so that their differentiation cannot be determined. Grading systems need to take these factors into account as well as the fact that some sarcomas always have a slow course and low metastatic potential and others are always aggressive.

Several grading systems are in clinical use (Coindre, 1993) as none has been universally accepted. As well as diagnostic category, factors commonly used are pleomorphism, mitotic index and necrosis. In some systems, these are assigned scores which are summed to give the final grade. Most systems have three grades, which relate to differences in survival.

Molecular genetic findings might relate to prognosis. For example, in alveolar rhabdomyosarcoma those tumours with t(1;13)(q36;q14) have a more favourable outcome than those with t(2:13)(q35–37;q14) (Kelly et al., 1997) and, in synovial sarcoma, a significantly longer metastasis-free survival period has been associated with patients whose localized tumour involved the *SSX2* gene rather than the *SSX1* gene (Kawai et al., 1998).

Some lesions, notably fibromatosis, are technically benign but can be relentlessly locally recurrent and infiltrative and thereby cause significant morbidity and mortality.

4.5 Pseudosarcomas and reactive conditions

4.5.1 *Reactions to injury*

(a) *Early reactions to injuries*

Tissue destruction is followed by the formation of granulation tissue, with ingrowth of inflammatory cells, endothelial cells and myofibroblasts. The latter display features of both smooth muscle cells and fibroblasts (Schürch, 1997) and have contractile and collagen synthetic functions; they play a major role in wound healing and resultant fibrosis or development of scar tissue which represents the late stage of reaction to trauma.

Diagnosis of malignancy can be difficult, both from benign neoplasms of similar differentiation and from a large group of tumours and tumour-like lesions, sometimes called pseudosarcomas. These can be mistaken for malignancies (particularly spindle-cell sarcomas), both clinically because of their rapid growth and microscopically by the presence of atypical cells and frequent mitoses. Any of the diagnostic categories can be involved, but the commonest are proliferations of fibroblasts or myofibroblasts. These include cutaneous fibrous histiocytomas, the keloids, fasciitis, and the majority of reactions to injury or to foreign substances.

Assessment of such lesions begins with consideration of clinical factors. Among these are the size and duration of the tumour (for example, a sarcoma is generally larger with a longer history, while fasciitis is smaller and of more rapid onset), and its location, including anatomical plane—cutaneous, subcutaneous or deep. Most pseudosarcomas and benign tumours, but only rarely sarcomas (predominantly myxofibrosarcoma, epithelioid sarcoma, malignant peripheral nerve sheath tumour and leiomyosarcoma), occur in the superficial soft tissues. Conversely, a mass located beneath the deep fascia, within or between muscles, is more likely to be a sarcoma. The plane in which the tumour is situated can also be determined by imaging (computerized tomography or nuclear magnetic resonance), which can additionally suggest the composition of the lesion.

Fasciitis

Soft-tissue myofibroblastic reactions include the various types of fasciitis, a term which includes a number of possibly unrelated conditions of which the type example is nodular fasciitis. Proliferative myositis, occurring within skeletal muscle, is closely similar and inflammatory pseudotumours in some visceral locations, including larynx, bladder and spermatic cord, also resemble nodular fasciitis conditions.

Nodular fasciitis (Meister *et al.*, 1978; Bernstein & Lattes, 1982; Montgomery & Meis, 1991) is a reactive condition characterized by its extremely rapid growth (more so than the usual sarcoma). There is sometimes a history of recent trauma. Nodular fasciitis occurs in relation to the superficial fascia, mainly on the upper limb and trunk in young adults, although cases arise elsewhere including head and neck. The lesion achieves its small size of 2–3 cm in a matter of days or weeks; only rarely are lesions larger or of longer duration (three to 12 months). This lesion has been reported in the dermis (Lai & Lam, 1993; Price *et al.*, 1993), and intravascular fasciitis (Patchefsky & Enzinger, 1981) and cranial fasciitis (Lauer & Enzinger, 1980) are well documented variants.

Most early cases display a zonation effect or maturation from the centre (hypocellular or hyalinized) to the periphery (hypercellular with inflammatory cells and blood vessels). In between, a loose myxoid area is populated by non-pleomorphic myofibroblasts loosely arranged in a 'tissue culture'-like manner in a variably myxoid stroma, with lymphocytes and red blood cells. Older lesions have a variety of patterns with storiform foci, interdigitating bundles and myxoid, hyalinized (especially in older lesions) or cystic areas, even in the same lesion. Most examples contain one or two mitoses per 10 high power fields ($\times$ 400); a lesion with large numbers of mitoses or abnormal forms should be viewed with caution and may represent a malignant process. Ultrastructurally, the cells are myofibroblasts and fibroblasts, in keeping with which immunohistochemistry demonstrates smooth muscle and muscle-specific actins (but not desmin or CD34).

Because of its rapid growth and mitotic activity, nodular fasciitis is often confused by both clinicians and pathologists with a sarcoma, particularly myxofibrosarcoma or leiomyosarcoma. It is, however, essentially a reactive and non-recurrent lesion.

Proliferative fasciitis and myositis

These two benign lesions, which occur at older ages than nodular fasciitis, are characterized by a fasciitis-like background containing clusters of ganglion-cell-like modified fibroblasts which have basophilic cytoplasm and a large nucleus with prominent nucleolus. The same changes may occur either in superficial soft tissues (proliferative fasciitis; Chung & Enzinger, 1975) or in skeletal muscle (proliferative myositis; Enzinger & Dulcey, 1967). Architecturally, proliferative fasciitis resembles nodular fasciitis, whereas proliferative myositis is characterized by a chequerboard infiltration of the connective tissue, separating muscle fibres. In both conditions, rounded basophilic ganglion-like cells form nodular aggregates within areas having the more traditional features of nodular fasciitis. The ganglion-like cells are considered to be modified fibroblasts (Meis & Enzinger, 1992).

Proliferative fasciitis (Enzinger & Dulcey, 1967) and myositis can be confused with malignancies, including carcinoma, melanoma or large-cell lymphoma in adults, and rhabdomyosarcoma or ganglioneuroblastoma in children. These are usually readily separable by the clinical picture and by immunohistochemistry.

Ischaemic fasciitis

This was first described as atypical decubital fibroplasia (Montgomery *et al.*, 1992), and subsequently it was termed ischaemic fasciitis (Perosio & Weiss, 1993). Predominantly affected are elderly patients who are physically debilitated or immobilized. The sites include soft tissues of the shoulder, posterior chest wall, sacrum, greater trochanter, buttock, thigh and arm, with a short history of three weeks to six months. Lesions are located in the deep subcutis and occasionally extend into the muscle, but extensive epidermal ulceration is absent. Somewhat similar appearances can be found in infected surgical wounds which fail to heal.

Microscopically, there is a lobular arrangement of zones of fibrinoid and coagulative necrosis with fibrin thrombi and spindle cells in a prominent myxoid stroma rimmed by ingrowing ectatic thin-walled vessels. The spindle cells are focally atypical with large hyperchromatic nuclei, or with prominent nucleoli and basophilic cytoplasm, resembling the cells of proliferative fasciitis. Fat necrosis is seen at the periphery. Two thirds are actin-positive, and half display CD34. Desmin is negative although one case had cytokeratin. An occasional case recurs but none has metastasized. This can be misdiagnosed as epithelioid sarcoma, myxoid malignant fibrous histiocytoma, myxoid chondrosarcoma or myxoid liposarcoma.

Somewhat similar atypical fibroblastic proliferations are seen in a variety of non-neoplastic circumstances, including trauma, ischaemia and following radiation therapy, presumably as a common reaction. For the pathologist, the importance lies in not over-diagnosing a sarcoma by misinterpreting the atypia (there are no abnormal mitoses) and necrosis.

INTRODUCTION

Non-neoplastic heterotopic ossifications

A number of possibly related reactive or benign neoplastic conditions of soft tissues are characterized by formation of osteoid or bone (Kilpatrick *et al.*, 1997). Because such lesions can be very cellular in the early stages, they may be misdiagnosed as sarcomas. They occur in muscle, and also sometimes in subcutis, fascia or periosteum, and are therefore variously termed myositis ossificans, ossifying fasciitis, florid reactive periostitis and fibro-osseous pseudotumour of digits. Collectively, they can be regarded as pseudomalignant osseous tumours of soft tissue. Many but not all cases have a definite history of trauma, so that they conceivably represent an exaggerated dystrophic response to tissue damage.

The type example is myositis ossificans (Enzinger & Weiss, 1995), which affects young adults, and especially the flexor muscles of the arm and the quadriceps muscles of the thigh. It appears within a few weeks and can form a mass exceeding 6 cm in diameter. Histologically, the developed lesion displays zonation, with a central nodular fasciitis-like vascular myofibroblastic proliferation, and peripheral progressively maturing bone. The growth of myositis ossificans is usually self-limiting, and it can spontaneously regress.

The principal differential diagnosis is from extraskeletal osteosarcoma, which can readily be misdiagnosed in the early stages, when there is very cellular tissue with immature bone. This can be particularly difficult in a small core needle biopsy. However, the infiltrative growth, nuclear atypia and abnormal mitoses of osteosarcoma are absent. Fibro-osseous pseudotumour of digits is somewhat similar, but is located in the subcutis, is not zoned and has an irregular multinodular growth pattern. Cartilage was present in two of 21 cases and showed maturation to bone without atypia (Dupree & Enzinger, 1986).

Bizarre parosteal osteochondromatous proliferation (BPOP, Nora's reaction; Nora *et al.*, 1983) is a lesion which is thought also to be related to trauma, but which might conceivably have an ischaemic etiology. It was described initially as involving the small tubular bones (proximal phalanges, metatarsals or metacarpals) of hands and feet, but a subsequent larger series (Meneses *et al.*, 1993) identified nearly half of the cases in long bones. Typically, a mass protrudes from the cortex of a bone into the adjacent soft tissue. Histologically, there is a cap of aggressive cytologically bizarre cartilage showing irregular ossification, with spindle cells in the inter-trabecular spaces of the bone.

BPOP requires distinction not only from other non-neoplastic soft-tissue lesions with bone formation such as the pseudomalignant osseous tumours of soft parts mentioned above (which generally lack atypia), but also from parosteal osteosarcoma. BPOP is smaller, has a lobular architecture, more slender, short and irregular bony trabeculae and differs in location and radiological features from the osteosarcoma, and it does not invade adjacent muscle.

Inflammatory pseudotumours

These arise in a variety of organs, including soft tissue, with or (mostly) without a history of trauma. They are composed of a variable mixture of bland-looking myofibroblastic and fibroblastic cells, chronic inflammatory cells and fibrous tissue. This is a heterogeneous group (Chan, 1996), comprising:

(1) Post-inflammatory repair reactions. A subgroup of these, histologically resembling spindle-cell sarcomas, has been described following surgical procedures or trauma, primarily in the urogenital tract, and especially in the bladder neck, prostate or vagina, and also in the buccal mucosa. They are sometimes termed post-operative spindle-cell nodules (Proppe *et al.*, 1984), but similar tumours can also arise spontaneously, especially in the lower urinary tract, where they have been given a variety of descriptive terms.

(2) Benign or low-grade malignant myofibroblastic tumours (including the inflammatory myofibroblastic tumour/inflammatory fibrosarcoma spectrum) (Meis & Enzinger, 1991; Coffin *et al.*, 1995).

(3) EBV-positive inflammatory follicular dendritic-cell sarcomas, especially in liver and spleen (Chan, 1997).

(4) Reactions to infectious agents. These are attributable to a variety of bacteria, including the specific situation of mycobacterial (*Mycobacterium avium-intracellulare* or *M. tuberculosis*) infection in patients with HIV (IARC, 1996) or other causes of immunosuppression.

(5) Reactive mediastinal spindle-cell tumours in anthracosis and anthrasilicosis (Argani *et al.*, 1998).

(b) Neoplasms associated with scar tissue

Exuberant scar tissue in the skin with dense bands of collagen is termed a keloid, and this must be distinguished from dermal sarcomas such as dermatofibrosarcoma protuberans which it clinically resembles. In spite of the intense cellular proliferation and extracellular matrix formation, characteristic of healing wounds, the process is self-limiting. Neoplasms described include squamous-cell carcinoma after burns, basal-cell carcinoma at smallpox vaccination sites (Kaplan, 1987), and sarcomas which arise rarely in longstanding scars (Drut & Barletta, 1975; Brand, 1982; Sherlock *et al.*, 1987; Gargan *et al.*, 1988). The latter have included malignant fibrous histiocytoma (Gargan *et al.*, 1988; Cocke & Tomlinson, 1993), osteosarcoma (Drut & Barletta, 1975), liposarcoma (Nishimoto *et al.*, 1996) and leiomyosarcoma (Can *et al.*, 1998). There are sporadic case reports of fibrosarcoma or malignant fibrous histiocytoma arising in surgical scars (Ju, 1966; Kanaar & Oort, 1969; Sherlock *et al.*, 1987). However, in view of the common occurrence of scars and the rarity of malignancies arising within them, a chance association cannot be ruled out.

Fibromatosis is a clonal proliferation of uniform, bland, evenly dispersed, parallel-aligned fibroblasts and myofibroblasts which produce excessive collagen (Lucas *et al.*, 1997). It is unrelated to trauma but can be histologically difficult to distinguish from scar tissue, especially in the early stages. Fibromatosis can arise in the superficial or deep soft tissues. Examples of the former include palmar, plantar and penile fibromatoses. The latter are desmoid tumours, which typically involve large muscle groups. A common location for desmoid tumours is the anterior abdominal wall, where they can arise in association with pregnancy. Fibromatosis occasionally has an increased familial incidence and some examples in the abdomen (mesentery) are associated with familial polyposis coli in Gardner's syndrome (Rodriguez-Bigas *et al.*, 1994). Desmoid tumours infiltrate locally and can recur, but do not metastasize. They need to be distinguished from scar tissue and nodular fasciitis, and from the closely similar low-grade fibromyxoid sarcoma (Evans, 1993), which has metastatic potential.

4.5.2 *Reactions to foreign material*

Foreign material invokes a variety of tissue reactions. In most instances there is inflammation, followed by encircling fibrosis with or without a foreign body giant cell reaction. In some cases, however, there are more specific morphological appearances, notably with reactions to particulates which can be phagocytosed by macrophages; these appearances can be mistaken for sarcomas. For example:

(*a*) Polyvinylpyrrolidone (PVP) (see IARC, 1999a), formerly used as a plasma expander, has continued to be inappropriately applied as a 'blood tonic' for intravenous injection. It can leak into adjacent tissues and result in the so-called PVP granuloma (Kuo *et al.*, 1997). This is a cellular pseudosarcomatous lesion with abundant extracellular material containing characteristic blue-grey vacuolated macrophages which display positive staining reactions to mucicarmine, colloidal iron and alkaline Congo red, and none with periodic acid–Schiff (PAS) stain and alcian blue. This lesion somewhat resembles myxoid liposarcoma but its cells lack the morphology of lipoblasts and it does not have the characteristic vascular pattern. Its history as well as the pathological findings are usually diagnostic (Hizawa *et al.*, 1984).

(*b*) Silicone, from prosthetic implants or cosmetic injections, can cause a variety of soft-tissue reactions, including the formation of a fibrous capsule (van Diest *et al.*, 1998). Synovial metaplasia has also been reported in about 10% of cases in relation to movement of the prosthesis. Free silicone, via injection or leakage, can induce foreign body giant cells, granulomas and a histiocytic tissue reaction in which the cells, with their ingested silicone, resemble lipoblasts, suggesting a diagnosis of well differentiated liposarcoma (Weiss, 1996). Leaked silicone can also reach draining lymph nodes and a lesion resembling Kikuchi's disease (histiocytic necrotizing lymphadenitis) has been observed (Sever *et al.*, 1996).

(*c*) There are a number of case reports of sarcomas arising in association with metallic (cobalt–chromium, aluminium oxide ceramic, stainless steel) surgical implants, either for fixation of a fracture or reconstruction (see Section 2C.1). However, specific diagnoses in some earlier reports are inadequately documented or might be changed if re-evaluated using current criteria and modern techniques.

(d) The extent of skin and soft tissue damage produced by shrapnel and bullets depends on the type of weapon and the firing distance. Military bullets are fully encased by metal and do not fragment in soft tissues. These bullets are delivered at high velocity and may pass intact through tissues, causing minimal damage. In contrast, hunting bullets expand upon contact with the target, causing extensive soft-tissue damage. Contact wounds produced by high-velocity rifles cause massive destruction, leaving residual powder soot and searing at the entrance site. When fired at greater distances, powder soot produces stippling or tatooing of the skin surface. Metallic balls released from shrapnel projectiles cause multiple soft-tissue wounds. In contrast to entrance wounds, exit wounds do not have a collar of abraded tissue. In general, bullets are not hot when fired. Searing of the skin at the site of a contact wound is caused by the flame of burning powder particles (Di Maio, 1985).

5. General issues in epidemiological research on implants and cancer

There has been relatively little epidemiological research on the association between implants and the occurrence of human cancer. Most of the evidence accumulated so far comes from case reports of malignancies occurring at or near the site of implant. Case reports can be used to identify potential risks but, due to their selective nature and the absence of a control group, they cannot quantify risk nor provide evidence of a cause–effect relationship. Moreover, reports of cancer formation at the site of an implant are extremely rare, in relation to the millions of individuals worldwide who have received implanted devices (Coleman, 1996). The more relevant studies for evaluating whether implants increase cancer risk are case–control and especially cohort studies.

For one form of implant, silicone breast implants, descriptive studies have been conducted to evaluate whether certain cancer incidence trends may be associated with the widespread introduction of these implants. Based on data from the United States Surveillance, Epidemiology and End Results (SEER) programme, no change in the incidence of malignant fibrosarcoma or other sarcoma of the breast was observed between 1973 and 1990 (May & Stroup 1991; Engel *et al.*, 1995), the period of time when breast implants have been in use. While the ecological nature of this type of analysis requires cautious interpretation, the rarity of sarcoma (particularly sarcoma of the breast) in humans suggests that even a few additional cases would lead to a detectable change in incidence.

There are a number of methodological difficulties in investigating the potential association between implants and subsequent cancer risk. These difficulties involve design issues such as selection of study populations, latency and length of follow-up, statistical power, and accuracy of exposure classification, as well as data analysis issues such as control for confounding and multiple hypothesis testing. All of these need to be evaluated before reported exposure–disease associations can be assessed for causality.

5.1 Identification and selection of study population

A primary concern in epidemiological studies of implanted devices is that patients receiving implants may have a lower baseline risk for cancer compared with the general population. This appears to be true for patients selected for hip and knee replacement, who have a better life expectancy than the general population, as they are also likely to have lower cancer morbidity and are encouraged to give up smoking (Holmberg, 1992; Visuri *et al.*, 1994, 1996). Similarly, women at low baseline risk for breast cancer may preferentially seek breast augmentation, and the presence or absence of breast cancer risk factors may influence the plastic surgeon's decision whether or not to perform augmentation (Brinton *et al.*, 1996; Deapen *et al.*, 1997; Kern *et al.*, 1997). These risk factors include family history of breast cancer, and there is some evidence that large breasts are a risk factor for breast cancer, although this was accounted for, in part, by obesity (Hsieh & Trichopoulos, 1991).

Similarly, rheumatoid arthritis is a common indication for hip or knee replacement and is believed to be associated with a higher incidence of certain types of tumour, including non-Hodgkin lymphoma and brain cancer, compared with the general population (Gridley *et al.*, 1993). Therefore, studies of hip or knee replacement in relation to cancer occurrence should either exclude patients with rheumatoid arthritis altogether or at least analyse those patients with rheumatoid arthritis separately (Gillespie *et al.*, 1996; Lewold *et al.*, 1996; Visuri *et al.*, 1996). An observed excess of cancer restricted to the rheumatoid arthritis group, particularly if it is independent of latency, would suggest an association with rheumatoid arthritis and not necessarily with the hip or knee implant itself (Lewold *et al.*, 1996).

With respect to breast augmentation, an additional concern is that women may undergo more intense pre-operative screening and will be deterred from receiving an implant if breast abnormalities are detected. However, this type of detection bias would tend to produce the largest reduction in breast cancer risk during the first year or two after implantation followed by an increased risk later on, a pattern which has not been consistently observed in the epidemiological studies to date (Brinton & Brown, 1997).

It has also been hypothesized that breast implants may interfere with physical breast examination or mammographic visualization of breast tumours, leading to delays in breast cancer diagnosis and worse prognosis among women receiving implants. However, a number of epidemiological studies suggest that women with implants do not present with more advanced stages of breast cancer or experience shorter survival (Birdsell *et al.*, 1993; Brinton *et al.*, 1996; Deapen *et al.*, 1997; Friis *et al.*, 1997).

5.2 Latency and length of follow-up

The observation periods in follow-up studies need to be long in order to evaluate thoroughly the long-term health consequences of implants. This is particularly true given the long latency and low incidence of several of the relevant types of cancer, as well as the increasing use of joint replacements at younger ages and the increasing length of time they are in place in the body.

Moreover, it is important to examine cancer risk by time since implantation and to exclude the first year or two of follow-up. Cancers which occur within a short latency period are likely to be coincidental or to represent a surveillance bias in the implant group (Nyrén et al., 1995). With respect to cancer occurrence, latency is of particular concern given the immunological changes hypothesized to occur along with deterioration of the breast implant capsule over time (Brinton & Brown, 1997), or the increase over time of metallic or non-metallic materials in other types of implants associated with deterioration (Coleman, 1996).

5.3 Statistical power

Many of the epidemiological studies conducted to date have a rather low statistical power to detect any increased risk of rare types of cancer, especially sarcomas (Gillespie et al., 1988; Visuri & Koskenvuo, 1991; Malone et al., 1992; Gabriel et al., 1994; Visuri et al., 1996; Friis et al., 1997). Only as larger cohorts of implant recipients are identified, and as more time has elapsed since implants were first used, can these risks be evaluated with adequate power. Moreover, low statistical power precludes adjustment for extraneous factors which could potentially confound an association between implants and cancer risk.

5.4 Exposure classification

In retrospective cohort studies, errors in recorded surgical procedures can produce underascertainment of exposure and underestimates of the risk associated with implants. However, this type of bias in exposure classification is likely to be minimal if based on registry data (Nyrén et al., 1995). In contrast, the accuracy of implant data is often questionable in case–control studies which rely on patient reports of previous hip or knee replacement or breast implant.

5.5 Multiple hypothesis testing

In epidemiological studies of implants in relation to a variety of malignancies, multiple comparisons (or multiple hypothesis testing) can produce artifactual increases or decreases in risk for site-specific cancers that are a result of chance alone. The occasional statistically significant finding requires cautious interpretation, given that it is often based on small numbers of cases and may reflect the problem of multiple comparisons. As a result, conclusions regarding the association between implants and specific types of cancer must be based on the collective evidence, taking into account consistency across studies and a plausible temporal sequence.

5.6 Control for confounding influences

A major difficulty may be inability to control adequately for implant recipient characteristics, which may be independently related to cancer risk and which may artificially increase or decrease the observed risk estimates. This is of particular concern in studies which use external reference groups or in record-linkage studies, in which the investigator does not have the opportunity to collect additional data on known or suspected confounding variables. For example, among breast augmentation recipients, the potential confounders include higher socioeconomic status, younger age at first birth, leanness, small breasts, and better access to medical care. Similarly, women who smoke cigarettes and who have a greater number of lifetime sexual partners appear more likely to seek breast augmentation and are independently at higher risk for lung or cervical cancer (Cook *et al.*, 1997; Deapen *et al.*, 1997; McLaughlin *et al.*, 1998). With respect to hip or knee replacement patients, potential confounders include immunosuppressive therapy, tobacco smoking, alcohol abuse, use of non-steroidal anti-inflammatory drugs and obesity.

1. EXPOSURE DATA

1A. Metallic Medical and Dental Materials

1A.1 Chemical and physical data

1A.1.1 *Metallurgy*

All metallic materials used for the fabrication of medical and dental devices are mixed in the molten state and poured into a mould for solidification. Some devices may be fabricated from parts moulded or cast in nearly their final shape; others are subjected to a series of thermomechanical processes to produce the final product from the initial ingot. Differences in the resulting microstructures can have significant effects on wear and corrosion rates. In order to understand what alloys were and are used, and how they may behave *in vivo*, it is therefore necessary to be aware of the physical metallurgy of the alloys used in implant surgery.

(a) Solidification and casting

As molten metal cools in a mould, solidification usually begins on the surface of the mould. If the mould is very hot, there are only a few locations where the solid begins to form (nucleate) and grow. If the mould is cold, there are many nucleation sites. At each site, atoms are laid down on the solid in an orderly crystalline manner. For most metallic alloy systems, the solid phase grows as an advancing front with side branches. This pattern resembles the leaf of a fern, and is referred to as dendritic growth. Solidification continues until growth areas meet and form a boundary. Each of these growth sites is called a crystal or grain, and each boundary is a crystal or grain boundary. On a microscopic scale, distinct regions can be identified as the dendrites, the interdendritic region and the grain boundary (Brick *et al.*, 1977). For dental castings, alloying elements are added to produce fine-grained non-dendritic structures.

The positional relationship between atoms is described by what is called a primitive cell or Bravais lattice. For example, atoms may arrange themselves with atoms at eight corners of a cube, with one in the middle; this is called the body-centred cubic lattice or structure. The most common crystal structures for surgical alloys are body-centred cubic, face-centred cubic and hexagonal close-packed. The principal base metals used for implants—iron, cobalt and titanium—undergo allotropic transformation during cooling, resulting in a change in crystal structure. Thus, for example, iron undergoes the phase transformation from liquid to a body-centred cubic solid structure, followed by additional transformations to face-centred cubic and then back to body-centred cubic during cooling (Jackman, 1981).

Metallic alloys are mixtures of several elements in a solid solution, sometimes with intermetallic compound precipitates. For elements of similar atomic charge, diameter and crystal structure, there is no limit to the solubility of one element in another and they therefore solidify as a single phase. For example, copper and nickel are fully soluble in each other. The melting temperature of nickel is higher than that of copper, so that the solid that forms first (the dendrite) will be richer in nickel and that which solidifies later will be richer in copper. Thus, implants in the 'as cast' condition may have a distinct dendritic structure, with differences in chemical composition on a macroscopic scale. Cast devices may be subjected to a subsequent heat treatment known as homogenization or solution annealing to allow atomic diffusion to produce a more uniform chemical composition.

Small differences in the atomic diameter of the two (or more) elements in a single-phase alloy or a two-phase alloy provide strengthening. The presence of large atoms in a lattice of smaller atoms produces a localized strain in the lattice so that they are under localized compression. Similarly, a few small atoms in a lattice of larger atoms will be under localized tension. These localized strains increase the strength of the metal by a mechanism known as solid solution strengthening.

Elements with markedly different properties or crystal structures have limited solubility. For example, carbon atoms are much smaller than iron atoms. In small quantities, carbon is soluble in iron, but at higher concentrations, it precipitates out as a second phase, such as graphite, or forms a carbide. A number of alloy systems use the precipitation of second phases as a strengthening mechanism known as precipitation hardening. In some alloys such as the cobalt alloys, carbides are advantageous with regard to wear and strength. In contrast, they have a detrimental effect on the corrosion resistance of stainless steel.

Carbon also influences the crystal structure of iron. At room temperature, iron has a body-centred cubic crystal structure and is known as α ferrite. When heated, it undergoes a phase transformation to a face-centred cubic structure and is known as γ-austenite. With further heating, it reverts to a body-centred cubic form (δ ferrite) before it melts. Since the spaces, or interstices, between atoms are larger in the face-centred cubic than in the body-centred cubic structure, the carbon atoms fit better in the face-centred cubic structure and thus have a higher solubility in this structure. This has several implications. At low concentrations, carbon increases the thermodynamic stability of the face-centred cubic structure. In other words, the presence of carbon lowers the temperature at which the body-centred cubic α ferrite converts to the face-centred cubic γ austenite and increases the temperature at which the latter converts back to body-centred cubic δ ferrite. Carbon also provides interstitial solid solution strengthening of iron (Brick *et al.*, 1977; Jackman, 1981).

(b) Mechanical forming of wrought alloys

Mechanical forming methods, combined with appropriate heat treatments, can be utilized to produce fine-grained alloys with homogeneous microstructures. Compositional differences associated with dendrites are decreased and formation of small, relatively strain-free grains results in enhancement of corrosion resistance. Hot and cold forging techniques can produce components with uniform composition and a wide range of strain-induced strengths (Jackman, 1981).

Point or line defects can occur in lattice structures of crystalline solids. When viewed as a two-dimensional grid, there is an occasional line of atoms that ends at what is called a dislocation. Above the dislocation, the atoms are in compression, while below it they are in tension. By pushing against the side of the dislocation line with a shear force, the position of the dislocation can move one line or plane at a time. Because of the mobility of dislocations, metals can be deformed plastically. When a metal solidifies, there are few dislocations. If the metal is then mechanically worked, as in pounding with a hammer or bending (like bending a paper clip), dislocations move around, and their number greatly increases. This is the mechanism of plastic deformation of metals. Increasing the number of dislocations, each with its localized stress field, makes it more difficult to implement more plastic deformation: the dislocations obstruct one another. Thus, a metal becomes stronger and harder by the mechanism of cold working (or work hardening). However, due to the high energy state of cold-worked metals, cold working tends to increase the corrosion rate of a metal (Brick *et al.*, 1977; Foley & Brown, 1979; Jackman, 1981).

1A.1.2 *Chemical composition of metals and alloys*
(a) *Specifications for surgical alloys*

Voluntary national and international consensus standard specifications for surgical alloys have been developed and widely adhered to since the early days of metallic implants. The International Organization for Standardization (ISO) and the American Society for Testing and Materials (ASTM) have played a central role in the development and promulgation of standards worldwide. While the actual compositions of alloys in specifications have changed somewhat over the years, these voluntary standards have generally guided the manufacturer's design of metallic implants.

(b) *Stainless steels*

Steel is an alloy of iron, carbon and other elements. In addition to mechanical strength, corrosion resistance is the most valuable feature of stainless steel, and the precipitation of carbon to form a two-phase alloy is undesirable, since the contact between two phases can lead to galvanic corrosion. One way to avoid precipitation of carbon is to keep the concentration of carbon low (typically in the 0.03–0.08% range). It is also important that the iron is in the face-centred cubic form, since the solubility of carbon is higher in this form (Williams & Roaf, 1973; Brick *et al.*, 1977; Foley & Brown, 1979).

A minimum of 12% chromium is added to make steel 'stainless', by the formation of a stable and passive oxide film. Since chromium has a body-centred cubic structure, the addition of chromium stabilizes the body-centred cubic form of iron. Carbon has a great affinity for chromium, forming chromium carbides with a typical composition of $Cr_{23}C_6$. This leads to carbon precipitation in the region surrounding the carbide, where the chromium concentration is depleted as it is taken up into the carbide, and thus the corrosion resistance of the steel surrounding the carbide is reduced. If the chromium content is depleted to below 12%, there is insufficient chromium for effective repassivation, and the stainless steel becomes susceptible to corrosion (see Section 5A.1). To be on the safe side, surgical stainless steel contains 17–19% chromium and the carbon content of surgical alloys is kept below 0.03–0.08%, depending upon the application (Bechtol et al., 1959; Williams & Roaf, 1973; Brick et al., 1977).

Nickel has a face-centred cubic structure and is added to stabilize the face-centred cubic austenitic form of iron so as to keep the carbon in solution. Stainless steel cutlery typically has an '18–8' composition (18% chromium and 8% nickel). Stainless steel implants typically contain 17–19% chromium, 13–15% nickel and 2–3% molybdenum, the latter being added to improve corrosion resistance, while carbon content is below 0.03%. The result is a homogeneous, single-phase, corrosion-resistant stainless steel alloy. While stainless steel has good corrosion resistance, the options for strengthening mechanisms have been limited to cold working (Brick et al., 1977).

The problem of carbide formation is especially important with welded stainless steel parts. If steel is heated to temperatures above 870°C, the carbon is soluble in the face-centred cubic lattice, while below 425°C, the mobility of the chromium is too low for the formation of carbide. However, if the peak temperature in the metal near a weld is in the 'sensitizing range' of 425–870°C, the chromium can diffuse within the solid and carbides can form. This can result in what is known as weld decay, or corrosion of the sensitized metal on each side of the weld. If the metal is heat-treated after welding, the carbides can be redissolved, and the metal is then quickly quenched to avoid reformation (Fontana & Greene, 1978; Foley & Brown, 1979).

Medical devices have generally been made with austenitic stainless steels designated by the American Iron and Steel Institute (AISI) as the '300 series'. The nomenclature used varies somewhat from country to country and between standards organizations, but there is now a trend towards using a Unified Numbering System (UNS). Reference here will be made to the UNS numbers, and the ASTM and ISO standards.

Table 7 shows the chemical composition of five alloys in the 300 series. There is increased nickel content and added molybdenum in S31600, while S30300 has an increased phosphorus content and a much higher sulfur content. The latter is referred to as free-machining stainless steel and has much lower corrosion resistance than the other alloys. While these standards are for instrument-grade stainless steel, some 302 or 304 stainless steels are used for items requiring spring-like properties, such as aneurysm clips. These are similar in composition to those used in the early history of implant surgery, as discussed below.

Over the past couple of decades, the specifications have been tightened. The original ASTM specifications for stainless steel for surgical implants (F 55 and F 56) were published in 1966. They indicated maximum concentrations of phosphorus and

Table 7. Specifications for stainless steels, AISI 300 series (wt %)[a]

Type[b]	Cr	Ni	Mo	Mn	Si	C	N	P	S
301	16–18	6–8	–	< 2	< 1	< 0.15	–	0.045	< 0.03
302	17–19	8–10	–	< 2	< 1	< 0.15	< 0.1	0.045	< 0.03
303	17–19	8–10	< 0.07	< 2	< 1	< 0.12	–	0.06	0.15–0.35
304	17–19	8–11	–	< 2	< 1	< 0.07	< 0.1	0.045	< 0.03
316	16.5–18.5	10.5–13.5	2–2.5	< 2	< 1	< 0.07	< 0.1	0.045	< 0.03

[a] Balance of composition in each case is iron (Fe)
[b] ISO and ASTM specifications:
ASTM F 899 Standard specification for Stainless Steel Billet, Bar, and Wire for Surgical Instruments; ISO 7153-1 Surgical Instruments - metallic materials – Part 1. Stainless steel (304 = S30400; (Fe73Cr18Ni8); 316 = S31600)
From ASTM (1998); ISO (1998)

sulfur of 0.03% and both < 0.08% ("316" stainless steel) and < 0.03% ("316L" stainless steel) of carbon. Since then, the high-carbon composition identified as grade 1 has been deleted, F 55 and F 56 specifications have been withdrawn and moved in 1971 to the new specifications F 138 and F 139 which are both called "316C".

Table 8 lists the composition of stainless steels used in implant applications according to the current ASTM and ISO specifications. Many of these specifications correspond to the wrought low-carbon S31673. ASTM separates the mechanical properties in individual standards for rolled, drawn, forging and fixation wire products. The casting alloy F 745 has a similar composition to S31673. There are also two slightly different nitrogen-strengthened wrought stainless steels, F 1314 and the matching standards ISO 5832-9 and ASTM F 1586.

(c) Cobalt–chromium alloys

Cobalt is a transition metal which has a hexagonal close-packed structure at room temperature, and a face-centred cubic structure above 417°C. The allotropic transformation on cooling to below this relatively low temperature takes place slowly and may not be complete in many alloy systems. The addition of some nickel and carbon can stabilize the face-centred cubic structure at room temperature. Cobalt metal is much more corrosion-resistant than iron, and therefore it can be used in a multiphase alloy for enhanced mechanical properties (Brick *et al.*, 1977; Planinsek, 1979).

Chromium is the primary alloying element in a wide variety of cobalt superalloys, being added primarily to give corrosion resistance. Chromium, tantalum, tungsten, molybdenum and nickel all enter the face-centred cubic structure and contribute to strengthening by solid-solution effects. Molybdenum and tungsten are significantly larger than cobalt, and are thus the elements most used for strengthening (Brick *et al.*, 1977).

Table 8. Specifications for implant-grade stainless steels (wt %)[a]

Type[b]	Cr	Ni	Mo	Mn	Si	C	N	P	S	Cu	Nb	V
F 138	17–19	13–15	2.25–3	<2	<0.75	<0.03	<0.10	<0.025	<0.01	<0.50	–	–
5832-1 D	17–19	13–15	2.25–3.5	<2	<1	<0.03	<0.10	<0.025	<0.01	<0.50	–	–
5832-1 E	17–19	14–16	2.35–4.2	<2	<1	<0.03	0.1–0.2	<0.025	<0.01	<0.50	–	–
F 745	17–19	11–14	2–3	<2	<1	<0.06	–	<0.045	<0.03	–	–	–
F 1314	20.5–23.5	11.5–13.5	2–3	4–6	<0.75	<0.03	0.2–0.4	<0.025	<0.01	<0.50	0.1–0.3	0.1–0.3
5832-9	19.5–22	9–11	2–3	2–4.5	<0.75	<0.08	0.25–0.5	<0.025	<0.01	<0.25	0.25–0.8	–

[a] Balance of composition in each case is iron (Fe)
[b] ISO and ASTM specifications:
ASTM F 138 Standard specification for 18 Chromium-14 Nickel-2.5 Molybdenum Stainless Steel Bar and Wire for Surgical Implants (S31673) (Fe64Cr18Ni14Mo2.5). Other standards with the same composition include ASTM F 139, F 621 and F 1350, also known as "316C".
ISO 5832-1 (composition D and E): Implants for Surgery - Metallic materials - Wrought stainless steel (S31673)
ASTM F 745 Standard specification for 18 Chromium-12.5 Nickel-2.5 Molybdenum Stainless Steel for Cast and Solution-Annealed Surgical Implant Applications (J31670)
ASTM F 1314 Standard specification for Wrought Nitrogen Strengthened-22 Chromium-12.5 Nickel-5 Manganese-2.5 Molybdenum Stainless Steel Bar and Wire for Surgical Implants (S20910) (Fe57Cr22Ni13Mn5Mo2.5)
ISO 5832-9 Implants for Surgery - Metallic materials - Wrought High Nitrogen Stainless Steel (S31675) (Fe63Cr21Ni10Mn3Mo2.5).
ASTM F 1586 corresponds to the same composition.
From ASTM (1998); ISO (1998)

Carbon is also an alloying element of major importance because of the formation and distribution of carbides. In the cast form, the alloy is made of solid-solution dendrites surrounded by interdendritic carbides, with intergranular carbides precipitated at the grain boundaries. The carbides may be in the form of M_7C_3, M_6C or $M_{23}C_6$, where M is chromium, molybdenum, cobalt and tungsten in various proportions, depending on heat treatment. Implants in the 'as cast' condition may have an extensive amount of very large intergranular carbides. Homogenization-anneal (1180°C) or solution-anneal (1240°C) heat treatments result in a more uniform structure and dramatic changes in carbide morphology, with their ultimate dissolution in the matrix leaving 'Kirkendall' holes. Porosity from casting or heat treatment may be reduced by hot isostatic pressing ('HIPping') of the casting (Bardos, 1979; Semlitsch & Willert, 1980).

Thermomechanical processes such as forging and powder metallurgical methods typically produce very fine microstructures, with a dispersion of fine carbides. Much research in the past decade has concentrated on refining these techniques, using carbides for control of grain growth during heat treatments and controlling the size and distribution of the carbide for optimum wear resistance (Semlitsch, 1992).

The cast cobalt–chromium–molybdenum (CoCrMo) alloy, first introduced in 1911 by Haynes as 'stellite' (the 'star' among the alloys, now referred to as Haynes-Stellite-21), had a nominal composition of 30% chromium and 5% molybdenum with some nickel and carbon. In 1926, an alloy of similar composition was patented under the name of Vitallium, and this has become one of the principal cobalt alloys used for implant applications. In the cast form, its specifications are designated F 75 and ISO 5832-4, as shown in Table 9. This is used for cast implants for osteosynthesis and arthroplasty. With minor changes in chromium and carbon content, forged and wrought versions of this alloy have been developed for high-stress applications, as in total hip replacements. The first-generation metal-on-metal total hips used in the 1960s were cast, whereas the second generation in use today are wrought (Schmidt et al., 1996).

Before the development of techniques for thermomechanically processing CoCrMo as a wrought alloy, a second alloy known as Haynes-Stellite-25, also known as wrought Vitallium, was introduced in 1952. This is a wrought alloy of cobalt, chromium, nickel and tungsten, with specifications F 90 or 5832-5 (Table 9). It has seen use primarily in intermedullary rods, side plates for stabilizing nails for femoral neck fractures, and some prosthetic heart valve frames.

Multiphase alloys have been developed in the search for stronger and corrosion-resistant alloys. For example, MP35N is an alloy of cobalt, nickel, chromium and molybdenum. In the solution-annealed condition, it has a face-centred cubic form which is very soft. With mechanical working, it undergoes a phase transformation to a hexagonal close-packed form, which appears as microscopically thin platelets that greatly increase its strength. Additional strengthening results from precipitation of Co_3Mo with ageing (Younkin, 1974). Other trade names for this alloy include Protasul-10 and Biophase. Its strength is excellent for total hip stems, but it is often used in conjunction with a cast cobalt–chromium–molybdenum head for improved

Table 9. Specifications for cobalt–chromium alloys (wt %)[a]

Type[b]	Cr	Ni	Mo	Mn	Si	C	Fe	Ti	W	N	P	S	Other
Cast alloy													
F 75	27–30	< 1.0	5–7	< 1.0	< 1.0	< 0.35	< 0.75	–	< 0.20	< 0.25	< 0.02	< 0.01	B < 0.01, Al < 0.3
5832-4	26.5–30	< 1.0	4.5–7	< 1.0	< 1.0	< 0.35	< 1.0						
Wrought alloy													
5832-12	26–30	< 1.0	5–7	< 1.0	< 1.0	< 0.35	< 0.75			< 0.25			
F 1537	26–30	< 1.0	5–7	< 1.0	< 1.0	< 0.35	< 0.75	–	–	< 1.0	–	–	
R31537	26–30	< 1.0	5–7	< 1.0	< 1.0	< 0.149	< 0.75			< 0.25			
R31539	26–30	< 1.0	5–7	< 1.0	< 1.0	< 0.35	< 0.75			< 0.25			Al < 1, La < 0.5
F 90	19–21	9–11	–	1–2	< 0.4	0.05–0.15	< 3	–	14–16	–	< 0.04	< 0.03	
F 562	19–21	33–37	9–10.5	< 0.15	< 0.15	< 0.025	< 1	< 1	–	–	< 0.015	< 0.01	B < 0.015
5832-6	19–21	33–37	9–10.5	< 0.15	< 0.15	< 0.025	< 1	< 1			< 0.015	< 0.01	
5832-8	18–22	15–25	3–4	< 1.0	< 0.5	< 0.05	4–6	0.5–3.5	3–4			< 0.01	
F 1058,1	19–21	14–16	6–8	1.5–2.5	< 1.2	< 0.15	bal	–	–	–	< 0.015	< 0.015	Be < 0.10, Co 39–41
F 1058,2	18.5–21.5	15–18	6.5–7.5	1.0–2.0	< 1.2	< 0.15	bal	–	–	–	< 0.015	< 0.015	Be < 0.001, Co 39–42
5832-7	18.5–21.5	14–18	6.5–8	1–2.5	< 1	< 0.15	bal				< 0.015	< 0.015	Be < 0.001, Co 39–42

Table 9 (contd)

bal, iron makes up the balance of the alloy content

[a] Balance of composition in each case is cobalt (Co), except for ASTM F 1058 and ISO 5832-7.

[b] ISO and ASTM specifications (including some common trade names):

ASTM F 75 Standard specification for Cast Cobalt-Chromium-Molybdenum Alloy for Surgical Implants (R30075) - ASTM F 1377 has the same composition. (R30075) (Co66Cr28Mo6). *Haynes-Stellite 21, Vitallium*®, *Zimalloy, Protasul*^{TM}*-1, Protasul*^{TM}*-2, Vinertia, Francabal, CCM*®

ISO 5832-4 Implants for Surgery - Metallic materials -Co-28Cr-6Mo Casting Alloy (R30075)

ASTM F 799 Standard specification for Cobalt-28 Chromium-6 Molybdenum Alloy Forgings for Surgical Implants

ISO 5832-12 Implants for Surgery - Metallic materials - Wrought Co-28Cr-6Mo Alloy (R31538)

ASTM F 1537 Standard specification for Wrought Cobalt-28 Chromium-6 Molybdenum Alloy for Surgical Implants (R31537-9). *FHS Vitallium*®, *GADS, Zimaloy Micrograin, Protasul*^{TM}*-20, CCM Plus*^{TM}

ASTM F 90 Standard specification for Wrought Cobalt-20 Chromium-15 Tungsten-10 Nickel Alloy for Surgical Implant Applications (Co55Cr20W15 Ni10). *Haynes-Stellite 25, Vitallium*®. ISO 5832-5 has a similar composition.

ASTM F 1091 Wrought Co-20Cr-15W-10Ni Alloy surgical fixation wire - ASTM F 90 has the same composition

ASTM F 562 Standard specification for Wrought Co-35Ni-20Cr-10Mo Alloy for Surgical Implant Applications (Co35Ni35Cr20Mo10) - ASTM F 688 and F 961 have the same composition.

ISO 5832-6 Implants for Surgery - Metallic materials - Wrought Co-35Ni-20Cr-10Mo Alloy. *Protasul*^{TM}*-10, MP35N, Biophase*

ISO 5832-8 Implants for Surgery - Metallic materials - Wrought Co-20Ni-20Cr-3Mo-3W-5Fe Alloy (R30563) - (Co49Cr20Ni20Fe5Mo3W3) - ASTM F563 has the same composition. *Syntacoben*

ASTM F 1058 Standard specification for Wrought Co-Cr-Ni-Mo-Fe Alloys for Surgical Implant Applications, grade 1: Co40Cr20Ni15Mo7Fe18 (R30003) and grade 2 (R30008). *Elgiloy* (grade 1)

ISO 5832-7 Implants for Surgery - Metallic materials - Forgeable and cold-formed Co-Cr-Ni-Mo-Fe Alloy (R30008). *Phymox*

From ASTM (1998); ISO (1998)

wear resistance. The heads are welded to the MP35N stems (Süry & Semlitsch, 1978; Richards Manufacturing Company, 1980; Semlitsch & Willert, 1980).

Two other cobalt alloys, Syntacoben and Elgiloy, have been developed as high-strength, corrosion-resistant materials for mechanical spring applications. Elgiloy is used as the stent material in some prosthetic heart valves and endovascular stents and as orthodontic wires.

(d) Titanium and titanium alloys

At room temperature, titanium has a hexagonal close-packed structure (the alpha form). At 882°C, it transforms to a body-centred cubic (beta) form. Alloys with an all-alpha structure develop good strength and toughness and have superior resistance to oxygen contamination at elevated temperatures, but have relatively poor forming characteristics. The all-beta structures display better formability and have good strength, but are more vulnerable to contamination from the atmosphere. Elements that stabilize the alpha structure are aluminium, carbon, boron, oxygen and nitrogen, while molybdenum, vanadium, manganese, chromium and iron stabilize the beta structure. Zirconium has properties very similar to titanium and thus enters a solid solution without any effect on phase (Brick et al., 1977; Knittel, 1983).

There are four grades of commercially pure (unalloyed) titanium (sometimes called CPTi), which contain small amounts of iron, nitrogen and oxygen. As the amounts of these other elements increase from grade 1 to 4, strength increases. The compositions of grades 1 and 4 are shown in Table 10.

The other common form of titanium for implant applications is known as Ti 6,4 (containing 6% aluminium and 4% vanadium), which has a two-phase structure with a dispersion of the beta form in the alpha phase. Heat treatment can have a significant effect on the phase morphology, from a very fine dispersion of beta particles to a very coarse plate-like structure. Another alloy, Ti 6,7 (containing 6% aluminium and 7% niobium), was developed due to concern regarding the toxicity of vanadium (Knittel, 1983; Semlitsch, 1992).

Recently there has been growing interest in the development of all-beta titanium alloys. The advantage of these alloys is reduced stiffness or elastic modulus, so that the material is mechanically more similar to bone (Brown & Lemons, 1996).

Titanium is very active electrochemically, lying between zinc and aluminium in the electromotive series. As a result, it reacts rapidly with oxygen (either gaseous or in an aerated solution) to form a very stable passive oxide film. With such a passive film, titanium is very resistant to electrochemical corrosion. However, it suffers from abrasive wear, and titanium total joint replacements have occasionally experienced catastrophic or 'run-away' wear (Knittel, 1983; Agins et al., 1988).

(e) Tantalum

Tantalum is a corrosion-resistant metal with a high atomic weight (180.95), density (16.69) and melting-point (3000°C), but relatively poor mechanical strength.

It is difficult to cast and form into devices, although electron beam refining and powder metallurgical methods can be used; ASTM and ISO standards exist for two forms designated R05200 and R05400 (Table 11). Due to its density, tantalum is used medically as a radiographic marker in polymeric and carbon devices. Fabricated tantalum is malleable and has been used for many years for repair of cranial defects (Black, 1994).

1A.1.3 *Chemical composition of dental casting alloys*

Three groups of precious-metal alloys are used specifically in dental castings: gold-based, palladium-based and silver-based alloys. Two main groups of non-precious metal (base metal) alloys are used: cobalt- and nickel-based. Commercially pure titanium, as described previously, is also used as a dental casting material. Within these groups, the alloys can be described by the weight percentages of their constituents in decreasing order, e.g., Au70Ag13.5Cu8.8 for an alloy with 70% gold, 13.5% silver and 8.8% copper. The classification of an alloy is determined by the components with the highest percentage. For example, Ag40Pd23In17 is a typical silver alloy, which may be referred to as a silver–palladium alloy or as a silver–palladium–indium alloy.

Standards for dental casting alloys are:
ISO 1562: Dental casting gold alloys
ISO 6871-1: Dental base metal casting alloys. Part 1: Cobalt-based alloys
ISO 6871-2: Dental base metal casting alloys. Part 2: Nickel-based alloys
ISO 8891: Dental casting alloys with noble metal content of at least 25% but less than 75%
ISO 9693: Dental ceramic fused to metal restorative materials

(a) *Gold-based alloys*

The classical dental gold alloy is a ternary alloy of gold, silver and copper, containing not less than 75% gold. Palladium and platinum are added to modify the melting point and increase the mechanical strength. Zinc is added to ease the castability, and small amounts of ruthenium, or other platinum group metals such as iridium or rubidium, in the range of 0.005 to 1% are believed to enhance the development of nucleation centres and thus produce a fine-grained structure throughout the alloy (Lanam & Zysk, 1982; Lloyd & Showak, 1984; Anusavice, 1996).

The alloys used for metal–ceramic reconstructions additionally need at least approximately 1% of non-precious metallic elements such as indium, tin or gallium to produce a slight oxide film on the surface of the dental substructure to achieve a metal–ceramic bond strength that surpasses the cohesive strength of the ceramic itself. If the gold content is decreased and replaced by palladium for economic reasons, the content of low-melting elements such as tin, indium and especially gallium has to be increased in order to lower the melting point of the alloy (Table 12) (Anusavice, 1996).

Table 10. Specifications for titanium and titanium alloys (wt %)[a]

Type[b]	Al	V	Nb	Mo	Zr	Fe	N	C	H	O	Other
Commercially pure titanium											
F 67-1	–	–	–	–	–	< 0.20	< 0.03	< 0.10	< 0.015	< 0.18	–
F 67-4	–	–	–	–	–	< 0.50	< 0.05	< 0.10	< 0.015	< 0.40	–
5832-2,1						< 0.10	< 0.012	< 0.03	< 0.0125	< 0.10	
5832-2,4						< 0.50	< 0.05	< 0.10	< 0.0125	< 0.40	
Titanium alloys											
F 136	5.5–6.50	3.5–4.5	–	–	–	< 0.25	< 0.05	< 0.08	< 0.012	< 0.13	–
F 1108	5.5–6.75	3.5–4.5	–	–	–	< 0.30	< 0.05	< 0.10	< 0.015	< 0.20	–
F 1472	5.5–6.75	3.5–4.5	–	–	–	< 0.30	< 0.05	< 0.08	< 0.015	< 0.20	Y < 0.005
5832-3	5.5–6.75	3.5–4.5	–	–	–	< 0.30	< 0.05	< 0.08	< 0.015	< 0.20	–
F 1295	5.5–6.5	–	6.5–7.5	–	–	< 0.25	< 0.05	< 0.08	< 0.009	< 0.20	Ta < 0.50
5832-11	5.5–6.5	–	6.5–7.5	–	–	< 0.25	< 0.05	< 0.08	< 0.009	< 0.20	Ta < 0.50
F 1713	–	–	12.5–14	–	12.5–14	< 0.25	< 0.05	< 0.08	< 0.012	< 0.15	
F 1813	–	–	–	10–13	5–7	1.5–2.5	< 0.05	< 0.05	< 0.02	0.08–0.28	

Table 10 (contd)

[a] Balance of composition in each case is titanium (Ti)
[b] ISO and ASTM specifications (including some common trade names):

ASTM F 67 Standard specification for Unalloyed Titanium for Surgical Implant Applications (R50250, 400, 550, 700). ASTM F1341 has the same composition. *Protasul^{TM}-Ti*

ISO 5832-2 Implants for Surgery - Metallic materials - Unalloyed Titanium (R50250, 400, 550, 700)

ASTM F 136 Standard specification for Wrought Titanium 6Al-4V Extra Low Interstitial Alloy for Surgical Implant Applications (R56401) (Ti90Al6V4).

ASTM F 620 has the same composition.

ASTM F 1108 Standard specification for Titanium 6Al-4V Alloy castings for Surgical Implants (R56406)

ASTM F 1472 Standard specification for Wrought Titanium 6Al-4V Alloy for Surgical Implant Applications (R56400)

ISO 5832-3 Implants for Surgery - Metallic materials - Titanium 6Al-4V Wrought Alloy (R56406)

ASTM F 1580 Standard specification for Titanium and Titanium-6% Aluminium-4% Vanadium Alloys Powders for Coatings of Surgical Implants (R50700 & R56406). *Tivanium, Protasul^{TM}-64WF*

ASTM F 1295 Standard specification for Wrought Titanium 6Al-7Nb Alloy for Implant Applications (R56700) (Ti87Al6Nb7)

ISO 5832-11 Implants for Surgery - Metallic materials - Wrought Titanium 6Al-7Nb alloy (R56700). *Protasul^{TM}-100*

ASTM F 1713 Standard specification for Wrought Titanium 13Nb-13Zr Alloy for Surgical Implants (R58130) (Ti74Nb13Zr13)

ASTM F 1813 Standard specification for Wrought Titanium 12 Molybdenum-6 Zirconium-2 Iron Alloy for Surgical Implants (R58120) (Ti78Mo12Zr6Fe2)

From ASTM (1998); ISO (1998)

Table 11. Specifications for tantalum for implant application (wt %)[a]

Type[b]	C	O	N	H	Nb	Fe	Ti	W	Mo	Si	Ni
R05200	<0.010	<0.015	<0.010	<0.0015	<0.100	<0.010	<0.010	<0.050	<0.020	<0.005	<0.010
R05400	<0.010	<0.030	<0.010	<0.0015	<0.100	<0.010	<0.010	<0.050	<0.020	<0.005	<0.010

[a] Balance of composition is tantalum (Ta)
[b] ASTM and ISO specifications:
ASTM F 560 Standard specification for Unalloyed Tantalum for Surgical Implant Applications (R05200, R05400). ISO 13782 corresponds to the same composition.
From ASTM (1998); ISO (1998)

Table 12. Composition of commonly used precious-metal dental cast alloys and metal-ceramic alloys (wt %)

Alloy type	Au	Pt + Pd	Ag	Cu	Other non-precious metals (e.g., Zn, Sn, In, Ga)
Gold-based alloys					
High gold cast alloys	71–96	0–5	3–14	0–10	1–12
High gold metal-ceramic alloys	70–92	6–20	0–11	0–6	0.2–6
Low gold cast alloys	50–69	4–10	8–25	0–12	3–14
Low gold metal-ceramic alloys	50–69	20–36	0–18	0–14	3–13
Palladium-based alloys					
Palladium-based alloys (PdAgSn)	0–16	50–78	7–40	–	8–14
Palladium-based alloys (PdCuCa)	0–6	76–80	0–7	4–15	18–22
Palladium-based alloys (PdSnGaIn)	0–2	80–85	0–6	0–6	12–18
Silver-based alloys					
Silver-based alloys (AgPd)	0–25	15–27	40–70	0–18	3–24

(b)   *Palladium-based alloys*

Palladium alloys contain 50–85% palladium (Table 12). The melting point of pure palladium (1552°C) is much too high for dental casting machines. High proportions of silver or copper, as well as other elements such as gallium, indium and tin have to be added in order to lower the melting point to 1200–1400°C. These non-precious metals also serve to form essential oxygen bridges at the surface for bonding to the veneering ceramic after appropriate heat treatment. In most cases, copper-free alloys are more corrosion–resistant (Lanam & Zysk, 1982; Anusavice, 1996).

(c)   *Silver-based alloys*

Silver-based alloys with a grey colour have a silver content between 50 and 70% and contain copper, palladium and sometimes gold (Table 12). A gold-coloured silver alloy type consists of approximately 40% silver, 23% palladium, 17% indium and some gold, copper and zinc. It is a heterogeneous alloy, with an orange-coloured palladium–indium phase and a silver-coloured phase. The mixture of these phases has a golden colour which explains the popularity of this alloy, despite its low resistance to corrosion and tarnishing (Anusavice, 1996).

(d)   *Cobalt- and nickel-based alloys*

These alloys (Table 13) are mainly used for removable partial dentures because of their high mechanical strength and stiffness. Nickel–chromium (NiCr) alloys are sometimes preferred over cobalt–chromium (CoCr) alloys by dental technicians because of their much easier casting properties and brilliant appearance, especially if 2% beryllium is added. The precious metal alloys have an inherent resistance to corrosion

Table 13. Composition of commonly used base metal dental casting alloys (wt %)

Alloy type	Co	Ni	Cr	Mo	Mn	W	Si	Fe	C	Other elements
Cobalt-based alloys	52–67	[a]	24–32	4–6	0–1	0–10	0–1.5	0–1	0–0.5	Ce 0.2; La 0.1; N 0.3
Nickel-based alloys	0.3–0.5	59–81	11–27	4–11	–	–	0–1.5	0–1.2	0.1	Be 0–2; Ce 0–0.2; Al 0.3

[a] The total cobalt + nickel + chromium content must be at least 85%, and cobalt must be ≥ 50%. 'Nickel-free' cobalt-based alloys must contain < 0.1% nickel.

because of their low reactivity to oxygen. In contrast, cobalt and nickel alloys contain metallic elements having a high affinity to oxygen, but the oxide film at the surface can protect against further corrosion. With a chromium content of around of 24% and a molybdenum content between 2 and 5%, the corrosion resistance can be similar to that of the precious-metal alloys (Planinsek, 1979; Tien & Howson, 1981; Anusavice, 1996). The drawback of the NiCr alloy with a high beryllium content is its very high corrosion rate compared with other CoCr or NiCr alloys (Geis-Gerstorfer & Pässler, 1993).

(e) *Copper-based alloys*

A copper alloy with typical composition Cu79.3Al7.8Ni4.3Fe4Zn3Mn1.6 and having gold-coloured appearance (trade name NPG = Non Precious Gold) but very low corrosion resistance is used mainly in the United States, South America and Eastern Europe because of its very low cost (Anusavice, 1996).

1A.1.4 *Dental amalgam*

To produce dental amalgam, mercury is mixed with an alloyed metallic powder consisting predominantly of silver and tin. Mercury comprises 40–50% of the amalgam, and the remainder is the alloy. The conventional alloy powder contains at least 65% silver, 29% tin and less than 6% copper. Other elements, such as zinc or gold are allowed in concentrations less than the silver or tin content. During the 1970s, high-copper alloys containing between 6 and 30% copper were developed. These alloys produce amalgams that are superior in many respects to the traditional low-copper amalgams. The amalgam is mixed by the dentist or the assistant to obtain a plastically formable mixture to be inserted in the tooth (IARC, 1993a; Anusavice, 1996).

1A.1.5 *Orthodontic metallic materials*

For orthodontic treatments, wrought base metal alloys are used for wires, brackets and bands. The types of alloy preferred in orthodontics can be divided into six groups according to their composition (Table 14) (Anusavice, 1996).

1A.1.6 *Analytical methods*

(a) *Measurement of composition of metallic alloys*

All ASTM metallic implant material specifications cite ASTM specifications for chemical analysis. These specifications describe a series of wet chemistry and photometric methods for determination of the alloy composition.

Specifically, the titanium alloy standards cite E 120 (Standard Test Methods for Chemical Analysis of Titanium and Titanium Alloys), the stainless steel and cobalt alloy standards cite E 353 (Standard Test Methods for Chemical Analysis of Stainless, Heat-Resisting, Maraging and Other Similar Chromium-Nickel-Iron Alloys) and E 354 (Standard Test Methods for Chemical Analysis of High-Temperature Electrical, Magnetic and Other Similar Iron, Nickel, and Cobalt Alloys).

Table 14. Composition of commonly used orthodontic materials

Alloy type	Typical composition	Applications
Stainless steel (type 301/302/304)	Fe74Cr17Ni7 (hard and spring hard)	Wires, brackets, bands
Manganese steel	Fe60.8Cr18Mn18Mo2	Wires, brackets
Cobalt–chromium–nickel alloys (Elgiloy®)	Co40Cr20Ni16 (soft and hard)	Wires
Nickel–titanium alloys	Ni52Ti45Co3 or Ni51Ti49	Wires
β-Titanium alloys	Ti78Mo11Zr6.5Zn4.5	Wires
Titanium (commercially pure)	Ti	Brackets

ISO material standards for stainless steel (5832-1 and 5832-9) cite a series of ISO standards for chemical analysis, and ASTM E 112 for determining average grain size. The other ISO TC-150 metal specifications do not cite chemical analysis test methods.

(b) *Measurement of metals in biological tissue and fluids*

ASTM F 561 (Practice for Retrieval and Analysis of Implanted Medical Devices, and Associated Tissues) contains detailed methods for chemical analysis of tissues by flame atomic absorption spectroscopy (flame AAS), graphite furnace atomic absorption spectroscopy (GFAAS), inductively coupled plasma optical emission spectroscopy (ICP-OES) or mass spectroscopy. Detection limits for metal analysis by flame AAS, GFAAS and ICP-OES are given in Table 15. Detection limits for elements in tissues depend upon, among other factors, the amount of specimen dilution during sample preparation.

1A.2 Production

Some metallic devices are formed by casting into the nearly final shape. Portions of the cast parts may be subjected to subsequent machining or polishing treatments. Some devices are used with the metal in the 'as cast' condition. In the case of certain devices or certain manufacturers, castings may be subjected to subsequent heat treatments.

Metallic devices can also be made by subjecting the original cast ingot to a series of mechanical rolling or drawing steps. After each process involving extensive cold working, the alloy is heated to anneal it or relieve stress. This results in the formation of new crystals with few dislocations. Suitable control of the temperature and time gives a soft, fine-grained metal that can be subsequently cold worked. Alternatively, the forming may be done with hot metal so that recrystallization occurs spontaneously after the rolling or drawing. Parts can also be formed mechanically by forging a piece from a nearly final form. Again, this can be done under hot or cold conditions (Jackman, 1981).

Metallic components can also be made using the techniques of powder metallurgy. A fine powder is usually made by melting the alloy and atomizing it. The powder is

Table 15. Comparison of detection limits[a] for selected analytical methods

Metal	Inductively coupled plasma optical emission spectroscopy	Flame atomic absorption spectroscopy	Graphite furnace atomic absorption spectroscopy
Aluminium	2	30	0.01
Beryllium	0.07	1	0.02
Chromium	2	3	0.01
Cobalt	1	4	0.02
Copper	0.9	1	0.02
Gallium	10	60	0.5
Indium	20	40	1
Molybdenum	3	20	0.02
Nickel	3	90	0.1
Palladium	4	10	0.3
Silver	0.8	2	0.005
Titanium	0.4	70	0.5
Vanadium	0.7	50	0.2
Zinc	0.6	0.5	0.001

[a] All values are shown as µg/L
From Gill (1993)

then compacted to a nearly final shape and subjected to controlled high temperature and pressure in sintering and HIPping processes (Bardos, 1979; Jackman, 1981).

The treatment of surfaces during manufacture can have a major effect on both wear and corrosion resistance. A wide variety of methods are used. Cast devices generally have a matte surface from the ceramic of the investment casting, or may be grit-blasted to remove residual cast material. Stainless steel implants are very often polished mechanically and then electropolished (Schneberger, 1981). Surfaces may also be treated by ion implantation, plasma or ion nitriding, or coated with hard ceramic-like materials for enhanced wear resistance. Bearing surfaces receive a very high degree of mechanical polishing, either by hand or by computer-controlled machines (Alban, 1981; Krutenat, 1981).

Since the early 1980s, a number of surface modifications have been used in total joint replacements to provide biological fixation by in-growth of bone into a porous or textured surface. Porosity can be created by sintering a layer of beads on the surface, diffusion-bonding a fibre metal mesh or micromachining to create a textured surface. Coatings are also applied by a variety of thermal spray techniques (Crowninshield, 1988).

In most cases, there is a final process of passivation (see Section 5A.1) in nitric acid. The term passivation may be a misnomer, since the surgical alloys are all self-passivating. The nitric acid treatment probably increases the passive film thickness and removes any metallic contamination on the surface. These processes are described in ASTM standard F 86 (Standard practice for surface preparation and marking of metallic surgical implants), adopted in 1984.

1B. Non-metallic Medical and Dental Materials

1B.1 Chemical and physical data

Non-metallic medical and dental materials are used extensively in soft-tissue and bone implants. Major classes of materials include synthetic polymers, ceramics and composites.

Synthetic polymers are widely used in applications such as breast and joint prostheses, heart valves, grafts, sutures and dental bridgework. Metallic implants can be coated with ceramic materials, carbon or hydroxylapatite. Ceramic materials may also serve as implants. Tooth-coloured dental materials are made from composite materials and ceramics.

1B.1.1 *Polymer chemistry*

Most polymers are synthesized using one of three reaction mechanisms:
- addition (chain reaction) polymerization
- coordination polymerization
- condensation (step reaction) polymerization

The three mechanisms are distinct in the way that the molecules interact to form polymer chains. More importantly, each requires different reaction conditions, catalysts and synthesis media, which in turn yield polymers with different properties (Borg, 1979; Paschke, 1981; Billmeyer, 1989; Lenz, 1989; Visser *et al.*, 1996).

In an addition reaction (or, more precisely, a chain reaction), the monomers contain at least one carbon–carbon double bond, and the reaction begins when an initiator breaks the double bond. Initiators include free radicals, cations, anions or stereo-specific catalysts. When an initiated monomer molecule reacts with the double bond of another monomer, a reactive site remains at the end of the polymer chain, which enables chain growth to continue. Reaction proceeds through the steps of initiation, propagation and termination to produce the final polymer molecules. The molecular weight distribution in the polymer is dependent on the initiator:monomer ratio and other reaction conditions, but the distribution is difficult to control with precision and is generally broad (Lenz, 1989; Visser *et al.*, 1996).

Coordination polymerization techniques allow control of the stereo-regularity of the polymers produced. Polymerization takes place through the interaction of monomer with specific catalysts via an intermediate coordination complex. The Ziegler-Natta catalysts are used in the production of linear stereo-regular polymers from a wide variety of monomers. This technology has made possible the production of plastics such as ultra-high molecular weight polyethylene (UHMWPE) and is therefore discussed in more detail later (Borg, 1979; Brydson, 1979; Paschke, 1981).

In condensation (or step reaction) polymerization, two monomers react to form a covalent bond, often with release of a small molecule such as water as a by-product. With reactions of this type, the molecular weight distribution is generally dependent only on the ratio of the two reacting species and the time of reaction. The distribution parameters are relatively easy to control, but long reaction times are generally required if products of high molecular weight are desired (Lenz, 1989; Visser et al., 1996).

Copolymerization refers to the combination of different monomer types to form copolymers that contain more than one type of repeating unit, in contrast to polymers which contain only one type of repeating unit, referred to as homopolymers. Depending on the reaction conditions and the reactivity of each monomer type, copolymers produced from addition polymerization may be random (-A-B-B-A-B-A-), alternating (-A-B-A-B-A-B-) or block copolymers (-A-A-A-B-B-B-). In the case of condensation polymerization, the nature of the copolymerization may be precisely controlled, a feature exploited in the production of polyurethanes, for example. Random copolymers exhibit properties that are approximately the average of those of polymers made separately from each of the two types of monomer units. Block copolymers tend to phase-separate into a monomer-A-rich phase and a monomer-B-rich phase, displaying properties unique to each of the homopolymers. This has a marked influence on material properties, including biological properties such as haemocompatibility and biocompatibility (Lenz, 1989; Visser et al., 1996).

Post-polymerization cross-linking is also possible for many polymers. This may be achieved by the addition of small quantities of trifunctional comonomers, or by introduction of chemical cross-links between functional groups in the polymer chain. Physical cross-links are also formed in some types of polymer, most notably the polyamides (Visser et al., 1996).

The amount and types of impurities present in plastics are clearly dependent not only on the method of manufacture, but also on the types of processing. Moreover, many additives are used as processing aids and to improve the properties of plastics. Plastics used in the medical device industry are usually complex combinations of polymer and other ingredients such as catalyst residues, antioxidants, processing aids, colorants, solvent residues, radio-opaque fillers, and trace impurities such as those that arise from polymerization by-products, sterilization or ingredient impurities. Attention is usually focused on the chemical and physical properties of the base polymer, but the formulation constituents, even if present in relatively small amounts, have a great influence on the chemical and physical properties of the materials (Sears & Touchette, 1989).

1B.1.2 *Synthesis and composition of polymers*

Table 16 lists the major polymer classes used in medical implants and dental materials and indicates their applications.

Table 16. Non-metallic medical and dental materials

Name	Abbreviation, common name and/or trade names	Structure	Applications
Polymers			
Polydimethyl-siloxane	Silicone, silastic	$\left[\begin{array}{c} CH_3 \\ -Si-O- \\ CH_3 \end{array} \right]_n$	Soft contact lenses. Intra-ocular lenses (IOLs), pacemaker lead insulation and components, breast prostheses, urinary and central venous catheters, implantable infusion systems, coatings
Polyurethanes	Pellethane, Biomer, Tecoflex	Pellethane: $\left[-O-\overset{O}{\overset{\|}{C}}-\overset{H}{\overset{\|}{N}}-R_2-\overset{H}{\overset{\|}{N}}-\overset{O}{\overset{\|}{C}}-O-R_1 \right]_n \left[-\overset{O}{\overset{\|}{C}}-\overset{H}{\overset{\|}{N}}-R_2-\overset{H}{\overset{\|}{N}}-\overset{O}{\overset{\|}{C}}-O-R_3 \right]_n$ $R_1 = -C_2H_4-$ $R_2 = -\bigcirc-CH_2-\bigcirc-$ $R_3 = -C_2H_4-O-C_2H_4-$	Central venous, angioplasty, balloon angioplasty and electrophysiology catheters, pacemaker lead insulation and components, heart valves, balloon heart assist devices, implantable infusion systems
Poly(methyl methacrylate)	PMMA, Perspex, Lucite, Acrylic	$\left[\begin{array}{c} CH_3 \\ -CH_2-C- \\ \| \\ C=O \\ \| \\ O-CH_3 \end{array} \right]_n$	Contact lenses, IOLs, bone cements, dental prostheses

Table 16 (contd)

Name	Abbreviation, common name and/or trade names	Structure	Applications
Poly(2-hydroxyethyl methacrylate)	PHEMA		Soft contact lenses, burn dressings, artificial cornea
Polydioxanone			Sutures
Poly(ethylene terephthalate)	PET, Dacron, Mylar, Terylene		Vascular grafts, heart valve sewing rings, haemofiltration, sutures
Polypropylene	PP		Sutures, IOL anchors (haptics)
Polyethylene	UHMWPE, PE		Prosthetic hip and knee components, hernia repair

Table 16 (contd)

Name	Abbreviation, common name and/or trade names	Structure	Applications
Polytetra-fluoroethylene	PTFE, EPTFE, Teflon, Gore-tex	$\left[\begin{array}{c} F\ \ F \\ -C-C- \\ F\ \ F \end{array}\right]_n$	Coatings, sutures, aneurysm clips, vascular grafts, dental applications
Polyamides	Nylons	$\left[\begin{array}{c} O=C-R_1-C-NH-R_2-NH \\ O \end{array}\right]_n$ $\left[\begin{array}{c} O=C \\ NH-R_1 \end{array}\right]_n$	Sutures, epidural catheters, dental bridge materials
Polylactide	PLA	$\left[\begin{array}{c} O=C-O \\ CH \\ CH_3 \end{array}\right]_n$	Bioresorbable sutures, pins and other items
Poly(glycolic acid)	PGA	$\left[\begin{array}{c} O=C-O \\ CH_2 \end{array}\right]_n$	Bioresorbable sutures, pins and other items

Table 16 (contd)

Name	Abbreviation, common name and/or trade names	Structure	Applications
Ceramics			
Aluminium oxide ceramics		Al_2O_3	Total joint replacement, dental crown and bridges, dental implants
Calcium phosphate ceramics	TCP	$Ca_3(PO_4)_2$	Bone void filler, implant coating
Hydroxyl-apatite ceramics	HA	$Ca_{10}(PO_4)_6(OH)_2$	Bone void filler, implant coating
Pyrolytic carbon		C	Heart valves, coatings
Zirconium oxide ceramics		ZrO_2	Total joint replacement, dental crown and bridges, dental implants
Composite materials[a]			Filling materials

From Brydson (1979); Jones et al. (1991); Ravaglioli & Krajewski (1992); Visser et al. (1996); Glantz (1998); Yoda (1998)
[a] See Section 5B of this monograph for more detailed description.

(a) Polydimethylsiloxane (silicone)

The name silicone is used for polymers having the general chemical structure shown in Table 16. The chemistry of these polymers and their production sequence are highly complex and many compounds are possible. The bulk of such materials are based on methylchlorosilanes and the gross differences in their physical properties are largely dependent on the functionality of the intermediate.

Dimethyl silicone fluids are made by the catalysed equilibration of dimethyl silicone stock with a source of a chain terminator. Silicone resins are highly cross-linked siloxane systems. The cross-links are introduced by the inclusion of trifunctional and tetrafunctional silanes at the early stages of manufacture (Hardman & Torkelson, 1989). Silicone gels comprise a complex mixture of lightly cross-linked silicone polymer permeated by silicone fluids with a wide range of molecular weight. Silicone gels and elastomers are manufactured by cross-linking of linear polymers of high molecular weight (~500 kDa) after fabrication. The degree of cross-linking determines the hardness of the elastomer or gel. The curing agents, normally peroxide free radical initiators such as benzoyl peroxide, 2,4-dichlorobenzoyl peroxide or *tert*-butyl perbenzoate, are added to the silicone polymer before fabrication, along with other compounding agents and fumed silica as a filler. Curing is achieved by heating the material to a high temperature. Other curing systems are available, particularly when monomers with reactive functional groups are incorporated into the dimethylsiloxane backbone (Brydson, 1979).

(b) Polyurethanes

The reaction between an isocyanate and an alcohol results in the formation of a urethane. If a compound containing two isocyanate groups (a diisocyanate) is made to react with another compound containing two hydroxyl groups (a diol or glycol), the polymer formed is generally called a polyurethane, even though the urethane bond is often the least common type of bond in the molecule.

Polyurethanes of medical interest are reaction products of three different molecules that are generally referred to as the diisocyanate, the macroglycol and the chain extender (also a diol, but sometimes a diamine) (see Table 17). The product comprises segmented molecular structures made up of soft (polyol) and rigid (isocyanate) domains (Figure 1) (Piskin, 1994; Visser *et al.*, 1996).

A large number of aliphatic and aromatic isocyanates are available for the production of polyurethanes, but only a few are used in practice. The most common aromatic diisocyanates used to make polyurethanes for industrial applications are mixtures of 2,4-toluene diisocyanate and 2,6-toluene diisocyanate (generally referred to as TDI). In medical applications, the diisocyanates most frequently used are methylene diisocyanate (MDI) and hydrogenated methylene diisocyanate (HMDI). The macroglycol (also called the soft segment) in medical polyurethanes may be based on polyester (these polyurethanes are known as poly(ester urethanes)), polycarbonate or alkyl diols, but the predominant macroglycols used in implantable polyurethanes are polyethers from ethylene,

Table 17. Chemical structure of some polyurethane intermediates

O=C=N—⟨C₆H₄⟩—CH₂—⟨C₆H₄⟩—N=C=O   4,4′-Methylene bisphenyl diisocyanate or methylene diisocyanate (MDI)

H₂N—⟨C₆H₄⟩—CH₂—⟨C₆H₄⟩—NH₂   4,4′-Methylene bisphenyl diamine or methylene dianiline (MDA)

O=C=N—⟨C₆H₁₀⟩—CH₂—⟨C₆H₁₀⟩—N=C=O   4,4′-Methylene biscyclohexane diisocyanate or hydrogenated methylene diisocyanate (HMDI)

2,4-Toluene diisocyanate (TDI)

2,4-Toluene diamine (TDA)

HO—(CH$_2$—CH$_2$—O—CH$_2$—CH$_2$)$_n$—OH   Polytetramethylene ether glycol (PTMEG or PTMO)

Table 17 (contd)

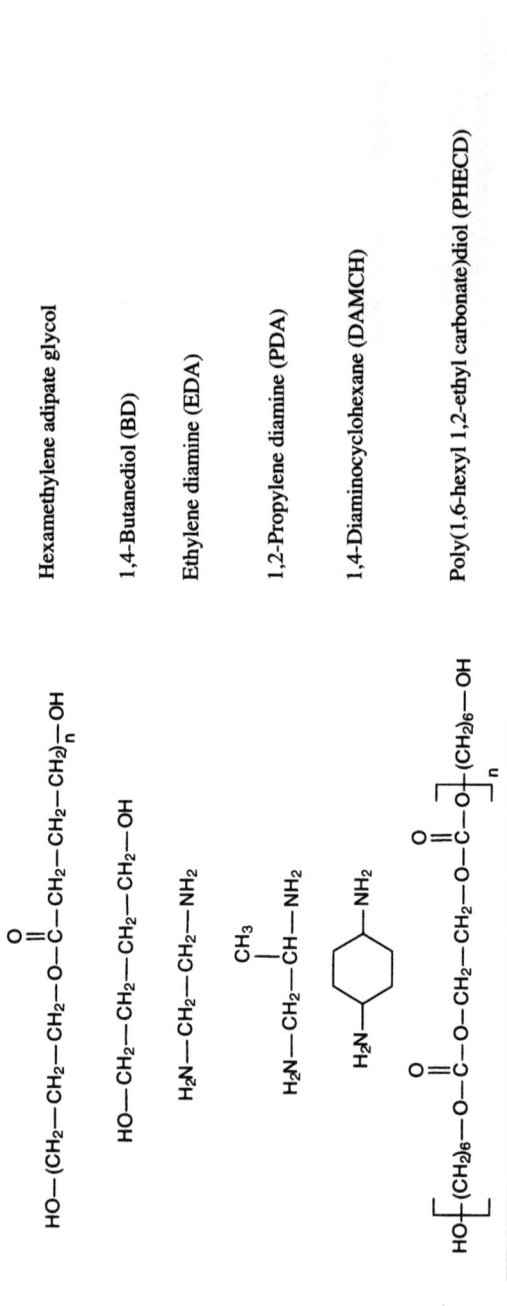

From Pinchuk (1994)

Figure 1. Two-stage polyurethane reaction where a rigid isocyanate (a) is reacted with an amorphous macroglycol (b) to form a prepolymer (c). The prepolymer is further reacted with a rigid chain extender (d) to form a segmented (mixture of hard and soft segments) polyurethane (e).

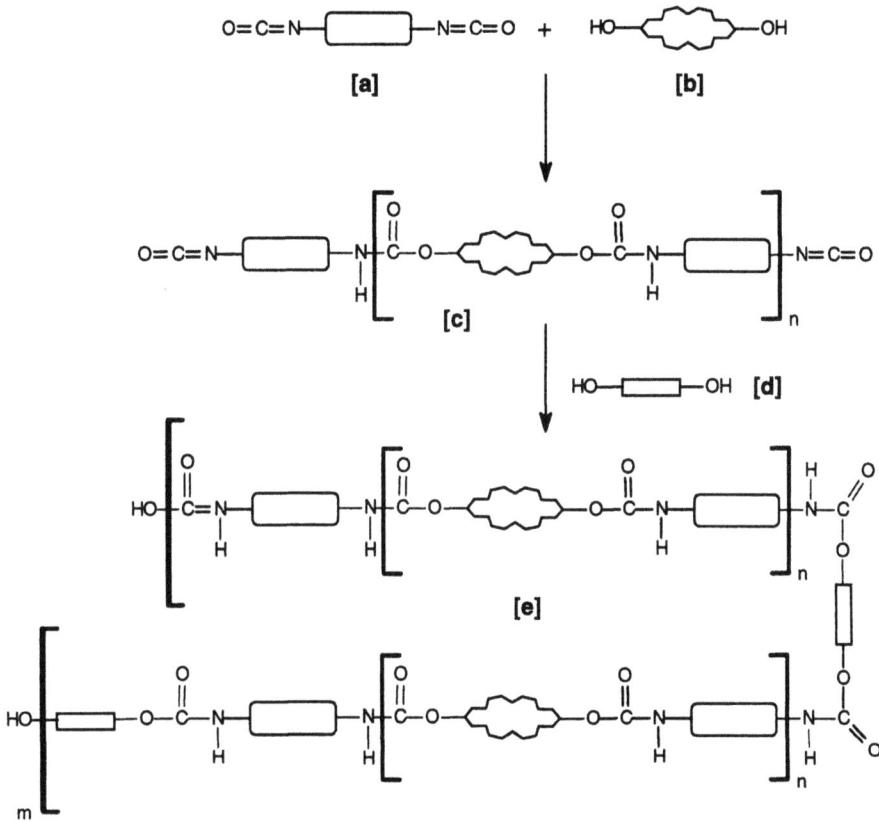

propylene and tetramethylene oxides. The polyether diol most often used in medical devices is poly(tetramethylene ether glycol) (PTMEG) of molecular weight ranging from 650 to 2000 Da. Polyurethanes based on MDI or HMDI and PTMEG or other polyether glycols are known as poly(ether urethanes) (Pinchuk, 1994; Piskin, 1994).

The degradation of poly(ester urethanes) used as backing materials in Même breast prostheses has received much attention and is discussed in detail in Section 5B of this monograph. The release of TDI from these polymers could be due either to incomplete conversion of TDI to polyurethane or to the easy hydrolysis of the ester linkage in the polymer, and would be facilitated by the high specific surface area of the foam backing. Poly(ester urethanes) are no longer used in implant applications (Pinchuk, 1994).

Environmental fatigue failure of poly(ether urethanes) has been attributed to oxidation of the ether groups in the ether segments. This degradation occurs through oxidative cleavage at the ether linkages and reduces the polymer molecular weight. Elution of methylene dianiline is insignificant with these types of product. As a result the trend is towards use of ether-free, or substantially ether-free polyurethanes. This can be achieved either by using alkyl macrodiols or by using polyether glycols based on monomers with longer alkyl chains (for example, polydecamethylene ether glycol) (Pinchuk, 1994; Piskin, 1994).

The polymer is prepared by combining the rigid isocyanate with the macroglycol to form a prepolymer of relatively low molecular weight. The isocyanate molecules are relatively mobile compared to the macroglycol, so that the latter tends to form a prepolymer 'capped' by isocyanate groups. This prepolymer is then combined with a rigid chain extender to form the final high molecular weight polymer. The chain extender and isocyanate provide the hardness. Catalysts such as stannous octanoate are sometimes used in the synthesis of polyurethanes (Ulrich, 1983; Pinchuk, 1994).

(c) *Polymethacrylates*

Polymethacrylates (IARC, 1979b) are produced by free radical polymerization of methyl methacrylate (yielding poly(methyl methacrylate) (PMMA)) or other methacrylates such as 2-hydroxyethyl methacrylate (yielding poly(2-hydroxyethyl methacrylate) (PHEMA)) (Table 16). These polymers are often called acrylics. In the case of PHEMA, the repeating monomeric unit is hydrophilic, so that the polymer is, in principle, water-soluble. In practice, in the presence of water the material is cross-linked to form a swollen rubbery network with a typical equilibrium water content of about 38% (Kine, 1981; Peppas, 1996; Visser *et al.*, 1996). In dental composites, a number of different polymethacrylates are used, some with two or more monomers.

PMMA is available in two forms. The first is a rigid, heat-cured, preformed material of high clarity that is widely used in intra-ocular lenses. The second is a cold-curing 'dough' that can be moulded and shaped into any form. The latter form is widely used in bone cements for orthopaedic applications (Ousterhout & Stelnicki, 1996).

Bone cements are prepared by mixing a PMMA powder containing initiator with a liquid monomer for several minutes. When the dough has reached an appropriate consistency, it is applied to the site of implantation, sometimes using a special applicator. The setting process is exothermic and temperatures exceeding 70°C may be reached. PMMA bone cements may contain barium sulfate as an additive, to give radio-opacity. A number of antibiotics have been included in commercial cements. Some residual monomer may remain in the polymer matrix after setting (Ousterhout & Stelnicki, 1996).

(d) *Poly(ethylene terephthalate)*

A vast number of polyesters, including poly(ethylene terephthalate) (PET), may be synthesized and a great many of these are fibre-forming. The most important, as a synthetic fibre and as a medical implant material, is PET. In textile form, this is used to manufacture vascular grafts, filter materials, heart valve sewing rings and sutures. PET textile fibres are known as Dacron and Terylene. Titanium dioxide may be used in small amounts to delustre the fibres (Davis, 1982; Piskin, 1994).

It is possible to synthesize PET using terephthalic acid or *para*-xylene as reagents, but it is difficult to obtain these in a pure enough form. Therefore PET is manufactured by the ester interchange (step reaction) polymerization of dimethyl terephthalate and ethylene glycol. The reaction is carried out in two stages. The first is ester interchange in the presence of catalysts such as antimony trioxide with cobalt acetate. This produces a polymer of low molecular weight which, in the second stage, is heated under progressive reduced pressure in order to achieve further condensation (Brydson, 1979; Davis, 1982).

(e) *Polyethylene, polypropylene and other polyolefins*

Polyethylene and polypropylene are products of free radical addition reactions. There are several types of polyethylene with widely diverse physical properties, generally defined in terms of density, molecular weight and linearity, for example low-density polyethylene (LDPE), high-density polyethylene (HDPE) and ultra-high molecular weight polyethylene (UHMWPE). Of these the most important for medical implant applications is UHMWPE, which can be produced only by the use of Ziegler–Natta catalysts (i.e., the Ziegler process). Polypropylene and other higher olefins such as diene rubbers also are manufactured only with the use of Ziegler–Natta catalysts. When used to polymerize higher olefin monomers, these catalysts offer the added advantage of allowing control of the polymer tacticity (Borg, 1979; Brydson, 1979; Crespi & Luciani, 1981; Kochhar & Kissin, 1981; Paschke, 1981).

Ziegler–Natta catalysts are complexes formed by interaction of alkyls of metals of Groups I–III in the periodic table with halides and other derivatives of transition metals of Groups IV–VIII. A typical Ziegler–Natta catalyst is a complex between aluminium alkyl and titanium halide. In general, the gaseous monomer is fed under low pressure into a reactor containing a liquid aliphatic hydrocarbon (C_4–C_8) diluent. The catalyst may be first prepared and fed into the reaction vessel or it may be prepared *in situ* by feeding the catalyst components into the main reactor. The reaction is carried out at temperatures below 100°C in the absence of oxygen and water, both of which deactivate the catalyst. The catalyst remains suspended and the polymer is precipitated from the solution as it is formed. At the end of the reaction, the catalyst is destroyed using ethanol, water or alkali. The decomposition of the catalyst and subsequent purification are important in order to reduce the amount of metallic fragments in the product (Brydson, 1979; Mills & Cusumano, 1979; Paschke, 1981).

(f) *Fluorocarbon polymers*

Fluorocarbons have extremely high thermal stability, are chemically inert, have low friction properties and extreme toughness and flexibility at low temperatures. To produce polytetrafluoroethylene (PTFE), tetrafluroethylene is usually polymerized with free radical initiators at elevated pressure in an aqueous medium. Redox initiation may also be used; persulfates and hydrogen peroxide have been employed as initiators (Brydson, 1979; Gangal, 1980).

PTFE has exceptionally high viscosity above its melting-point (342°C). This prevents use of the techniques commonly applied for processing of thermoplastics. Granular PTFE product is processed using fabrication techniques similar to those used with ceramics and powder metallurgy. A powder is preformed, usually at room temperature, sintered at a temperature (370–390°C) above the melting-point, and then cooled. Preforming is the process of compressing a sieved powder that has been evenly loaded into a mould. Granular polymer may be extruded, at very low rates, by means of both screw and ram extruders (Brydson, 1979; Gangal, 1980).

Because PTFE parts require sintering, this material suffers from severe wear and particle shedding in joint replacement applications (Charnley & Cupic, 1973). The process of expanding thin sheets of PTFE produces a microporous material known as Gore-Tex® (Costantino, 1994).

PTFE is also available in the form of coagulates consisting of particle agglomerates with an average diameter of 450 µm, made up of primary particles 0.1 µm in diameter. Products with improved tensile strength and flexibility may be made using these agglomerates, but they are not easily fabricated using the techniques described above. Instead, this type of PTFE starting material is first mixed with 15–25% of lubricant (petroleum ether or a non-volatile oil) and extruded. The lubricant is then evaporated and the extrudate is sintered. Only thin-section extrudates can be made using this method. Thin-wall tubing and tape are manufactured using these methods (Brydson, 1979; Gangal, 1980).

There are several tetrafluoroethylene copolymers that retain most of the physical and chemical characteristics of PTFE but are more easily processed by conventional techniques. Also polychlorotrifluoroethylene has good chemical resistance (although not as good as that of PTFE) and is easily processed using conventional techniques. However, these variants have not been widely applied in medical implants.

(g) *Polyamides*

Of the many possible methods for preparing linear polyamides, only three are of commercial importance:

Reaction of diamines with dicarboxylic acids via a 'nylon salt'

$$n\ HO-\underset{\underset{O}{\|}}{C}-R_1-\underset{\underset{O}{\|}}{C}-OH\ +\ n\ H_2N-R_2-NH_2\ \longrightarrow\ n\ HO-\underset{\underset{O}{\|}}{C}-R_1-\underset{\underset{O}{\|}}{C}-O^-\ H_3\overset{+}{N}-R_2-NH_2$$

$$*\!-\!\!\left[\!-O-\underset{\underset{O}{\|}}{C}-R_1-\underset{\underset{O}{\|}}{C}-O-NH-R_2-NH-\right]_n\!\!-\!* \ +\ 2n\ H_2O$$

Self condensation of an ω-amino acid

$$n\ H_2N-R_1-\overset{O}{\underset{\|}{C}}-OH \longrightarrow *-\left[NH-R_1-\overset{O}{\underset{\|}{C}}-O\right]_n-* + nH_2O$$

Opening of a lactam ring

$$n\ R\overset{N}{\underset{C=O}{\diagdown|}} \longrightarrow *-\left[NH-R-\overset{O}{\underset{\|}{C}}-O\right]_n-*$$

An example of the first route is the preparation of nylon-6,6, which is made by the reaction of hexamethylene diamine with adipic acid. The first 6 indicates the number of carbon atoms in the diamine and the second the number of carbon atoms in the dicarboxylic acid. Thus nylon-6,10 is made by reaction of hexamethylene diamine with sebacic acid. When a single number is used, for example nylon-6 or nylon-11, the material must have been prepared either by the self-condensation of an ω-amino acid or by lactam ring-opening (Putscher, 1982).

Additives used in nylons may include heat and light stabilizers, plasticizers, lubricants, filler pigments and fungicides. With the exception of pigments, additives are incorporated by the polymer manufacturer, and only limited information on additives is normally available. Heat stabilizers include syringic acid, phenyl-β-naphthylamine, mercaptobenzothiazole and mercaptobenzimidazole. Light stabilizers include carbon black and various phenolic materials. Plasticizers are comparatively uncommon but sulfonamides such as *n*-butylbenzene sulfonamide and blends of *ortho-* and *para*-ethylbenzene sulfonamides are known to be in use in medical device materials (Saunders, 1982; Welgos, 1982).

(h)   Bioresorbable materials

Materials of many types have been investigated for use as bioresorbable polymers, including polyhydroxybutyrate (PHB), polyhydroxyvalerate (PHV) and their copolymers, polycaprolactone, polyanhydrides, poly(α-amino acids) and polyphosphazenes. However, only a small number have been approved for clinical trials on humans and only three—polylactide (or poly(lactic acid); PLA), poly(glycolic acid) (PGA) and polydioxanone (PDS)—are used in a limited range of implant applications, mainly for sutures (Piskin, 1994; Kohn & Langer, 1996).

PGA and PLA are synthesized by catalytic ring-opening polymerization of their respective glycolides (glycolic acid, lactic acid). The ring-opening process is very similar in each case, so that the production of copolymers of glycolic acid and lactic acid is analogous to that of the homopolymers. Polymers of high molecular weight are produced by polymerization at high temperature using tin, zinc and antimony catalysts, the most commonly used being stannous acetate. Low molecular weight polymers may be produced by heating aqueous solutions of the monomers at low temperatures without catalysts (Piskin, 1994; Athanasiou *et al.*, 1995). PGA is highly crystalline (up to 50% crystallinity), has a high melting-point (224–226°C) and is slightly soluble in few organic solvents. PGA sutures have been available under the trade name of Dexon® since 1970 (Piskin, 1994; Kohn & Langer, 1996).

PGA degrades rapidly, typically over a period from hours to several weeks depending mainly on the initial molecular weight, morphology (amorphous/crystalline phases) and surface-to-volume ratio. PLA is more hydrophobic than PGA and degrades more slowly (from weeks to years). Therefore, PGA/PLA copolymers have been developed to extend the range of applications (Piskin, 1994; Kohn & Langer, 1996). Degradation occurs via hydrolysis of the ester linkages. *In vivo*, enzymes are thought to enhance the rate of degradation (Ashammakhi & Rokkanen, 1997).

PGA/PLA copolymers are used in sutures, screws, plates and rods, which are fabricated using techniques such as injection moulding, extrusion, solution casting and compression moulding (Athanasiou *et al.*, 1995; Ashammakhi & Pokkanen, 1997).

1B.1.3 *Ceramics*

Ceramics are composed of atoms that are ionocovalently bound into compound forms. The resulting atomic immobility makes ceramics poor conductors of heat and electricity. Because ceramics have melting-points that are generally above 1000°C, it is very expensive to melt them and because they are brittle, it is impossible to cold-work ceramics. The same factors confer a high degree of environmental stability (Davis, 1979; Hare, 1979a,b).

Many of the more common ceramics are metal oxides. Three metal oxide ceramics used as implant materials are alumina (Al_2O_3) and zirconia (ZrO_2) which are used for orthopaedic and dental applications, and silica (SiO_2) which is used as a very fine, high surface area filler for silicone elastomers (Black, 1992; Andreopoulos & Evangelatou, 1994; Anusavice, 1996).

Ceramics are typically strong and hard, which gives them excellent wear resistance. However, grain boundary impurities often lead to failure and grain excavation in situations of wear or abrasion. One method of toughening ceramics is to engineer the grains and grain boundaries so that a crack tends to go through the boundary and be deflected by the grain. Another approach is to develop compounds such as partially-stabilized zirconia with yttria or magnesia, in which a phase transformation is induced by stress and crack propagation is prevented (Hare, 1979b; Piconi *et al.*, 1998).

Non-oxide ceramics used as implant materials include synthetic analogues of the bone mineral phase. The two more commonly used are tricalcium phosphate (TCP) and hydroxylapatite (Table 16). Both materials stimulate new bone formation *in vivo* and are used as coatings to stabilize joint and tooth root replacements. Hydroxylapatite has the slower dissolution rate, especially when in the form of a fully dense solid block. Porcelain used for dental full crowns and metal–ceramic reconstructions is mainly composed of feldspar (70–80%), quartz (17–30%) and kaolin (0–3%) (Ravaglioli & Krajewski, 1992).

Carbon is also used as a single-element ceramic material. Several forms of pyrolytic carbon can be fabricated by pyrolysis of organic gases such as methane or of polymer blocks or fibres. The most common form is referred to as low-temperature isotropic (LTI) carbon, which is used as a wear-resistant, blood-compatible coating on cardiovascular devices such as heart valves and heart valve occluders (Björk, 1985).

Carbon fibres are made by pyrolysing polymer fibres. These have been used in fibre form for replacement or repair of ligaments or tendons, and for reinforcing composite materials (Barry *et al.*, 1995).

1B.1.4 *Composite materials*

Carbon fibre composites of several types have been developed. Short 'chopped' fibres are mixed with thermoplastic polymers and can be moulded. Long or 'continuous' fibre composites may have many layers of fibres all oriented in the same direction, or in alternating perpendicular orientations. Chopped carbon fibre composites with UHMWPE have been used for bearing surfaces of total joint replacements. Long-fibre composites have been investigated for fracture fixation and as the femoral component of total hip replacements (Black, 1992; Zhang *et al.*, 1996).

Composite materials used for dental restoration are composed of an inorganic component and an organic matrix (polymer). Three groups of materials exist: resin-based material with an inorganic filler (often termed 'composite'), resin-reinforced glass polyalkenoate cement, and the so-called 'compomer'. Compomer (which is derived by combining the two words composite and ionomer) is a mixture of resin-based material and a glass polyalkenoate cement in which the resin-based material is the main constituent (Blackwell & Käse, 1996).

1B.2 Production and use

1B.2.1 *Production*

A very wide variety of polymers and ceramic materials are used in medical implants and dental applications. In addition, the physical properties of these materials are determined not only by their composition but also by the processing and fabrication methods.

Custom-made devices in dentistry are made by dental technicians, and the limited control of these processes available in a laboratory setting may lead to increased levels of residual substances in the device.

In general, fabrication of objects of definite shape or form from non-metallic materials involves deformation of the material or a material precursor followed by setting of the final shape by some means. Methods employed include:

(i) deformation of polymer melts followed by cooling;
(ii) deformation of polymers in the rubbery state followed by cooling;
(iii) deformation of a solution or a suspension followed by evaporation or drying;

(iv) deformation of a low molecular weight polymer or a polymer precursor followed by cross-linking, curing or polymerization;

(v) machining operations.

Melt processing can be further subdivided into extrusion, injection moulding and calendering. In extrusion, the material is pumped through a die to give a product of constant cross-section. In injection moulding, the polymer melt is pumped into a mould of the desired shape. Calendering is a process in which sheet or film is produced by passing the molten material first between heated rollers and later between cooling rollers. Resins which are to undergo melt processing usually contain additives such as mould-release agents, antioxidants and other processing aids. Cooling (setting) of extrudates is carried out by quenching in water or air. Injection moulds include cooling mechanisms, such as water jacketing, to cool the material as it is injected (Brydson, 1979; Gangal, 1980; Kine, 1981; Paschke, 1981; Richardson, 1982; Peppas, 1996; Vissel *et al.*, 1996).

In some cases, it is more efficient not to process a melt, but to heat the material until a 'rubbery state' is achieved and then form the material by application of high or reduced pressure or by mechanical action. With the pressure methods, the material is either sucked or blown onto the sides of a mould (blow moulding) and then cooled. When mechanical pressure is used, the material is preheated and stamped—a process similar to forging. These techniques are not generally used to produce medical implants (Richardson, 1982; Welgos, 1982).

Solution processes are used mainly for coating, film casting and fibre spinning. The products are of thin cross-section, which allows the diffusion of solvents out of the polymer matrix. Fibre spinning from polymer solutions is not generally used to produce medical fibres (Richardson, 1982).

Casting from polymer solutions is used to make silicone breast prosthesis shells and other membranes. Essentially, the process involves casting the polymer solution onto an appropriately shaped mandril, allowing the solvent to evaporate from the resultant film and then peeling the film away.

Some products such as certain contact and intra-ocular lenses are formed before polymerization. In such cases, the monomer, or a mixture of the monomer, polymers and curing agents (cross-linking agents), is made to react inside a vessel or mould of the desired shape. As mentioned above, PMMA bone cements are also prepared according to this principle, although, in this situation, the 'fabrication' is performed *in situ* by the surgeon (Ousterhout & Stelnicki, 1996).

Some materials, in particular intra-ocular and certain contact lenses, are machined into their final shape. In these cases, the monomer is polymerized in bulk to form polymer 'buttons' which are subsequently shaped using a lathe.

Ceramics for most biomedical applications are prepared from a high-purity powder. Appropriate amounts of such powders are mixed together into a batch, which is then processed and formed into a shape that is similar to the final part. This unfired ceramic (called a 'green body') is then sintered at a temperature at which the powder coalesces into a hard material in which the particles have fused together to form grains of crystalline material with amorphous boundaries that often include higher levels of any impurities. The sintered parts are machined into their final shape by grinding and polishing methods.

Ceramic coatings can be applied with a variety of thermal spray techniques. These use materials such as hydroxylapatite in a powder form that is fed into a chamber in which a rapidly expanding hot gas is used to heat the powder to near its melting temperature and projects it towards the material to be coated. Each particle impacts (or 'splats') on the surface to form a primarily mechanically interlocked coating of splats. Coatings can also be applied by sol-gel techniques in which the device is dipped into a solution of the ceramic material.

Pyrolytic coatings are typically formed from graphitic bodies with a shape and dimensions close to those of the final device. These are placed in a fluidized bed in which an up-flow of gas causes the particles to float. A hydrocarbon gas, such as methane, is heated to a pyrolysing temperature and carbon is deposited on the parts as layers of carbon crystals. Each crystal has an orientation independent of the others, hence the name isotropic. The crystals have a plate-like structure known as turbostratic. Coating is typically done at temperatures below 1500°C, so the product is called low-temperature isotropic pyrolytic carbon with a turbostratic microstructure. Such coatings are often alloyed with silicon for increased strength. Parts are then given a high mechanical polish to produce the very smooth, wear-resistant surfaces needed for heart valves.

One of the most common carbon fibres starts as extruded fibres of polyacrylonitrile. These are subjected to a series of heating and pyrolysis steps to convert the polymer first into an aromatic ring structure and then to the hexagonal crystal structure of carbon. A range of mechanical properties can be obtained, depending on the final pyrolysis temperature. The fibres are coated with an organic sizing to prevent sticking and clumping. The sizing is removed before use.

Carbon fibre composite production depends on the fibre form and matrix. Chopped fibres are mixed with the polymer matrix and extruded as pellets. These are used for injection or compression moulding. Long fibres can be laid up in pre-impregnated sheets. For thermoplastics, these sheets are laid in stacks and moulded by heat compression. Fibres can also be mixed with thermosetting resins, catalysts or other components and polymerized. Parts can be moulded in final form, or machined from large blocks.

1B.2.2 *Use*

Silicone gel-filled breast implants consist of a silicone elastomer shell that encases different volumes of silicone gel. The gel is a mixture of silicone oils dispersed in a lightly cross-linked silicone matrix, and the shell is manufactured by slip casting an uncross-linked, linear silicone fluid containing a curing agent and fumed silica onto a bulb-shaped mandril, as described above.

After the shell is filled with gel, the opening is closed using a patch of silicone elastomer which is cured onto the shell. The final coat of the silicone shell may be texturized by a variety of proprietary processes. It is believed that textured implants are less susceptible to encapsulation. In the past, some implants were covered or backed with a polyurethane foam or polyester patches, but this is no longer a commercial process. Silicone-shell breast implants may also be filled with saline, vegetable oils or polysaccharide hydrogels (Duffy, 1990; Szycher et al., 1991).

Intra-ocular lenses consist of an optical component (the lens or optic) made from PMMA, silicone or, to a lesser extent, hydrogel, supported by an outer PMMA or polypropylene 'strand' shaped into a 'C' or a 'J', known as a haptic. The haptics are inserted into holes on the sides of the optic and glued into place. The optic is either machined or cast from appropriate moulds, depending on the material used and the manufacturer's preference. The haptic is made using extrusion methods followed by rubbery-state shaping (Nagamoto & Eguchi, 1997; Yoda, 1998).

1C. Composite Medical and Dental Implants

1C.1 Description of devices

1C.1.1 *Generic orthopaedic joint replacements*

Implants for joint replacement (joint arthroplasty) have evolved over the years from devices that were inserted between the articulating cartilage surfaces to devices that require removal and replacement of the total joint. Inter-positional devices began as films or cups made of metals or plastics. These required minimal tissue removal, and it was assumed that they would stimulate cartilage repair. As a next stage, surface replacements were developed in which one surface, typically the cartilage of the femoral head of the hip, was removed and replaced with a cup fixed to the bone. As an extension of this concept, the replacement of one component or hemi-arthroplasty of the hip required surgical removal of the femoral head and neck and replacement with a device with a ball that articulated with the intact cartilage of the acetabulum, and a stem in the medullary canal of the femur (Williams & Roaf, 1973; McElfresh, 1991).

Total joint replacement uses implants which replace both sides of a joint. These are generally composed of a ball-and-socket, as in the total hip replacement configuration, or concave–convex surfaces, as in a total knee replacement. An exception to this is the finger or toe joint replacement, which typically is a one-piece, elastomeric, flexible hinge device. Elbow replacements are also typically a hinge-type device.

There are several levels of total knee replacement. The knee is often described as having three joints: two femoral condyle–tibial plateau joints and one patellar–femoral joint. The term 'unicompartmental replacement' pertains to the replacement of one condyle and its tibial plateau. A tricompartmental prosthesis consists of a femoral component, a tibial component and a patellar component. Such rolling-sliding devices depend on the ligamentous attachments to stabilize the knee. In the event that the medial and lateral collateral ligaments have been destroyed, as in multiple revisions or tumours, a hinge-type total knee replacement is used (Williams & Roaf, 1973; McElfresh, 1991).

A number of mechanisms are used for the fixation of joint prostheses, some of which result in significant modifications of the microstructure of the metal. The first-order division is between 'press-fit' and 'cemented'. Early devices were inserted after surgical removal of tissues as necessary and by pressing the device over the joint or into the medullary canal. These devices were anchored to the bone due to the matte finish or roughness of the surface, or by the bone growing into large fenestrations of the device. More recently, a variety of methods have been developed to achieve biological fixation, by the use of porous coatings or textured or roughened surfaces (see Section 1B.2.1). Cemented devices are stabilized by the insertion of poly(methyl methacrylate) bone cement that has been kneaded into a dough-like state, followed by insertion of the stem of the prosthesis into this bed of dough. Within 10–15 min, the cement hardens due to in-situ polymerization. A total joint replacement in which one component is press fit, while another is cemented, is termed a hybrid (Williams & Roaf, 1973; McElfresh, 1991).

Joint replacements may be either 'modular' or 'monoblock' types. A modular device is manufactured and shipped to the surgeon in several parts. Usually, there is some type of tapering press-fit or pin-locking mechanism. For example, a modular total hip replacement may have a femoral stem with a tapered cone, which can fit several different heads, which have tapered bores. The polyethylene acetabular liner could be modular and pressed into one of several types of metal shells or cups. These are assembled by the surgeon during the operation so as to give the optimal fit. Modularity also leads to optimization of material properties; for example, a femoral ball head material with excellent wear resistance (cobalt alloy or ceramic) can be combined with a stem material selected for greater strength or from a titanium alloy for greater flexibility. In contrast, a monoblock is implanted as received. The term 'monoblock' does not necessarily mean that the device is cast in one piece. The large balls of the hip hemiarthroplasties are cast as parts and welded together to create a hollow sphere on a stem. Some monoblock total hip stems are made by welding a stem of one cobalt alloy to a ball head of another cobalt alloy (Süry & Semlitsch, 1978; Richards Manufacturing Company, 1980; Semlitsch, 1992).

1C.1.2 *Orthopaedic fracture fixation devices*

Devices for bone fracture fixation (osteosynthesis) are often classified as 'spinal' or 'fracture fixation'. Simple pins and wires are used in both situations. There are a multitude of 'screws' used for fixation of bone. Many of these bear names either of the designer or of the anatomical location for which they were designed. Screws may be used to fix two fragments of bone directly (with either one or several screws) or they may be used to fix a plate-like device to the bone. Spinal devices may be assembled from several screws, pins and locking devices.

Various types of plate for fracture fixation are available. The simplest are essentially strips of metal with several holes for screws. Holes may be circular with conical or spherical countersink shapes, or they may be oval in shape or slotted. The differences depend on the surgical application but can also affect the degree of stability between screw head and plate hole, and thus the amount of corrosion and fretting. Most plates are designed to be bent and twisted by the surgeon so as to fit the contours of the bone. Multi-component plates have been developed for specific anatomical situations, such as fractures of the femoral neck and maxillofacial reconstruction. There exist a variety of sliding nail and screw devices for insertion into the femoral neck, with a side plate screwed to the femur (Williams & Roaf, 1973).

1C.1.3 *Cardiovascular devices*

Heart valves are classified as mechanical or bioprosthetic, depending upon whether they are made from synthetic materials or materials of biological origin; they all open and close passively. Mechanical valves have a ring structure which is attached to a textile sewing ring used to sew the valve to the heart, and a seating portion for the occluder to close the valve. There is also a containment system to keep the occluder in the valve. The classic was a Starr-Edwards model, with a polyester sewing ring, a cobalt alloy seating ring and wire cage, and a silicone rubber ball occluder. Bioprosthetic valves have leaflets made of chemically fixed bovine or porcine material which open and close against each other. Many have a textile sewing ring attached, and some have a metal wire frame or 'stent' to hold the leaflets in a proper position (Morse & Steiner, 1985).

There are a number of other cardiovascular uses for metals and alloys. Pacemakers often have the body sealed in a titanium canister and leads made of one of the cobalt alloys. Endovascular grafts, patches and stents may have metallic components as spring elements, fabric supports or for securing the anastomosis. Metals are also used as staples to seal a vascular anastomosis or skin incision.

1C.1.4 *Dental materials*

Dental metallic materials are used for fillings, prosthetic devices (crowns, bridges, removable prostheses), dental implants and orthodontic treatment. Prosthetic devices replace the tooth crown when tooth substance or the whole tooth is lost due to caries, periodontal disease, fracture, injury or other reasons. Dental implants may be placed subperiosteally or in the jaw bone; the latter method has now almost universal application. Dental implants anchor the so-called superstructure, e.g., a crown, bridge or a removable prosthesis. Orthodontic metallic appliances exert forces on teeth in order to move them into a desired position in patients having malocclusion. During the finishing of metallic dental materials in the mouth, it is possible for particles from the devices to be introduced into the soft tissue.

In the early years of development, a variety of materials such as tantalum (e.g., Tantal), niobium, CoCr alloys (e.g., Vitallium) and stainless steels were used in dental implants. However, the most successful experiences have been with titanium, either commercially pure or as its alloys (e.g., Ti 6,4), as specified in ISO 5832 and ASTM F 67 and F 136; see Section 1A.1.2). These materials are mainly used for endosseous implants (Brånemark, 1983; Anusavice, 1996).

The main differences between the various implants provided by different manufacturers are their shape, size and surface structure or coating. Early designs of dental implants included a variety of blade-like devices. Current designs employ screw-shaped or nonthreaded cylinders. A rough surface is considered to promote bone growth in order to induce a direct bond between the implant and the hard tissue. To achieve this, flame or plasma-spraying techniques are used to generate a thin porous layer of titanium oxide on the implant surface; sandblasting and etching are used to roughen the implant surface directly (Anusavice, 1996).

1C.2 Numbers of implants used

Comprehensive data on the numbers of medical and dental devices implanted worldwide are not available. Selected data from surveys, registries and published estimates are presented in this section, for illustrative purposes.

A National Health Interview Survey in the United States sampled 47 485 households in 1988. A Medical Device Implant Supplement identified the number of individuals with implants in their bodies. From these surveys, it was estimated that there were a total of 14 999 000 implants in the United States in 1988. Of these, 6 515 000 (43.4%) were orthopaedic implants. A quarter of the latter (1 625 000) were total joints, including 816 000 total hip replacements and 521 000 total knee replacements. The remaining 4 890 000 orthopaedic devices (75.1%) were fixation devices, with 646 000 upper-extremity implants, 2 690 000 lower extremity, 563 000 torso and 991 000 other locations (Moore *et al.*, 1991).

A 1992 survey report for the British market reported that 40 000 total hips per year were implanted in the United Kingdom. A total of 62 types were identified on the British market listing of total hips used in the United Kingdom in 1994. The stainless steel Charnley (ISO 5832-9, introduced in 1964) had over 20% of the market. Eight others were listed as having 5–20% of the market. These were Stanmore (cemented, polished stem, monoblock, made of cobalt alloy or Ti 6,4); CPT (cemented, Exeter concept, polished stem, modular, stainless steel); Exeter (modular, polished stem, stainless steel); Ultima (developed from Howse II, modular, smooth stem, cemented Ti 6,4); Elite (developed from Charnley, ISO 5832-9, modular); Harris precoat (cemented, modular, wrought CoCr); ABG (hydroxylapatite-coated, cementless, modular, titanium alloy); Omnifit-HA (hydroxylapatite-coated, cementless, modular, titanium alloy) (Murray *et al.*, 1994).

The Swedish Hip Registry was established in 1978. Its 1993 report stated that over 800 000 total hip replacements were performed worldwide each year. From 1978 until 1990, a total of 92 675 primary total hip replacements were reported to the Swedish Hip Registry. The number of implants per 100 000 inhabitants per year in 1988 was 101 in

Sweden, 54 in the United Kingdom, 108 in France, 116 in Belgium and 64–80 in the United States (in 1989). The incidence in 1991 in Sweden was up to 131 (Malchau et al., 1993). As reported in the 1998 registry, the vast majority of implanted hips were cemented. The five most frequently used hip systems for primary total hip replacement, all of which are cemented, are shown in Table 18 (Malchau & Herberts, 1998).

Table 18. Number of primary hip implants in Sweden during the period 1979–1996

Type	Metal	1979–86	1987–96	Total
Charnley	Stainless steel	16 054	28 525	44 579
Lubinus	CoCr	16 538	24 243	40 781
Exeter	Stainless steel	4 246	12 146	16 392
Scan Hip		920	5 310	6 230
Müller	CoCr	1 721	2 137	3 858
Total cemented		50 564	88 266	138 830
Uncemented		1 217	3 748	4 965
Hybrid		233	4 182	4 415
Grand total		52 014	96 196	148 210

Lubinus includes SPI, SP II and IP models; Exeter includes matte and three polished models.
From Malchau & Herberts (1998)

The total number of primary total knee implantations in Sweden from 1976 through 1992 was 30 003. The vast majority of these were made of CoCrMo alloy (Knutson et al., 1994).

The number of heart valves implanted worldwide as of 1985, for some of the more common types, were as follows: Starr-Edwards with HS-21 (F 75) cage and silicone ball, 170 000; and Starr-Edwards with hollow F 75 ball occluders, 53 500. Since 1969, 35 000 Hancock Bioprosthetic valves have been implanted and, since 1975, 125 000 Carpentier-Edwards bioprosthetic valves with Elgiloy (F 1058) frames have been implanted. A total of 100 000 Lillehei-Kaster and Medtronic-Hall valves with carbon occluders and titanium (F 67) frames and 80 000 all-carbon St Jude valves had been implanted (Morse & Steiner, 1985).

According to a 1998 market survey report, in 1990, 64% of all valves being implanted worldwide were mechanical. In 1996, 153 000 or 74% of all valves sold were mechanical and 54 000 were tissue or bioprosthetic valves. The all-carbon St Jude was then the leading valve worldwide, with a total of 725 000 having been implanted. The CarboMedics bileaflet valve is a pyrolytic carbon valve, of which over 200 000 had been implanted, while 125 000 of the all-carbon Sorin Biomedica had been implanted worldwide. About 150 000 Medtronic Hall valves were made with carbon occluders and a Ti 6,4 frame. The first tissue valve was implanted in France by Dr Carpentier in 1965. As of 1995, about 75 000 Carpentier-Edwards bovine pericardial and 250 000 porcine tissue valves with Elgiloy stents had been implanted (Dorland, 1998).

For cardiac pacemakers, the estimate from the Medical Device Implant Supplement yielded an annual implantation rate of 232 per million in the United States in 1988, 238 per million in western Europe in 1986 and 279 per million in Canada in 1989. The prevalence of cardiac pacemakers in the United States was 2.6 per 1000 inhabitants and the age-adjusted prevalence in men was 1.5 times that in women in 1988 (Silverman et al., 1995).

In 1990, 200 million dental restorative procedures were performed in the United States, including 96 million dental amalgam fillings (Working Group on Dental Amalgam, 1997). More than 12 million dental restorations were placed within the General Dental Service of the National Health Service for England and Wales in 1996 (Committee on Toxicity of Chemicals in Food, Consumer Products and the Environment, 1997). The worldwide annual use of gold for dental devices in 1993 and 1994 was 65 tonnes, which represents more than 65 million dental cast crowns (Beck et al., 1995).

It has been estimated that PET was used to produce 186 800 vascular grafts, 56 200 fabrics, patches and mesh (of the sort that are used in heart valve sewing rings) and 26 633 million sutures in 1992. It was also estimated that 309 900 vascular grafts and 126 600 surgical patches were produced using expanded PTFE in that year (Aronoff, 1995).

It was estimated that in 1991 over 100 000 women were electing to undergo breast implant surgery in the United States annually (Szycher et al., 1991) and that between 1 and 2 million women (Anon., 1992) had received breast implants in the United States between 1962 and 1992. These figures have been revised by Terry et al. (1995), who estimated that 894 206 women received cosmetic breast implants between 1963 and 1988 in the United States.

It has been estimated that 1 400 000 intra-ocular lenses were implanted in the United States in 1990 (Ratner et al., 1996).

There is increasing use of composites in dentistry. Data from the United States indicate that composite materials are now selected for dental fillings as often as dental amalgam (Mjör & Moorhead, 1998).

1C.3 Regulations and guidelines

In Europe, the Active Implantable Medical Devices Directive regulates all implantable powered devices, including cardiac pacemakers and implantable defibrillators. Other implantable medical and dental devices are regulated by the Medical Device Directive. The Directives require that any product should receive premarketing approval by a third party, the so-called Notified Bodies. Approval by a Notified Body in any one of the European Economic Agreement (EEA) member countries implies that the device may be marketed in all of these countries. The European Commission, in seeking to achieve uniform implementation of the Medical Device Directive across Europe, requested that Project Groups be set up to develop guidance for breast implants and dental amalgam (De Giovanni, 1995; Polyzois et al., 1995; Tinkler, 1995).

In the United States, medical and dental devices are evaluated by the Food and Drug Administration (FDA). The Safe Medical Devices Act of 1990 and the Medical Device Amendments regulate the premarketing review and postmarket surveillance (Monsein, 1997a,b).

In Japan, all medical and dental devices are regulated under the Pharmaceutical Affairs Law by the Ministry of Health and Welfare. This law indicates the principles of regulation, and details of regulatory procedures and guidelines are promulgated in the Ministry of Health and Welfare notifications. Medical and dental implantable devices require premarketing approval by the Ministry.

In Australia, the Therapeutic Goods Administration (TGA) is responsible for the certification of medical and dental devices, according to the Therapeutic Goods Act 1989 and the Australian Medical Device Requirements – Version 4 (DR4). Among other devices, breast protheses, active implantable devices and intra-ocular lenses require premarketing evaluation (Therapeutic Goods Administration, 1998).

Biocompatibility evaluation of medical and dental devices is preferably done according to ASTM F 748 (Standard practice for selecting generic biological test methods for material and devices), or the ISO 10993 series of standards (Biological evaluation of medical devices). One standard (ISO 10993-1, Evaluation and testing) gives the framework for the evaluation and selection of test methods, and the other ISO 10993 standards suggest methods for in-vitro and in-vivo testing. For carcinogenicity testing of new materials with which there is no experience or information on their potential carcinogenicity when used as a long-term implant, ISO 10993-3 (Tests for genotoxicity, carcinogenicity and reproductive toxicity) can be used as a guideline. This document has a flowchart attached which clarifies an admissible approach.

STEP 1: Three types of in-vitro testing are suggested:
(i) a bacterial mutagenesis test (e.g., the *Salmonella* reverse mutation assay or Ames test)
(ii) a mammalian cell mutagenesis test, either: (*a*) Chinese hamster ovary cells hprt locus test, (e.g., ASTM E1262) or (*b*) mouse lymphoma $tk^{+/-}$ test, (e.g., ASTM E1280)
(iii) a chromosomal aberration test (e.g., Preston et al., 1981).

STEP 2: If the results from all of the above tests are negative, the material can be said to have no genotoxic potential. If any results are positive, then:

If the results from (i) or (ii) are positive, perform either: (1) an in-vivo unscheduled DNA synthesis test (e.g., ASTM E1398) or (2) a mouse spot test.

If the results from (iii) are positive, perform either: (1) a short-term micronucleus test *in vivo* (e.g., ASTM E1263) or (2) a metaphase analysis in bone marrow in-vivo test.

STEP 3: If results from tests called for in step 2 are negative, the material is classified 'in-vitro mutagenic'. If the results from tests called for in Step 2 are positive, the material is classified as 'mutagenic'. As a final test, a long-term carcinogenicity test *in vivo* (e.g., ASTM F1439) may be performed.

Specific test methods for dental devices are also given in the international standard ISO 7405 (Dentistry – Preclinical evaluation of biocompatibility of medical devices used in dentistry – Test methods for dental materials). Requirements for medical devices are also given in the ASTM standards.

1D. Other Foreign Bodies

1D.1 Introduction

Foreign bodies introduced directly through a puncture of the skin may include materials from occupational explosions or accidents. However, the principal categories of penetrating objects that remain in contact with tissue for long periods of time, other than those that are surgically implanted, are of two types: (1) bullets and pellets from the use of firearms; and (2) shrapnel (artillery) and shell fragments arising from wartime explosions.

Non-metallic objects of various types have been described and associated with 'accidental' intrusions into the body including materials such as glass, wax, oils and plastics. These materials have been reported, for example, in the pleural cavity, breast, thumb, abdominal cavity, leg, larynx and colon (Thompson & Entin, 1969; Pennisi, 1984; Jennings *et al.*, 1988; Maier & Beck, 1992). However, no systematic exposure data are available on these objects.

1D.2 Bullets and pellets

The nature of bullets and pellets and their metallic composition have evolved with the use of different alloys and the introduction of outer jackets to enhance delivery, body penetration and tissue destruction. Originally, bullets consisted simply of lead spheres. Lead still remains commonly used in bullets and pellets since it spreads out in soft tissues, creating extensive tissue damage. Some bullets, pellets and projectiles have contained alloys of other metals such as nickel, tungsten, bismuth and tin. The advent of rifled barrels and high-velocity weapons led to the use of new fabrication methods and still other metals in bullets and shot.

Modern bullets fall into two categories: lead bullets and metal-jacketed bullets. Lead has been traditionally used for small-bore bullets, such as .22 calibre rimfire ammunition and for revolver cartridges. Metal-jacketed bullets are used in high-velocity rifles and automatic pistols. Lead bullets are composed of lead with small amounts of tin or antimony added to increase the hardness of the alloy. Some lead bullets are coated with a very thin layer (0.1 µm) of copper or copper alloy known as 'gilding', which hardens and lubricates the bullet. Copper gilding is used extensively in .22 calibre high-velocity rimfire ammunition.

Jacketing is now used in bullets for high-velocity rifles to prevent fragmenting or melting of the lead. Jacketed bullets are also used in semiautomatic pistols to prevent deposition of lead in the action or barrel and jams that may result when large numbers of lead bullets are fired. A variety of jacketed bullets exist. Some have a lead or steel core covered by an outside jacket of gilding material (such as copper or zinc); others are gilded metal-clad steel, cupro-nickel or aluminium. The most common military bullets have a lead or mild steel core covered by a full metal jacket. The high-velocity rifle ammunition used for hunting as well as for high-velocity revolvers and automatic pistols generally consists of partially metal-jacketed bullets with the tip open to expose the lead core. The Silver-Tip® bullets contain a very light covering of aluminium over the tip of the lead. Although the composition and construction of bullets vary, for most ammunition lead still remains the main component (Di Maio, 1985).

The chemical and physical properties of metallic lead are summarized in IARC (1980) and by the Agency for Toxic Substances and Disease Registry (1988).

Pellets or shot are used in shotguns and vary with the type of game hunted. However, the pellets are of four basic types: drop or soft shot (essentially pure lead), chilled or hard shot (lead hardened by the addition of antimony), plated shot (lead shot coated with a thin coat of copper or nickel) and steel shot. The pellets vary in size from small birdshot to larger buckshot or shotgun slugs that are used for hunting larger animals such as deer and bear (Di Maio, 1985).

In the United States, the use of lead shot or balls for waterfowl hunting has been banned since 1991, and steel shots are now the only approved shot for such activities. Guidelines established in the United States indicate that metals or alloys used as shot formulations must be tested for their acute toxicity, as well as for corrosion and chronic and reproductive toxicity (United States Fish & Wildlife Services, 1989).

1D.3 Shell fragments

Until recently, most shrapnel (artillery) and shell fragments penetrating and implanting in the body consisted of metallic alloys with a high percentage of iron and steel and minor amounts of other metals, such as tungsten (Blakely, 1952).

With the introduction of depleted uranium for civilian applications in the 1960s and 1970s and for military applications in the early 1980s (as a dense protective armour for vehicles and as a component of armour-piercing missiles), metallic shell fragments consisting of depleted uranium have evolved as a potential health concern. The number of persons exposed so far to depleted uranium fragments is small and the duration of the exposure is short relative to normal latency periods for carcinogenesis. However, future human exposures to depleted uranium fragments in military actions should be envisaged.

Naturally occurring uranium is typically composed of 99.284% ^{238}U, 0.711% ^{235}U, and 0.005% ^{234}U. Depleted uranium is the by-product of the uranium-enrichment process used to develop high-grade uranium capable of sustaining chain reactions needed for reactor fuel or for nuclear weapons. This enrichment process depletes or lowers the weight concentration of the more radioactive ^{234}U and ^{235}U isotopes, thus raising the proportion of the lower specific activity ^{238}U from 99.2 to 99.8%. The mixture of isotopes in the depleted uranium is approximately 99.8% ^{238}U and 0.20% ^{235}U. Only trace levels of other uranium isotopes (0.0003% ^{236}U and 0.001% ^{234}U) are present. Thus, depleted uranium has a much lower specific activity (0.4 μCi/g) than natural uranium (0.7 Ci/g), and its chemical toxicity predominates over the radiation effects when it is taken into the body in a soluble form.

All uranium radioisotopes are radioactive and emit α particles. The half-lives are quite long, 4.5×10^9 years for ^{238}U and 2.5×10^5 years for ^{235}U. Some of the daughter products emit β and γ rays as well. Natural uranium is widely present in the environment and is present in many food products. The chemical and physical properties of depleted uranium are reviewed in AEPI (1995) and by the Agency for Toxic Substances and Disease Registry (1998).

Depleted uranium has several commercial applications, including its use in neutron detectors, radiation detection and shielding for medicine and industry, shielding in shipping containers for radiopharmaceuticals and other radioisotopes, components of aircraft parts (e.g., inertial guidance devices and gyro compasses), in petroleum exploration (boring bars, damping weights, etc.), as counterbalance weights in radar antennae, satellites, missiles and other craft, and as X-ray targets. However, the major use of depleted uranium has been for military applications. It has been incorporated into both projectiles and armour by the military of the United States and other countries because of its density, availability and low relative cost. According to the Agency for Toxic Substances and Disease Registry (1998), the major uses for depleted uranium in 1978 were in military applications (71.8%), counterweights (11.4%), radiation shielding (13.6%), and chemical analysis (3.2%).

By far the greatest potential for 'implantation' of depleted uranium is related to military operations, especially fragments from depleted uranium contained in missiles and shells and in vehicle shielding. When depleted uranium burns, as happens when an anti-tank armour-piercing shell strikes a tank with depleted uranium plating, much of the metal is oxidized into small respirable particles and some into metal shards or fragments. These respirable particles, if inhaled or ingested, can exert toxic effects on various organ systems. The metal fragments of depleted uranium can also inflict tissue injuries and, when left in the body, serve as depots of metal species that may translocate over time.

The first military action in which depleted uranium was involved was the 1991 Gulf War, primarily by United States military units. To date, 33 cases with implanted depleted uranium fragments have been identified among American military personnel participating in the Gulf War.

isotopes used to develop high-grade uranium capable of sustaining chain reactions needed to reach criticality for nuclear weapons. The enrichment process depleted even layers the weight concentration of the more radioactive ^{234}U and ^{235}U isotopes, thus raising the proportion of the lower specific activity ^{238}U. Thus 99.2 to 99.8% the mixture of isotopes in the depleted uranium is approximately 99.8% ^{238}U and 0.20% ^{235}U only trace levels of other uranium isotopes (0.0005% ^{234}U and 0.001% ^{236}U) are present. Thus depleted uranium has a much lower specific activity (0.4 µCi/g) than natural uranium (0.7 Ci/g), and its chemical toxicity predominates over the hazards from its radiation. Whereas it is taken into the body in soluble form.

All uranium radioisotopes are radioactive and emit α particles. The half-lives of ^{238}U, ^{235}U, ^{234}U are 4.5×10^9 years, 7×10^8 and 2.5×10^5 years, respectively. As a result of the slow decay of ^{238}U, there is also a very low rate of spontaneous fission.

2. STUDIES OF CANCER IN HUMANS

2A. Metallic medical and dental materials

2A.1 Case reports

The pathology of the cases illustrated in the reports summarized in this section was reviewed by the Working Group and the diagnoses were deemed reliable.

Compilations of the published case reports describing malignant tumours at the site of the metallic implants are presented in Tables 19 (14 cases) (static orthopaedic metallic implants) and 20 (two cases) (joint prostheses).

A total of 16 case reports of local sarcoma or lymphoma at the site of metallic implants have been found in the medical literature. The time lapse between implantation and tumour diagnosis for these cases varied from a few months to 30 years. The ranges were 1.2–30 years for static orthopaedic implants (14 cases) but the majority were less than 10 years (seven cases) and 3.5 and five years for joint endoprostheses (two cases). Almost all case reports relating to tumours at the site of static implants involved the femur. The implanted materials (where reported) were stainless steel or cobalt–chromium alloys. The number of cases appears to be small in comparison with large numbers of implanted metallic devices. Reporting of individual cases is not systematic, so the actual number of occurrences is likely to be greater.

2A.2 Analytical studies

In a case–control study of soft-tissue sarcoma by Morgan & Elcock (1995) described in the chapter on 'composite implants' (see Section 2C.2.1b), a subgroup analysis of metal implants was performed, that yielded an odds ratio of 0.8 (95% confidence interval (CI), 0.3–1.5).

A case–control study in Australia (Ryan et al., 1992) studied the relationship between dental amalgam containing mercury (see IARC, 1993a), diagnostic dental X-rays (IARC, 2000) and subsequent development of brain tumours. The study included 170 cases of brain tumours (110 gliomas, 60 meningiomas) and 417 general population controls. There was a decreased odds ratio of 0.5 (95% CI, 0.3–0.9) for glioma and an odds ratio of 1.0 (95% CI, 0.4–2.5) for meningioma associated with amalgam fillings for at least one year.

Table 19. Malignant tumours at the site of static non-articulating orthopaedic metallic implants

Reference	Implant	Metal	Age at implantation/sex	Preoperative diagnosis	Site	Histopathology	Years between implantation and diagnosis	Remarks
McDougall (1956)	Plate and screws	Plate: stainless steel, 74% Fe 18% Cr, 8% Ni screws: 88% Fe, 12% Cr	12/M	Fracture	Humerus, diaphysis	Ewing's sarcoma	30	Extensive corrosion of plate and screws (difference in potential between plate and screws of 80 mV)
Bürkle de la Camp (1958)	Medullary nail	NR	22/M	Complicated fracture	Femur, great trochanter	Alveolar sarcoma	3	
Delgado (1958)	[Egger's plate (Hughes et al., 1987) and screws]	NR	37/M	Fracture	Tibia, diaphysis	Unclassified sarcoma [probably osteosarcoma (McDonald, 1981)]	3	
Dube & Fisher (1972)	Sherman (stainless steel) plate and screws	(Plate and 8 screws: stainless steel 316: 18% Cr, 10% Ni, 3% Mo 2 screws: stainless steel 304: 20% Cr, 9% Ni	58/M	Non-union of a fracture (bilateral fracture)	Tibia, diaphysis of both legs	Haemangio-endothelioma	26	Fixed with bone graft, 2 loose screws, corrosion of 2 plate screw holes (the other tibia was also fixed with bone graft, and two screws)
Monkman et al. (1974)	Nail plate	NR	57/M	Fracture	Proximal femur	Chondrosarcoma (grade 3)	2	

Table 19 (contd)

Reference	Implant	Metal	Age at implantation/sex	Preoperative diagnosis	Site	Histopathology	Years between implantation and diagnosis	Remarks
Tayton (1980)	Sherman plate and six screws	CoCr (Vitallium)[a]	4/F	Congenital hip dislocation	Proximal femoral diaphysis	Ewing's sarcoma	7.5	Bilateral osteotomies and plate fixation. Removal of plates and screws one year later
McDonald (1981)	Plate and screws	CoCr (Vitallium)[a]	31/M	Fracture	Tibia, diaphysis	Histiocytic type lymphoma	17	Tumour infiltrating the bone
Dodion et al. (1983)	1 Strycker screw + 1 Knowles screw, 1 McLaughlin plate and 5 Phillips screws	CoCr (Vitallium)[a]	49/M	Fracture of the femoral neck	Femur (neck)	Immunoblastic lymphoma	1.2	Deep infection
Lee et al. (1984)	Plate and screws	NR	30/M	Open femur fracture	Femur, diaphysis	Malignant fibrous histiocytoma	14	Removal of plate and screws and bone grafting for suspected osteomyelitis 4 months before diagnosis
Hughes et al. (1987)	One Sherman screw	CoCr[b]	14/M	Slipped proximal femoral epiphysis	Femur, neck	Malignant fibrous histiocytoma	29	Single screw
Ward et al. (1990)	Smith-Petersen nail	Stainless steel (Ni, Co, Cr, Mo, Fe)	56/F	Fracture of the femoral neck	Femur, neck	Osteosarcoma	9	

Table 19 (contd)

Reference	Implant	Metal	Age at implantation/sex	Preoperative diagnosis	Site	Histopathology	Years between implantation and diagnosis	Remarks
Khurana et al. (1991)	Hansen Street intramedullary nail	Stainless steel (17–19% Cr, 12–14% Ni, 2–3% Mo, 2% Mn; Fe)	25/M	Gunshot fracture	Proximal femoral diaphysis	Malignant fibrous histiocytoma	14	
Scully et al. (1991)	Staples	Stainless steel 316 (18% Cr, 10% Ni)	8/M	Morquio's syndrome, genu valgum	Distal femoral diaphysis	Osteosarcoma	10	Bilateral femoral osteotomies
Kumar (1996)	Two staples	NR	7/M	Post-poliomyelitic deformity	Distal femoral diaphysis (knee)	Osteosarcoma	9	

[a] Vitallium, 58.4% min. Co; 27–30% Cr; 5–7% Mo; 2.5% max. Ni; 1% max. Mn; 0.75% max. Fe
[b] CoCr = cobalt–chromium alloy, composition not stated
NR, not reported

Table 20. Malignant tumours at the site of joint endoprosthesis (metal only)

Reference	Prosthesis	Metal	Age at implantation/sex	Preoperative diagnosis/site	Histopathology	Years between implantation and diagnosis	Remarks
Castleman & McNeely (1965)	Moore prosthesis	NR	49/M	Old fracture of the femoral neck (hip)	Giant cell sarcoma (malignant)	3.5	Nail and plate for 8 months before the prosthesis ('fatty' tumour excised from the knee 14 years before implantation)
Penman & Ring (1984)	Ring	Stem-head alloy: CoCr Cup: CoCr Fixation: Uncemented	75/F	Osteoarthritis THA	Osteosarcoma	5	

THA, total hip arthroplasty
NR, not reported

2B. Non-metallic Medical and Dental Materials

2B.1 Case reports

2B.1.1 *Cancer following silicone implants for the breast*

Published case reports describing malignant tumours at the site of plastic implants (silicone) are summarized in Tables 21–24.

Table 21 lists 15 cases of breast cancer reported following cosmetic augmentation with silicone injections. Injection of liquid silicone into breasts for cosmetic purposes was an illicit practice performed until about 1970 (Morgenstern *et al.*, 1985). It was frequently followed by short- and long-term complications, including inflammation, sinusitis, contractures and deformities. Table 22 summarizes nine cases of breast cancer reported following cosmetic breast augmentation using silicone prostheses. Considering the large number of women with silicone implants (mainly in the United States), the number of case reports seems to be rather low. The reported cases are in general of younger age than the age distribution of breast cancer diagnosis observed in Western populations. This may reflect the younger age of most patients at the time of breast implantation and the relatively short time period during which this procedure has been in widespread use.

Six cases of breast cancer and four cases of Paget's disease of the nipple were reported after reconstructive operation generally following mastectomy. Few data are available on other risk factors in these cases (Table 23).

Table 24 summarizes six cases of lymphoma after implantation of silicone in the breast or fingers. Eighteen female cases of multiple myeloma were reported from a nationwide multiple myeloma registry in the United States (Rabkin *et al.*, 1996). One additional male case of multiple myeloma after penile implant was reported by Tricot *et al.* (1996). In addition, one case of desmoid tumour was reported by Schuh & Radford (1994).

2B.1.2 *Sarcomas at the site of vascular grafts*

Eight cases of sarcomas involving a graft have been reported (Table 25). Most patients were operated on for aortic aneurysms. Histopathological examination showed three cases of malignant fibrous histiocytoma, two angiosarcomas and three fibrosarcomas.

2B.2 Analytical studies

2B.2.1 *Cohort studies*

Six cohort studies of cancer among women undergoing cosmetic implants of silicone prosthesis have been reported and are summarized in Table 26.

A record-linkage cohort study in California, United States, included 3182 Caucasian women, resident in Los Angeles County, who had been treated for cosmetic breast enlargement between 1953 and 1980 (Deapen *et al.*, 1986, 1997). Patients' records were

Table 21. Breast cancer after cosmetic augmentation with silicone injection in women

Reference	Age at injection	Histopathology	Interval between silicone injection and cancer diagnosis (years)	Remarks
Lewis (1980)	26	Inflammatory carcinoma	7	
Morgenstern et al. (1985)	48	Infiltrating ductal [adeno]carcinoma	20	Family history of breast cancer
Morgenstern et al. (1985)	45	Infiltrating ductal [adeno]carcinoma	14	
Morgenstern et al. (1985)	30	Infiltrating ductal [adeno]carcinoma	19	
Morgenstern et al. (1985)	19	Infiltrating ductal [adeno]carcinoma	15	
Morgenstern et al. (1985)	24	Infiltrating ductal [adeno]carcinoma	16	
Morgenstern et al. (1985)	21	Metaplastic squamous and pseudosarcomatous carcinoma	16	Family history of breast cancer
Morgenstern et al. (1985)	46	Infiltrating ductal [adeno]carcinoma	13	
Morgenstern et al. (1985)	30	Infiltrating ductal [adeno]carcinoma	17	
Morgenstern et al. (1985)	32	Poorly differentiated adenocarcinoma	6	
Timberlake & Looney (1986)	30	Poorly differentiated adenocarcinoma	12	
Maddox et al. (1993)	30	Poorly differentiated invasive ductal [adeno]carcinoma	5	
Ko et al. (1995)	27	Adenocarcinoma	25	Oestrogen and progesterone replacement therapy for previous 8 yrs
Ko et al. (1995)	39	Intraductal carcinoma	22	
Talmor et al. (1995)	45	Squamous cell carcinoma	25	

Table 22. Breast cancer after cosmetic augmentation with silicone prostheses in women

Reference	Prosthesis composition	Age at implantation	Histopathology	Interval between silicone implant and cancer diagnosis (years)	Remarks
Gottlieb et al. (1984)	Gel-filled	29	Invasive lobular carcinoma	3	
Gottlieb et al. (1984)	Gel-filled	39	Invasive ductal carcinoma	4	
Morgenstern et al. (1985)	Silicone	35	Infiltrating ductal [adeno]carcinoma	7	Family history of breast cancer
Morgenstern et al. (1985)	Silicone	36	Infiltrating ductal [adeno]carcinoma	12	
Morgenstern et al. (1985)	Silicone	39	Infiltrating ductal adenocarcinoma	5	
Bingham et al. (1988)	Silicone gel-filled	32	Ductal [adeno]carcinoma	13	Mother had Paget's disease
Silverstein et al. (1990)	Silicone gel-filled	54	Ductal [adeno]carcinoma	12	
Paletta et al. (1992)	240 mL style 2100 Heyer Schulte silicone gel	37	Squamous cell carcinoma originating from the posterior implant capsule	15	
Kitchen et al. (1994)	240 mL style 2100 Heyer Schulte silicone gel	37	Squamous cell carcinoma	15	

abstracted from 35 private practices (out of a total of about 100 in the county at that time). Subjects receiving reconstructive implants after mastectomy, either for prophylactic purposes or for cancer treatment, were excluded. Subjects moving out of the county were excluded from the time of the last contact as residents. The mean age of subjects at implantation was 37.4 years. Eighty-six per cent of the prostheses used were silicone gel or silicone/saline and the remainder (14%) were 'other' or 'unknown' types. Sixty patients received polyurethane-coated silicone implants and nine more from the 'unknown' group were believed to have received polyurethane devices also. Cohort members were followed up through record linkage with the local population-based tumour registry—the Los Angeles County Cancer Surveillance Program—from the time of surgical implantation (or 1 January 1972, whichever was later) until 31 December 1991. A total of 37 439 person–years were accumulated, with a median duration of follow-up of 14.4 years. Great effort was made to identify subjects moving

Table 23. Breast cancer and Paget's disease of the nipple after silicone implantation for medical indication in women

Reference	Prosthesis composition	Age at implantation	Preoperative diagnosis	Histopathology	Interval between silicone implant and cancer diagnosis (years)	Remarks
Hoopes et al. (1967)	Silastic prosthesis, (RT V 53G2, Dow Corning) then 3 yrs later Silicone liquid no. 360 injection 0.5 years before diagnosis	37	NR	Infiltrating lobular carcinoma	3	
Bowers & Radlauer (1969)	Silastic prosthesis	46	Fibrocystic disease, subcutaneous mastectomy	Ductal [adeno]-carcinoma	3	Prosthesis under pectoralis major muscle
Bowers & Radlauer (1969)	Silastic prosthesis	44	Fibrocystic disease, subcutaneous mastectomy	Scirrhous adeno-carcinoma	1.5	
Dalinka et al. (1969)	Silastic prosthesis	38	Fibrocystic disease, mastectomy	Carcinoma (not specified)	3	
Frantz & Herbst (1975)	Cronin silastic prosthesis	30	Postirradiation atrophy of the breast	Poorly differentiated adenocarcinoma	2.5	Irradiation of the breast at the age of 3–15 months for haemangioma

Table 23 (contd)

Reference	Prosthesis composition	Age at implantation	Preoperative diagnosis	Histopathology	Interval between silicone implant and cancer diagnosis (years)	Remarks
Mendez-Fernandez et al. (1980)	Silicone gel prosthesis	45	Fibrocystic disease of the breast, subcutaneous mastectomy	Paget's disease plus infiltrating duct cell adenocarcinoma	8	
Pennisi (1984)	Silicone injections	20	Pectus excavatum	Ductal adeno-carcinoma	23	Family history of breast cancer
Shearman & Watts (1986)	Silicone prosthesis	4	Subcutaneous mastectomy for spheroidal cell cancer	Paget's disease	1.5	
Shearman & Watts (1986)	Silicone prosthesis	50	Subcutaneous mastectomy for intraductal carcinoma	Paget's disease	1.5	
Shearman & Watts (1986)	Silicone prosthesis	46	Subcutaneous mastectomy for adenocarcnoma	Paget's disease	4	

NR, not reported

Table 24. Lymphomas and myelomas following implantation of silicone prosthesis

Reference	Prosthesis composition	Age at implantation/sex	Indication for implantations	Histopathology	Interval between silicone implant and cancer diagnosis (years)	Remarks
Digby (1982)	Silastic Swanson finger prostheses	47/F	Rheumatoid arthritis	Undifferentiated large cell lymphoma	9	Implant fracture. Other hand was also prosthetized.
Murakata & Rangwala (1989)	Silastic finger joints	59/F	Rheumatoid arthritis	Immunoblastic lymphoma	9	
Cook et al. (1995)	Replicon polyurethane-covered silicone implant	50/F	Sequel after mastectomy for ductal carcinoma	Follicular mixed lymphoma	6	
Duvic et al. (1995)	Même polyurethane-coated silicone	35/F	Augmentation mammoplasty	Cutaneous T-cell lymphoma	3	
Duvic et al. (1995)	Polyurethane-coated Dow-Corning silicone implants	24/F	Eczematous eruption	Cutaneous T-cell lymphoma	11	
Duvic et al. (1995)	Dow-Corning silicone implants	33/F	Augmentation mammoplasty	Cutaneous T-cell lymphoma	20	
Rabkin et al. (1996)	Breast silicone implant	38–75/F (at diagnosis)		18 cases of multiple myeloma	2–25	Probably reported also by Silverman et al. (1996) and by Tricot et al. (1996).
Tricot et al. (1996)	Penile silicone implant	67/M	Unknown	Multiple myeloma	1 month	Reports also nine female cases that are probably included in Rabkin et al. (1996).

Table 25. Malignant tumours at the site of vascular grafts in men[a]

Reference	Prosthesis	Site	Age at implantation	Preoperative diagnosis	Histopathology	Interval between operation and diagnosis (years)
Burns et al. (1972)	Teflon-Dacron	Thigh	21	Traumatic rupture of the superficial femoral artery after an accident	Fibrosarcoma (or angiosarcoma)	10.5
O'Connell et al. (1976)	Woven Dacron 19 mm	Abdominal aorta	59	Aortic aneurysm	Fibrosarcoma	0.3
Weinberg & Maini (1980)	Woven Dacron 26 mm	Thoracic, abdominal aorta	47	Thoracic-abdominal aortic aneurysm	Malignant fibrous histiocytoma	1.2
Fehrenbacher et al. (1981)	Woven Dacron	Abdominal aorta	55	Aortic aneurysm	Angiosarcoma	12
Paterson et al. (1989)	Double-velour Dacron 20 mm	Descending thoracic aorta	57	Aortic aneurysm	Malignant fibrous histiocytoma	0.5
Weiss et al. (1991)	Woven double-velour Dacron	Infrarenal aorta	52	Aortic aneurysm	Angiosarcoma	4
Raso et al. (1993)	Dacron 8 mm	Superficial femoral artery	76	Aneurysm	Fibrosarcoma	0.2
Fyfe et al. (1994)	Dacron	Descending thoracic aorta	66	Acute aortic dissection	Malignant fibrous histiocytoma	4

[a] The insertion of vascular grafts requires the application of sutures, an additional implanted material

Table 26. Cohort studies of cancer following implantation of silicone breast prostheses

Reference (use)	Country	Exposed cohort size	Reference population	Design	Follow-up	Cancer site	No. of cases among exposed	SIR (95% CI)
Deapen et al. (1997) (cosmetic)	United States	3182	Population tumour registry (Los Angeles County)	Record linkage, tumour registry	37 439 person–years; implant 1953–80; follow-up through 1991	Breast	31	0.6 (0.4–0.9)
Bryant & Brasher (1995) (cosmetic)	Canada	10 835	Population tumour registry (Alberta Province)	Record linkage, tumour registry	89 219 person–years; implant 1973–86; follow-up through 1990	Breast	45	0.8 (0.6–1.1)[a] 0.9 (0.6–1.2)[b] 0.7 (0.3–1.3)[c]
Friis et al. (1997) (cosmetic)	Denmark	1135	National tumour registry	Record linkage, tumour registry	[9525] person–years; implant 1977–92; follow-up through 1993	All cancers Lung Breast Ovary Melanoma Skin, other Non-Hodgkin lymphoma Sarcomas Other	27 2 8 3 1 5 1 1 6	1.1 (0.7–1.6) 1.5 (0.2–5.3) 1.0 (0.4–2.0) 2.5 (0.5–7.3) 0.7 (0.0–3.7) 1.6 (0.5–3.7) 2.2 (0.0–12.0) 2.7 (0.0–14.9) 0.7 (0.3–1.5)

Table 26 (contd)

Reference (use)	Country	Exposed cohort size	Reference population	Design	Follow-up	Cancer site	No. of cases among exposed	SIR (95% CI)
Gabriel et al. (1994) (mixed)	United States	534 cosmetic 125 reconstructive 90 prophylactic	1498 community controls	Medical record review	5847 person–years; implant 1964–91; follow-up through 1991	Cancers other than breast	13	1.1 (0.6–2.1)
						Cosmetic	8	1.0 (0.4–2.1)
						Reconstructive	2	1.3 (0.3–4.4)
						Prophylactic	3	1.5 (0.4–4.3)
McLaughlin et al. (1998) (cosmetic)	Sweden	3473	National tumour registry	Record linkage, tumour registry	35 644 person–years; implant 1965–93; follow-up through 1993	All cancers	74	1.1 (0.8–1.3)
						Large bowel	3	0.7 (0.1–2.0)
						Lung	7	2.7 (1.1–5.6)
						Skin	5	0.9 (0.3–2.0)
						Breast	18	0.7 (0.4–1.1)
						Cervix	10	1.9 (0.9–3.5)
						Ovary	6	1.3 (0.5–2.8)
						Brain	4	1.1 (0.3–2.9)
						Non-Hodgkin lymphoma	1	0.6 (0.0–3.5)
						Myeloma	1	2.6 (0.1–15)
						Leukaemia	3	2.7 (0.6–7.8)
Kern et al. (1997) (cosmetic)	United States	680	Control cohort ($n = 1022$)	Record linkage, tumour registry	[Cases: 3128 Controls: 5519] person–years; implant 1980–93; follow-up through 1993	Breast	4	0.7 (0.2–2.2)[d]
						Other cancers	4	0.2 (0.1–0.6)

Table 26 (contd)

Reference (use)	Country	Exposed cohort size	Reference population	Design	Follow-up	Cancer site	No. of cases among exposed	SIR (95% CI)
Petit et al. (1994) (breast cancer)	France	146 women with breast cancer and silicone implant	146 women with breast cancer without silicone implant	Mortality, second primaries	Implantation 1965–83; average follow-up: 12.5 years	Second primary breast cancer	12	1.1 (0.5–2.7)
						Death from breast cancer	15	0.5 (0.3–1.0)
						Distant metastases	19	0.5 (0.3–0.8)
						Local recurrence	13	0.5 (0.3–1.1)
						Second primary cancers, other sites	5	0.8 (0.2–2.5)

SIR, standardized incidence ratio; CI, confidence interval
[a] Calculated taking into account an induction period of one year
[b] Calculated taking into account an induction period of five years
[c] Calculated taking into account an induction period of 10 years
[d] Analysis led to underestimation of the relative risk

out of the county during the study period, through extensive record linkages with the motor vehicle, voter registration, telephone, property tax and marriage files. Thirty-one patients were diagnosed with breast cancer (three *in situ* and 28 invasive) during the study period versus 49.2 expected. The standardized incidence ratio (SIR) was 0.6 (95% CI, 0.4–0.9) (Deapen *et al.*, 1997). The authors also reported on malignancies other than breast cancer (Deapen & Brody, 1995). In total, 45 cancers other than breast cancer were observed, compared with 50 expected (SIR, 0.9; 95% CI, 0.7–1.2). Among other sites, increased risk was observed for lung cancer (SIR, 2.1; 95% CI, 1.1–3.7; $n = 12$) and cancer of the vulva (SIR, 5.3; 95% CI, 1.7–12.3; $n = 5$). Furthermore, five cases of endometrial cancer (SIR, 0.7; 95% CI, 0.2–1.7) and four cases of invasive cervical cancer (SIR, 1.4; 95% CI, 0.4–3.5) were reported. [The Working Group noted that no information on potential confounding variables was available and that information on socioeconomic status was limited to a crude score based on census-tract of residence. The Working Group also noted that no allowance was made for length of induction period.]

A record-linkage cohort study in Canada identified women with breast implants from the records of the insurance payment claims of Alberta Health Care (Berkel *et al.*, 1992; Bryant *et al.*, 1994; Bryant & Brasher, 1995). After excluding women treated for reconstructive breast surgery, a cohort of 11 676 women was identified who received cosmetic breast implants within the province from 1973 through 1986. Approximately 85% of the subjects were treated with silicone gel prostheses and the remainder with saline-filled prostheses. No polyurethane-covered implants were in use in Alberta during the study period. Bryant & Brasher (1995) identified 45 breast cancer cases diagnosed between 1973 and 1990 in the cohort (five *in situ*) out of a total of 10 835 women contributing 89 219 person–years at risk. The SIRs were estimated as 0.8 (95% CI, 0.6–1.0) for all breast cancers and 0.7 (95% CI, 0.5–1.0) for invasive breast cancers only. When time between first implant and cancer diagnosis (induction period) was considered, the SIRs for induction periods of one year, five years and 10 years were 0.8 (95% CI, 0.6–1.1), 0.9 (95% CI, 0.6–1.2) and 0.7 (95% CI, 0.3–1.3), respectively. These estimates did not change appreciably in analyses restricted to invasive cancers only. [The Working Group noted the absence of information on potential confounding factors.]

A record-linkage cohort study in Denmark identified 1135 women who underwent cosmetic breast implant surgery between 1977 and 1992, through the nationwide Hospital Discharge Register (McLaughlin *et al.*, 1994, 1995a; Friis *et al.*, 1997). The mean age at implantation was 31 years (range, 13–64) and the average follow-up was 8.4 years (maximum, 17 years). A total of 27 cases of cancer were identified among cohort members through record linkage with the Danish population-based tumour registry. Breast cancer was the most common cancer (eight cases observed versus 7.8 expected), with an SIR of 1.0 (95% CI, 0.4–2.0). No departure from expected values was observed for any other cancer site. Four breast cancer cases developed 10 or more years after implant surgery (SIR, 1.7; 95% CI, 0.4–4.2). The authors reported that the reproductive histories of women with implants were similar to those of the general Danish population.

A historical cohort study in the United States identified all 749 women residents in Olmstead County, Minnesota, whose medical records indicated breast augmentation performed for cosmetic reasons (534 patients) or following mastectomy, either for breast cancer (125 patients) or for prophylactic purposes among high-risk subjects (90 patients) between 1964 and 1991 (Gabriel et al., 1994). Exposed subjects were followed up through 1991, corresponding to 5847 person–years (mean, 7.8 years per case). Of the 1840 devices implanted in these patients, 78.3% were silicone gel, 5.2% were saline, 6.7% were combination silicone gel/saline and 9.6% were polyurethane-coated. Community controls were 1498 women who had undergone a medical evaluation within two years of the date of implantation of one of the exposed subjects (two controls per exposed subject). Eight cases of cancer (other than breast) were identified among the 534 cosmetic implant patients, corresponding to a rate ratio of 1.0 (95% CI, 0.4–2.1). Among the 125 patients with post-cancer reconstructive implants, two cases of cancer at sites other than breast were identified, corresponding to a rate ratio of 1.3 (95% CI, 0.3–4.4). Among the 90 prophylactic implant patients, there were three cases of non-breast cancer, corresponding to a rate ratio of 1.5 (95% CI, 0.4–4.3).

A nationwide systematic record-linkage cohort study in Sweden included all 3473 women listed in a national hospitalization register with surgical procedures for cosmetic breast augmentation during the period 1965 through 1993 (McLaughlin et al., 1995a,b, 1998). Patients with a cancer diagnosis before or up to one month after the date of implant and those who died or emigrated before the start of follow-up were excluded. Median age at implant was 30 years. Median duration of follow-up was nine years (maximum, 29 years). After accumulating 35 644 person–years at risk, 74 cases of cancer at any localization were identified versus 70.3 expected, giving an SIR of 1.1 (95% CI, 0.8–1.3). The SIR for breast cancer, the most common cancer in this population, was 0.7 (95% CI, 0.4–1.1). The second most common occurrence was cervical cancer, with an SIR of 1.9 (95% CI, 0.9–3.5). The only appreciable departure from expectation was observed in relation to lung cancer (seven cases), with an SIR of 2.7 (95% CI, 1.1–5.6). There was no significant excess for any other cancer site, including non-Hodgkin lymphomas (one case), multiple myeloma (one case) and leukaemia (three cases versus 1.1 expected). The authors reported no difference in stage of breast cancer at diagnosis, compared with the general population. [The Working Group noted the absence of information on any potential confounding factors, including tobacco smoking, and the absence of analysis by latency.]

A cohort study in the United States used the statewide hospital discharge data of the State of Connecticut to identify 680 women who received cosmetic breast augmentation silicone prostheses between October 1980 and September 1993 (Kern et al., 1997). The mean age at implantation was 34 years. The exposed patients thus identified were compared with a reference cohort of 1022 women with a hospital discharge of sterilization by endoscopic tubal ligation during the period October 1981 through September 1985. Incident cases of all cancers among subjects in the exposed and control cohorts were identified by record linkage with the statewide Connecticut Tumor Registry. The mean follow-up times for the exposed and control cohorts were 4.6 and 5.4 years, respectively. Four cases of breast cancer and four cases of other malignancies (one skin, one colon and two lung cancers) were observed among the exposed patients, whereas nine cases of breast cancer and 28 cases of all other malignancies were observed among the unexposed group. The corresponding rate ratios were 0.7 (95% CI, 0.2–2.2) for breast cancer and 0.2 (95% CI, 0.1–0.6) for all other cancers combined. [The Working Group noted the absence of information on any potential confounders and that the statistical analysis that was performed led to underestimation of the relative risk.]

A study in France included 146 patients treated at the Gustave Roussy Cancer Institute between 1965 and 1983 for breast cancer with mastectomy followed by breast reconstruction with silicone gel prostheses (Petit et al., 1994). These patients were compared with 146 controls with breast cancer treated at the same hospital with mastectomy without breast reconstruction. Exposed cases and cancer controls were individually matched by age and year at diagnosis, stage, histological type of cancer, grade and nodal status. The average follow-up time to identify second primaries was 12.5 years. The relative risk (RR) for second primary breast cancer was 1.1 (95% CI, 0.5–2.7), whereas the risk of second primary cancer at all other sites was 0.8 (95% CI, 0.2–2.5). There were reduced risks for death from breast cancer (RR, 0.5; 95% CI, 0.3–1.0), distant metastases (RR, 0.5; 95% CI, 0.3–0.8) and local recurrence (RR, 0.5; 95% CI, 0.3–1.1) among the women with silicone implants.

2B.2.2 *Case–control studies* (Table 27)

A case–control study reported as a research letter was performed in the State of Washington, United States (Malone et al., 1992). Two groups of subjects were part of the study, one comprising 684 breast cancer cases and 816 population controls aged 21–44 years and the second 406 breast cancer cases and 339 population controls aged 50–64 years. Controls were residents of the same area as the cases and were identified through random-digit dialling. Exposure was assessed by telephone interview. In the younger group, six cases and nine controls reported a history of cosmetic breast augmentation implants, corresponding to a relative risk of 0.8 (95% CI, 0.3–2.2). In the older group, one case and six controls reported breast augmentation implants, giving a relative risk of 0.2 (95% CI, 0.1–1.3). [The Working Group noted that very limited information on study design and methods was available.]

A population-based case–control study on the role of silicone implants in breast cancer included two metropolitan areas in the United States (Atlanta, Georgia, and Seattle/Puget Sound, Washington) and five counties in central New Jersey (Brinton et al., 1996). In Seattle and New Jersey, cases were restricted to women under 45 years of age at diagnosis, while in Georgia the upper age limit was 54 years. All eligible

Table 27. Case–control studies of breast cancer incidence following cosmetic surgical implantation of breast prostheses

Reference	Country	Exposure	Outcome	No. of cases	No. of controls	No. (%) of cases receiving breast prosthesis	No. (%) of controls receiving breast prosthesis	Adjustment	Odds ratio (95% CI)
Malone et al. (1992)	United States	Silicone	Breast cancer	1090	1155	7 (0.6%)	15 (1.2%)		0.8 (0.3–2.2) (age 20–44) 0.2 (0.1–1.3) (age 50–64)
Brinton et al. (1996)	United States	Silicone	Breast cancer	2174	2009	36 (1.7%)	44 (2.2%)	Study site, age, race, body size, familial risk, previous mammography	0.6 (0.4–1.0) 0.5 (0.3–1.0) (age ≥ 35 at implant) 0.5 (0.2–0.9) (≥ 10 years after implant)

CI, confidence interval

breast cancer cases diagnosed within the study area during the period from May 1990 to December 1992 were identified through a rapid ascertainment system by agreement with the local population-based tumour registries. Controls were selected through random-digit dialling (90.5% response rate) and matched to the cases on area of residence and age. Personal interviews collected a broad range of data on potential risk factors for breast cancer and detailed information on history of breast surgery, including aspirations, biopsies, lumpectomies and enlargement or reduction operations. Complete interviews were obtained from 2174 cases (85.2% of eligible) and 2009 controls (78.1% of eligible). A total of 36 cases (1.7%) and 44 controls (2.2%) reported a history of cosmetic breast augmentation, giving a relative risk of 0.6 (95% CI, 0.4–1.0), after adjustment for race, body size, family history of breast cancer and history of mammography, in addition to matching factors. The decrease in risk was seen for subjects who underwent surgery at age 35 years or older (relative risk, 0.5; 95% CI, 0.3–1.0) and in those 10 or more years after implantation (relative risk, 0.5; 95% CI, 0.2–0.9).

2C. Composite Medical and Dental Implants

2C.1 Case reports

2C.1.1 *Orthopaedic implants*

Compilations of the published case reports describing malignant tumours at the site of implants are presented in Tables 28 (three cases, joint prosthesis, metal with bone cement) and 29 (32 cases, joint prosthesis, metal and polyethylene with bone cement). Reports of metastatic tumours found at the site of a joint implant are presented in Table 30 (seven cases).

The time lapse for these cases varied from a few months to 15 years, with the majority being less than 10 years. Metastases from other sites to the proximity of a prosthesis have been discovered within lapse times of from two months to two years (seven cases, see Table 30). Almost all case reports relating to tumours at the site of static implants have involved the femur. The implanted materials (where reported) were stainless steel, cobalt–chromium alloys (rarely with alumina) or titanium, in combination with polyethylene and cements (generally poly(methyl methacrylate) (IARC, 1979b)).

The number of cases appears to be small in comparison with the estimated number of implanted devices worldwide (see Section 1C.2). Reporting of individual cases is not systematic, so that the actual number of occurrences is likely to be greater.

2C.1.2 *Cardiac pacemakers*

Thirteen cases of breast cancer and one case of plasmacytoma in the vicinity of cardiac pacemakers have been reported (Table 31). The median age at implantation was 64 (43–83) years and the median latent period four (1–18) years. A case of metastasis

Table 28. Malignant tumours at the site of joint endoprosthesis (metallic with bone cement)

Reference	Prosthesis	Composition 1) Stem-head alloy 2) Cup	Age at implantation/ sex	Preoperative diagnosis	Histopathology	Years between implantation and diagnosis	Remarks
Rushforth (1974)	McKee-Farrar THR	1) CoCr 2) CoCr (Visuri et al., 1996)	62/F	Radiation necrosis of the femoral head	Osteosarcoma of pelvis	0.5	3 insertions of radium (2500 rad) for carcinoma of cervix + external irradiation (mid-point dose of 2000 rad). Cancer possibly due to irradiation. Loose acetabular part
Arden & Bywaters (1978)	McKee-Farrar THR	1) CoCr 2) CoCr (Visuri et al., 1996)	56/M	Osteoarthritis	Fibrosarcoma, femur	2.5	
Swann (1984)	McKee-Farrar THR	1) CoCr 2) CoCr (Vitallium) cemented	63/M	Osteoarthritis	Malignant fibrous histiocytoma, femur	4	

THR, total hip replacement

Table 29. Malignant tumours at the site of joint endoprosthesis (metal/polyethylene with or without bone cement)

Reference	Prosthesis	Composition 1) Stem-head alloy 2) Cup 3) Fixation 4) Additional implants	Age at implantation/sex	Preoperative diagnosis	Histopathology	Years between implantation and diagnosis	Remarks
Wines (1973)	Charnley THA	1–2) Not stated 3) PMMA cement	NR	Osteoarthritis	Bladder cancer, transitional cell carcinoma, WHO grade III, adjacent to extrapelvic	0.25	PMMA may have been released into the pelvis [the tumour may have preceded implantation]
Bagó-Granell et al. (1984)	Charnley-Müller THA	1–2) Not stated 3) PMMA cement 4) Trochanteric wires	75/F	Osteoarthritis	Malignant fibrous histiocytoma	2	Other hip, Charnley-Müller THA 2 years before
Weber (1986)	Variable axis TKA	1) CoCrMo (Vitallium) 2) Polyethylene 3) PMMA cement	76/F	Osteoarthritis	Epithelioid sarcoma (or malignant fibrous histiocytoma)	4.5	Distal femoral intramedullary enchondroma or bone infarct before operation
Ryu et al. (1987)	2 screws Hip	Uncemented THA (aluminium oxide acetabulum + femoral head with CoCrMo alloy)	52/M	Osteoarthritis secondary to fracture-dislocation	Soft-tissue fibrosarcoma	1.2	Ceramic prosthesis 12 years after implant of two screws
Vives et al. (1987)	Charnley-Müller THA	1) CoCr 2) Polyethylene 3) PMMA cement	67/M	Coxarthrosis	Malignant fibrous histiocytoma	2	

Table 29 (contd)

Reference	Prosthesis	Composition 1) Stem-head alloy 2) Cup 3) Fixation 4) Additional implants	Age at implantation/sex	Preoperative diagnosis	Histopathology	Years between implantation and diagnosis	Remarks
Lamovec et al. (1988)	Charnley-Müller THA	1) Stainless steel 2) Polyethylene 3) PMMA cement	50/M	Osteoarthritis secondary to congenital hip dislocation	Synovial sarcoma at THA site	12	
Lamovec et al. (1988)	Charnley-Müller THA	1–2) NR 3) Cemented	55/F	NR	Osteosarcoma	10	
Martin et al. (1988)	Charnley-Müller THA	1) CoCr 2) Polyethylene 3) PMMA cement	66/F	Osteoarthritis secondary to congenital dislocation of the hips	Telangiectatic osteosarcoma	10.5	Other hip, THA 1 month later, type not known
Tait et al. (1988)	Charnley-Müller THA	1) NR 2) [Polyethylene] 3) Cemented 4) Trochanter wires	45/F	Osteoarthritis	Malignant fibrous histiocytoma, gluteal region	11	
van der List et al. (1988)	1) Charnley-Müller 2) Revision, with bone autograft, Müller prosthesis 11 years later THA	1) CoCrMo 2) Polyethylene 3) PMMA cement	61/F	Osteoarthritis secondary to congenital hip dysplasia	Malignant epithelioid haemangioendothelioma, femur/acetabulum	12	Other hip, Charnley-Müller THA in the same year and revised with Müller THA 3 years later

Table 29 (contd)

Reference	Prosthesis	Composition 1) Stem-head alloy 2) Cup 3) Fixation 4) Additional implants	Age at implantation/ sex	Preoperative diagnosis	Histopathology	Years between implantation and diagnosis	Remarks
Haag & Adler (1989)	Weber-Hüggler THA	1) CoCrNi (Protasul 10) 2) Polyethylene 3) PMMA cement	59/F	Osteoarthritis	Malignant fibrous histiocytoma	10	Other hip, Weber-Hüggler THA, 1 year before
Mazabraud et al. (1989)	McKee-Farrar THA	1) CrNiCo 2) Polyethylene 3) PMMA cement	60/M	Osteoarthritis	Epidermoid carcinoma	4.5	Previous femoral osteotomy (type of implant not reported); 1.5 years earlier, chronic sinus present at second surgery
Brien et al. (1990)	Charnley THA	1) Stainless steel 2) Polyethylene 3) Cemented	50/F	Osteoarthritis secondary to hip dysplasia	Osteosarcoma	8	Both hips had same treatment
Harris (1990)	Charnley THA	1–3) NR	65/F	Osteoarthritis secondary to Maffucci's syndrome	Chondrosarcoma	3	Enchondromata of the upper femur. Other hip THA 11 years earlier

Table 29 (contd)

Reference	Prosthesis	Composition 1) Stem-head alloy 2) Cup 3) Fixation 4) Additional implants	Age at implantation/sex	Preoperative diagnosis	Histopathology	Years between implantation and diagnosis	Remarks
Troop et al. (1990)	1) Charnley-Müller, 2) Aufranc-Turner 3 years later, 3) Aufranc-Turner (long stem) 2 years later, 4) Sivash-Russin-Cr-Co cemented (long stem) Noiles (SRN) 3 years later, 5) Cemented titanium SRN, femoral allograft, cemented Arthropore acetabular, constraining ring 3 years later THA	1) Titanium 2) [Polyethylene] 3) Cemented	24/M	Traumatic osteoarthritis	Malignant fibrous histiocytoma	15	Deep infection, removal of wires and prosthesis in second phase – loosening

Table 29 (contd)

Reference	Prosthesis	Composition 1) Stem-head alloy 2) Cup 3) Fixation 4) Additional implants	Age at implantation/sex	Preoperative diagnosis	Histopathology	Years between implantation and diagnosis	Remarks
Nelson & Phillips (1990)	Müller THA	1) CoCr 2) Polyethylene 3) Cemented	62/F	Post-traumatic osteoarthritis	Malignant fibrous histiocytoma	10	Revision with porous-coated femoral and bipolar acetabular component with allograft 3 months before diagnosis
Himmer et al. (1991)	Guepa TKA	1–2) Metal 3) Cemented	61/F	Osteoarthritis	Angiosarcoma	13	Distal femoral fracture, cerclage fixation 6 years before angiosarcoma appearance
Eckstein et al. (1992)	Richards TKA	1) [CoCr] 2) [Polyethylene] 3) [Cemented] 4) Plates, screws for fixation of tibial tuberosity	76/M	Osteoarthritis	Fibrosarcoma	4	Post-operative deep infection, osteomyelitis
Jacobs et al. (1992)	Cobalt alloy-UHMM polyethylene cementless THA	1) CoCrMo ASTM F-75 2) Polyethylene 3) Uncemented	65/M	Osteoarthritis	Malignant fibrous histiocytoma	0.5	

Table 29 (contd)

Reference	Prosthesis	Composition 1) Stem-head alloy 2) Cup 3) Fixation 4) Additional implants	Age at implantation/ sex	Preoperative diagnosis	Histopathology	Years between implantation and diagnosis	Remarks
Solomon & Sekel (1992)	Charnley-Müller THA	1–2) NR 3) cemented	48/F	Necrosis of the femoral head	Malignant fibrous histiocytoma	7	Preoperative histiocytic non-Hodgkin abdominal lymphoma, radiotherapy to the hip joint
Rock (1993)	Porous-coated anatomic TKA	1) [CoCr] 2) [Polyethylene] 3) [Cemented]	55/M	NR	Osteosarcoma	1.2	
Rock (1993)	Porous-coated anatomic THA	1) NR 2) [Polyethylene] 3) Uncemented	71/M	NR	Malignant fibrous histiocytoma	8	
Aboulafia et al. (1994)	1) Uncemented, CoCr alloy, 2) Acetabular revision 1 month later, 3) Acetabular revision 2 months later, 4) Porous coated, CoCr 7 months later THA	1) CoCr 2) Polyethylene 3) Uncemented	63/F	Rheumatoid arthritis, displaced femoral neck fracture	Malignant fibrous histiocytoma	2	Deep infection, needing removal of the prosthesis, revision and irrigation. Recurrent dislocations

Table 29 (contd)

Reference	Prosthesis	Composition 1) Stem-head alloy 2) Cup 3) Fixation 4) Additional implants	Age at implantation/ sex	Preoperative diagnosis	Histopathology	Years between implantation and diagnosis	Remarks
Iglesias et al. (1994)	NR TKA	1) Titanium 2) Polyethylene 3) Cemented	72/F	Rheumatoid arthritis (diabetes)	Malignant fibrous histiocytoma	4	Condylar CoCrMo prosthesis of the other knee at age 67
Theegarten et al. (1995)	Charnley-Müller THA	1) NR 2) Polyethylene 3) Cemented	59/F	Coxarthrosis	Malignant fibrous histiocytoma	15	Loose
Mathiesen et al. (1995)	Lord THA	1) CoCrMo ASTM F-75 2) Polyethylene 3) Uncemented	58/M	NR	Malignant fibrous histiocytoma	5	
Bell et al. (1997)	NR Femoral prosthesis	1) CoCr 2) Polyethylene 3) PMMA cement	55/F	Osteoarthritis resulting from congenital hip dysplasia	Malignant fibrous histiocytoma	7	Loose femoral part
Cole et al. (1997)	1) Premier bipolar prosthesis (titanium/ uncemented) 2) Rx-90, Biomet THA, 16 months later	1) CoCr 2) Polyethylene 3) Stem cemented, cup uncemented	59/F	Fracture of the femoral neck	Malignant fibrous histiocytoma	2	

Table 29 (contd)

Reference	Prosthesis	Composition 1) Stem-head alloy 2) Cup 3) Fixation 4) Additional implants	Age at implantation/ sex	Preoperative diagnosis	Histopathology	Years between implantation and diagnosis	Remarks
Langkamer et al. (1997)	Müller THA	1–3) NR	75/F	NR	Leiomyosarcoma	2	
Langkamer et al. (1997)	Müller THA	1) Stainless steel FeCrNi 2) [Polyethylene] 3) Cemented	73/M	Osteoarthritis	Malignant fibrous histocytoma	2	
Langkamer et al. (1997)	Charnley THA	1) NR 2) Polyethylene 3) Cemented 4) Trochanteric wires, stainless steel	77/F	NR	Leiomyosarcoma	3.5	Cemented THA 16 years earlier
Langkamer et al. (1997)	Charnley THA	1) Stainless steel FeCrNi 2) Polyethylene	67/F	Subcapital fracture of the femoral neck	Malignant fibrous histocytoma	2	Kinematic knee prosthesis 7 years earlier, prosthesis removed 11 months later for infection

PMMA, poly(methyl methacrylate)
CoCr, cobalt–chromium alloy
THA, total hip arthoplasty
TKA, total knee arthroplasty
NR, not reported

Table 30. Metastatic tumours in patients with joint endoprosthesis

Reference	Prosthesis	1) Alloy 2) Cup/tibial plate 3) Fixation	Age at implantation/ sex	Preoperative diagnosis	Histopathology	Interval between implantation and metastasis
Katzner & Schvingt (1983)	THA, type NR	1) NR 2) [Polyethylene] 3) Cemented	67/M	Coxarthrosis	Renal cell carcinoma	2 years
Kernohan & Hall (1985)	Stanmore THA	1) NR 2) [Polyethylene] 3) Acrylic cement	69/M	Osteoarthrosis	Lung cancer, squamous-cell carcinoma	4 months
Kim & Yun (1986)	Bipolar hip hemiarthroplasty	1) Not reported 3) Cemented	73/F	Subcapital fracture of the femoral neck	Adenocarcinoma of the lung	10 months
Kolstad & Högstorp (1990)	Freeman-Samuelsson TKA	1–3) NR	75/M	Gonarthrosis	Adenocarcinoma of the stomach	2 months
Kahn & Blazina (1993)	Staples for osteotomy TKA	1–3) NR	70/F	Gonarthrosis	Adenocarcinoma of the breast	Unknown
Jeffery & McCullough (1995)	1) Cemented THA, type NR, 2) Revision surgery 4 months later with uncemented femoral component		66/F	Osteoarthritis	Adenocarcinoma of the breast	7 months
Pellengahr et al. (1997)	1) Unicondylar knee prosthesis, 2) TKA, 15 months later, 3) cemented titanium prosthesis	1–3) Not reported	68/F	Gonarthrosis	Non-Hodgkin lymphoma	2 years

THA, total hip arthroplasty
TKA, total knee arthroplasty
NR, not reported

Table 31. Malignant tumours at the site of cardiac pacemakers

Reference	Type of pacemaker	Age at implantation/sex	Pre-operative diagnosis	Histopathology	Interval (years) between implantation and cancer diagnosis	Remarks
Zafiracopoulos & Rouskas (1974)	Vitatron Pacemaker generator epicardial electrode	61/F	Complete A-V block	Scirrhous breast carcinoma	2	
Zafiracopoulos & Rouskas (1974)	Vitatron Pacemaker generator intracardiac electrode	64/F	Complete A-V block	Scirrhous breast carcinoma	4	
Hamaker et al. (1976)	Medtronic Model 5841 for 4 years, then titanium-covered pulse generator Medtronic Model 5942	43/M	After aortic valvuloplasty, complete A-V block	Plasmacytoma in the s.c. pocket of the pacemaker	5	
Biran et al. (1979)	Medtronic Model 5942	62/F	A-V block	Intraductal carcinoma of the breast	2	Operated and irradiated carcinoma of opposite breast 22 years earlier
Biran et al. (1979)	Medtronic Model 5942	64/F	A-V block	Breast adenocarcinoma + Paget's disease	1.5 months	
Dalal et al. (1980)	Vitatron MIP 43RT	71/F	NR	Breast adenocarcinoma	3	
Dalal et al. (1980)	Vitatron MIP 43RT	75/F	NR	Breast adenocarcinoma	2	

Table 31 (contd)

Reference	Type of pacemaker	Age at implantation/sex	Pre-operative diagnosis	Histopathology	Interval (years) between implantation and cancer diagnosis	Remarks
Magilligan & Isshak (1980)	1) Unknown type of generator for 6 years 2) Medtronic 5950 pacemaker	83/F	A-V dissociation	Infiltrating adenocarcinoma in the pacemaker pocket	8	Twenty-five months before pacemaker pocket cancer, a simple mastectomy was performed outside the pacemaker for infiltrating adenocarcinoma of the breast
Fraedrich et al. (1984)	1) Medtronic Xytron pacemaker for 3 years, then 2) Cordis Stanicor pacemaker	78/M	A-V block	Soft-tissue sarcoma in the subpectoral pocket. Metastasis of a malignant fibrous histiocytoma, situated in the lower pulmonary lobe	4	
Liczkowski & Barnbeck (1984)	NR	50/F	NR	Breast carcinoma simplex, partim medullary	6	
Liczkowski & Barnbeck (1984)	NR	54/F	NR	Breast carcinoma solidum simplex	3	
Rasmussen et al. (1985)	Unipolar Cordis Stanicor mercury zinc pacemaker	74/M	Bradycardia	Papillary adenocarcinoma of the breast	1	Purulent ulceration, change of battery

Table 31 (contd)

Reference	Type of pacemaker	Age at implantation/sex	Pre-operative diagnosis	Histopathology	Interval (years) between implantation and cancer diagnosis	Remarks
Bhandarkar et al. (1993)	1) Cordis Omni pacemaker for 6 years, then 2) Cordis 337A VVI pacemaker	70/F	Sinus bradycardia, cardiac pauses	Breast adeno-carcinoma	13	
Bhandarkar et al. (1993)	1) Teletronics VVI model 120B pacemaker for 10 years, then 2) Optima MP 580 VVI generator	72/F	NR	Breast adeno-carcinoma	12	
Rothenberger-Janzen et al. (1998)	Leptos VVI 01-A	72/F	Sick sinus syndrome	Intraductal adeno-carcinoma of the breast	18	Replacement of the generator 3 and 14 years after insertion

A-V, auriculo-ventricular
s.c., subcutaneous
NR, not reported

of a malignant fibrous histiocytoma from the contralateral lung, next to the pacemaker pocket was described by Fraedrich et al. (1984).

2C.2 Analytical studies

Undifferentiated carcinomas, melanomas, and some types of lymphoma may be confused histologically with soft-tissue sarcomas. The specific diagnosis of lymphomas relies on the use of immunological markers (Fisher, 1999) in combination with flow cytometry or immunohistochemistry. These techniques were not routinely used in diagnostic pathology until 1980 to 1985.

2C.2.1 *Orthopaedic implants*

(a) *Cohort studies*

The incidence of malignant tumours at any site after joint replacement has been examined in 14 cohorts. The results are summarized in Table 32. For the majority of these studies, information on confounding variables was not available. Also, the exact nature of the exposure to biomaterials was unavailable in most studies, as cohorts included individuals exposed to a range of implant types. Latency data beyond 16 years of exposure were unavailable.

A cohort study performed in New Zealand included 1358 persons in five New Zealand hospitals and one private surgical practice who had had a total hip replacement implanted between 1966–73 (Gillespie et al., 1988). They were followed up from the date of operation until cancer diagnosis, death or end of the observation period (1983). Overall, 14 286 person–years were accumulated. Persons from surgical registers were linked manually with national death registers, electoral rolls and the cancer registry. Expected numbers of cases were calculated using national cancer data from the cancer registry. For cancers at all sites combined, the SIR was 0.9 [95% CI, not reported]. For breast cancer, a decreased SIR was observed (SIR, 0.4; 95% CI, 0.1–0.8). SIRs for other cancers were 0.9 [95% CI, not reported] for bronchus and lung, 0.6 (95% CI, 0.4–1.0) for colorectal and 1.7 (95% CI, 1.1–2.6) for lymphatic and haematopoietic cancers. No information on other cancers was given. The excess of lymphomas was largely seen in the first year after implantation.

A cohort study performed in Stockholm County, Sweden (Mathiesen et al., 1995) examined a population that was to a large extent included within the cohort studied by Nyrén et al. (1995). It included persons who had had a primary total hip replacement, hemiarthroplasty or revision hip arthroplasty implanted between 1974 and 1988. The numbers of the different types of prosthesis implanted are not known but the original Charnley stainless-steel prosthesis was most commonly used, with a substantial number of chromium–cobalt prostheses such as the Müller, CAD, HD2 and others. Less than 5% were uncemented implants. The cohort was assembled using in-patients from the care register of Stockholm County. Cases were obtained by linkage to the Swedish Cancer Registry, the Stockholm County Council Regional Cancer Registry and to the national Register of Causes-of-Death. The cohort also included persons with

Table 32. Cohort studies of cancer incidence following orthopaedic implants

Reference	Country	No. in cohort	Type of controls	Exposure	Cancer site	No. of cases	SIR (95% CI)
Gillespie et al. (1988)	New Zealand	1358	National register	14 286 person–years; implant 1966–73, follow-up to end of 1983. Mixed cohort, some metal on metal prosthesis (Gillespie et al., 1996)	All cancers	164	0.9 (NR)
					Colon/rectum	21	0.6 (0.4–1.0)
					Breast	6	0.4 (0.1–0.8)
					Bronchus/lung	26	0.9 (NR)
					Lymphoma/haematopoietic	21	1.7 (1.1–2.6)
Mathiesen et al. (1995) (large overlap with Nyrén et al., 1995)	Sweden	10 785	National register	58 437 person–years; implant 1974–88, follow-up to end of 1989. Mixed cohort THA	All cancers	881	0.96 (0.90–1.03)
					Upper gastro-intestinal tract	67	0.9 (0.7–1.1)
					Colon/rectum	117	0.95 (0.78–1.14)
					Liver/gall-bladder/pancreas	77	0.9 (0.7–1.2)
					Respiratory	12	1.0 (0.5–1.7)
					Lung	56	0.8 (0.6–1.0)
					Breast	103	0.9 (0.7–1.0)
					Female reproductive system	80	1.2 (0.9–1.5)
					Male reproductive system	112	1.2 (1.0–1.4)
					Urinary tract	63	0.8 (0.7–1.1)
					Skin + melanoma	56	1.2 (0.9–1.5)
					Brain	20	0.9 (0.5–1.4)
					Thyroid	23	1.3 (0.8–1.9)
					Bone/connective tissue	5	0.9 (0.3–2.0)
					Lymphoma/haematopoietic	62	0.9 (0.7–1.1)

Table 32 (contd)

Reference	Country	No. in cohort	Type of controls	Exposure	Cancer site	No. of cases	SIR (95% CI)
Nyrén et al. (1995)	Sweden	39 154	National register	327 922 person–years; implant 1965–83, follow-up to end of 1989. Mixed cohort, may have included some metal on metal prostheses during the earlier years (Gillespie et al., 1996) THA	All cancers	4572	1.03 (1.00–1.06)
					Stomach	189	0.8 (0.7–0.9)
					Colon	415	1.0 (0.9–1.1)
					Rectum	202	0.95 (0.82–1.09)
					Liver	188	1.1 (0.9–1.2)
					Pancreas	156	0.9 (0.8–1.0)
					Lung	303	0.98 (0.87–1.09)
					Breast (male + female)	525	1.0 (0.9–1.1)
					Cervix	40	1.0 (0.7–1.3)
					Uterus	94	0.9 (0.8–1.1)
					Ovary	120	1.1 (0.9–1.4)
					Prostate	638	1.1 (1.0–1.2)
					Kidney	191	1.3 (1.1–1.5)
					Melanoma	98	1.2 (1.0–1.5)
					Other skin	213	1.1 (1.0–1.3)
					Brain	116	1.2 (1.0–1.4)
					Thyroid	29	1.0 (0.7–1.4)
					Bone	6	1.4 (0.5–3.1)
					Connective tissue	28	1.1 (0.7–1.6)
					Lymphoma	133	0.99 (0.83–1.17)
					Myeloma	80	1.2 (0.9–1.4)
					Leukaemia	107	1.0 (0.8–1.2)

Table 32 (contd)

Reference	Country	No. in cohort	Type of controls	Exposure	Cancer site	No. of cases	SIR (95% CI)
Lewold et al. (1996)	Sweden	14 551: osteoarthritis, 10 120 rheumatoid arthritis, 4431	National register	66 622 person–years; implant 1975–89, follow-up to end of 1990. Polyethylene on metal only	*Osteoarthritis*		
					All cancers	483	0.86 (0.7–0.9)
					Upper gastro-intestinal tract	40	0.95 (NR)
					Colon	33	0.7 (0.5–0.9)
					Rectum	21	0.8 (0.5–1.2)
					Liver/gall-bladder/pancreas	47	1.1 (NR)
					All respiratory tract	20	0.5 (0.3–0.7)
					Breast	64	0.9 (0.7–1.1)
					Female reproductive system	45	1.0 (0.8–1.4)
					Prostate	58	1.0 (0.8–1.3)
					Urinary	38	0.8 (0.6–1.1)
					Skin	25	0.9 (0.6–1.3)
					Brain	13	0.9 (0.5–1.5)
					Thyroid	16	1.1 (0.6–1.8)
					Bone/connective tissue	4	1.0 (0.3–2.5)
					Lymphoma	14	0.8 (0.5–1.4)
					Myeloma	10	1.1 (0.5–2.0)
					Leukaemia	18	1.4 (0.9–2.2)

Table 32 (contd)

Reference	Country	No. in cohort	Type of controls	Exposure	Cancer site	No. of cases	SIR (95% CI)
Lewold et al. (1996) (contd)					*Rheumatoid arthritis*		
					All cancers	215	0.8 (0.7–0.9)
					Upper gastrointestinal tract	11	0.6 (NR)
					Colon	9	0.4 (0.2–0.8)
					Rectum	3	0.2 (0.1–0.7)
					Liver/gall-bladder/pancreas	15	0.9 (NR)
					All respiratory tract	15	0.8 (0.4–1.3)
					Breast	30	0.7 (0.5–0.9)
					Female reproductive system	23	0.8 (0.5–1.2)
					Prostate	14	0.7 (0.4–1.2)
					Urinary	19	0.9 (0.6–1.4)
					Skin	18	1.3 (0.8–2.1)
					Brain	15	1.8 (1.1–3.0)
					Thyroid	1	0.4 (0.0–2.4)
					Bone/connective tissue	1	0.5 (0.0–2.8)
					Lymphoma	14	1.8 (1.0–2.9)
					Myeloma	3	0.7 (0.1–2.1)
					Leukaemia	5	0.9 (0.3–2.1)

Table 32 (contd)

Reference	Country	No. in cohort	Type of controls	Exposure	Cancer site	No. of cases	SIR (95% CI)
Visuri et al. (1996)	Finland	579	National register	9092 person–years; implant 1967–73, follow-up to end of 1993. Metal on metal only (McKee-Farrar THA)	All cancers	113	0.95 (0.79–1.13)
					Stomach	9	0.8 (0.4–1.5)
					Colon	5	0.7 (0.2–1.6)
					Rectum	7	1.3 (0.5–2.7)
					Liver	1	0.6 (0.01–3.2)
					Gall-bladder	3	1.2 (0.2–3.4)
					Pancreas	9	1.6 (0.7–3.0)
					Larynx	1	1.2 (0.03–6.8)
					Lung	7	0.4 (0.2–0.9)
					Breast	10	0.8 (0.4–1.5)
					Uterus	7	2.0 (0.8–4.2)
					Ovary	1	0.3 (0.01–1.9)
					Prostate	15	1.5 (0.9–2.5)
					Kidney	3	0.9 (0.2–2.7)
					Urinary tract	1	0.2 (0.01–1.3)
					Melanoma	2	1.2 (0.2–4.4)
					Skin	3	0.7 (0.2–2.1)
					Brain	1	0.5 (0.01–2.6)
					Thyroid	1	0.9 (0.02–5.2)
					Non-Hodgkin lymphoma	2	0.9 (0.1–3.3)
					Hodgkin's lymphoma	1	2.2 (0.1–12.4)
					Myeloma	2	1.1 (0.1–3.8)
					Leukaemia	7	2.3 (0.9–4.8)

Table 32 (contd)

Reference	Country	No. in cohort	Type of controls	Exposure	Cancer site	No. of cases	SIR (95% CI)
Visuri et al. (1996)	Finland	1585	National register	19 846 person–years; implant 1973–85, follow-up to end of 1993. Polyethylene on metal only THA	All cancers	212	0.8 (0.7–0.9)
					Stomach	10	0.4 (0.2–0.8)
					Colon	14	0.8 (0.5–1.4)
					Rectum	11	0.9 (0.4–1.6)
					Liver	2	0.5 (0.1–1.7)
					Gall-bladder	7	1.3 (0.5–2.6)
					Pancreas	15	1.2 (0.7–1.9)
					Larynx	2	1.0 (0.1–3.6)
					Lung	18	0.5 (0.3–0.7)
					Breast	22	0.8 (0.5–1.3)
					Cervix	1	0.4 (0.0–2.2)
					Uterus	5	0.7 (0.2–1.6)
					Ovary	3	0.5 (0.1–1.4)
					Prostate	28	1.0 (0.6–1.4)
					Kidney	11	1.3 (0.6–2.3)
					Other urinary	11	0.9 (0.5–1.7)
					Melanoma	3	0.7 (0.2–2.1)
					Brain	6	1.1 (0.4–2.4)
					Thyroid	2	0.9 (0.1–3.1)
					Connective tissue	1	0.7 (0.0–3.8)
					Non-Hodgkin lymphoma	1	0.2 (0.0–1.0)
					Hodgkin's lymphoma	1	1.1 (0.0–6.1)
					Myeloma	5	1.1 (0.4–2.7)
					Leukaemia	4	0.6 (0.2–1.6)

Table 32 (contd)

Reference	Country	No. in cohort	Type of controls	Exposure	Cancer site	No. of cases	SIR (95% CI)
Paavolainen et al. (1999) (partial overlap with Visuri et al., 1996)	Finland	31 651	National register	199 996 person–years Polyethylene on metal only THA	All sites	2367	0.90 (0.87–0.93)
					Lip	28	1.2 (0.8–1.7)
					Oral cavity and pharynx	14	0.7 (0.4–1.2)
					Oesophagus	23	0.7 (0.4–1.0)
					Stomach	132	0.8 (0.7–0.9)
					Colon	145	0.9 (0.7–1.0)
					Rectum	103	0.9 (0.7–1.1)
					Liver	35	0.9 (0.6–1.3)
					Gall-bladder	42	0.9 (0.6–1.2)
					Pancreas	93	0.8 (0.7–1.0)
					Larynx	13	0.8 (0.4–1.4)
					Lung, bronchus	222	0.7 (0.6–0.8)
					Breast	293	0.98 (0.87–1.09)
					Cervix	12	0.9 (0.5–1.6)
					Uterus	47	1.0 (0.7–1.3)
					Ovary	38	1.0 (0.7–1.3)
					Prostate	158	1.1 (0.9–1.2)
					Kidney	86	1.0 (0.8–1.2)
					Bladder, ureter	119	1.0 (0.9–1.2)
					Melanoma	51	1.1 (0.8–1.4)
					Other skin	105	1.0 (0.8–1.2)
					Brain, nervous system	59	1.0 (0.8–1.3)
					Thyroid gland	25	1.0 (0.7–1.5)
					Bone	3	1.1 (0.2–3.1)
					Soft tissue	10	0.7 (0.3–1.3)
					Non-Hodgkin lymphoma	75	0.9 (0.7–1.1)
					Hodgkin's disease	8	1.2 (0.5–2.4)
					Multiple myeloma	40	1.0 (0.7–1.4)
					Leukaemia	50	0.9 (0.7–1.2)

Table 32 (contd)

Reference	Country	No. in cohort	Type of controls	Exposure	Cancer site	No. of cases	SIR (95% CI)
Gillespie et al. (1996)	USA	1034 knee replacement	Matched within same database	Implant 1972–84. Mixed cohort may contain small number of metal on metal; generally contains metal on polyethylene prosthesis	Lymphoma or leukaemia	2	0.5 (0.1–0.9)[a]
		1005 hip replacement	Matched within same database		Lymphoma or leukaemia	8	0.7 (0.3–1.4)[a]
Gillespie et al. (1996)	Scotland	7749 knee or hip replacement	Matched within same database	69 397 person-years; implant 1981–83. Mixed cohort may contain small number of metal on metal; generally contains metal on polyethylene prosthesis	Lymphoma or leukaemia	60	1.1 (0.8–1.5)[a]

Table 32 (contd)

Reference	Country	No. in cohort	Type of controls	Exposure	Cancer site	No. of cases	SIR (95% CI)
Fryzek et al. (1999) (finger/hand arthroplasty cohort)	Denmark	858	National register	7664 person–years; implant 1977–92. Follow-up to the end of 1995	All cancers	88	1.0 (0.8–1.2)
					Digestive organs	18	0.9 (0.5–1.5)
					Respiratory system	11	1.0 (0.5–1.9)
					Breast	15	1.1 (0.6–1.8)
					Female genital system	7	0.7 (0.3–1.5)
					Skin	18	1.2 (0.7–1.9)
					Lymphohaematopoietic	10	2.1 (1.0–3.8)
					Other cancers	9	0.7 (0.3–1.4)
Fryzek et al. (1999) (temporo-mandibular arthroplasty cohort)	Denmark	389	National register	2365 person–years implant 1977–92. Follow-up to the end of 1995	All cancers	27	1.1 (0.8–1.7)
					Digestive organs	4	0.8 (0.2–2.2)
					Respiratory system	3	1.1 (0.2–3.1)
					Breast	5	1.2 (0.4–2.9)
					Female genital system	5	2.0 (0.6–4.7)
					Skin	5	1.2 (0.4–2.7)
					Lymphohaematopoietic	0	
					Other cancers	5	2.1 (0.7–4.9)

Table 32 (contd)

Reference	Country	No. in cohort	Type of controls	Exposure	Cancer site	No. of cases	SIR (95% CI)
Olsen et al. (1999) (hip replacement cohort)	Denmark	22 997	National register	180 000 person–years. Follow-up to end of 1993 Mixed cohort may contain small number of metal on metal	All cancers	3304	0.94 (0.91–0.98)
					Buccal cavity and pharynx	53	0.9 (0.7–1.2)
					Oesophagus	31	0.9 (0.6–1.2)
					Stomach	71	0.6 (0.5–0.8)
					Colon	281	0.84 (0.75–0.95)
					Rectum	153	0.9 (0.8–1.1)
					Liver	45	1.3 (0.9–1.7)
					Biliary tract	33	0.9 (0.6–1.3)
					Pancreas	105	1.0 (0.8–1.2)
					Larynx	17	0.6 (0.4–1.0)
					Lung	322	0.73 (0.66–0.82)
					Breast	289	1.0 (0.9–1.2)
					Cervix	37	1.0 (0.7–1.4)
					Uterus	84	1.2 (1.0–1.5)
					Ovary	75	1.3 (1.0–1.6)
					Prostate	280	1.0 (0.9–1.2)
					Testis	6	2.0 (0.7–4.3)
					Kidney	87	0.9 (0.7–1.1)
					Bladder	219	0.95 (0.83–1.09)
					Melanoma	80	1.5 (1.2–1.8)
					Epidermis	555	1.03 (0.95–1.12)
					Brain	55	1.0 (0.7–1.3)
					Thyroid	6	0.6 (0.2–1.4)
					Bone	4	2.0 (0.5–5.2)
					Connective tissue	10	1.2 (0.6–2.2)
					All haematopoietic	226	1.1 (1.0–1.3)
					Non-Hodgkin lymphoma	86	1.2 (1.0–1.5)
					Hodgkin's disease	8	1.3 (0.6–2.5)
					Myeloma	38	1.0 (0.7–1.3)
					Leukaemia	94	1.1 (0.9–1.4)

Table 32 (contd)

Reference	Country	No. in cohort	Type of controls	Exposure	Cancer site	No. of cases	SIR (95% CI)
Olsen et al. (1999) (knee replacement cohort)	Denmark	4771	National register	31 000 person–years. Follow-up to end of 1993 [Polyethylene on metal only]	All cancers	574	0.97 (0.89–1.06)
					Buccal cavity and pharynx	4	0.5 (0.1–1.2)
					Oesophagus	2	0.4 (0.0–1.3)
					Stomach	8	0.5 (0.2–0.9)
					Colon	59	1.0 (0.7–1.2)
					Rectum	26	0.9 (0.6–1.4)
					Liver	7	1.2 (0.5–2.5)
					Biliary tract	9	1.3 (0.6–2.5)
					Pancreas	23	1.2 (0.8–1.8)
					Larynx	1	0.3 (0.0–1.7)
					Lung	47	0.8 (0.6–1.0)
					Breast	83	1.2 (1.0–1.5)
					Cervix	10	1.2 (0.6–2.2)
					Uterus	28	1.7 (1.1–2.4)
					Ovary	9	0.7 (0.3–1.2)
					Prostate	28	1.0 (0.7–1.5)
					Testis	0	
					Kidney	10	0.7 (0.3–1.2)
					Bladder	37	1.2 (0.8–1.9)
					Melanoma	15	1.5 (0.9–2.5)
					Epidermis	90	1.0 (0.8–1.2)
					Brain	7	0.7 (0.3–1.4)
					Thyroid	3	1.6 (0.3–4.7)
					Bone	0	
					Connective tissue	2	1.4 (0.2–5.1)
					All haematopoietic	32	0.9 (0.6–1.3)
					Non-Hodgkin lymphoma	13	1.0 (0.5–1.7)
					Hodgkin's disease	2	2.0 (0.2–7.3)
					Myeloma	6	0.9 (0.3–1.9)
					Leukaemia	11	0.8 (0.4–1.4)

THA, total hip arthroplasty
NR, not reported
[a] RR

rheumatoid arthritis (8.3%). Non-Swedish citizens with no available record linkage data were excluded from the study, as well as persons with a primary total hip replacement implanted earlier than 1974 or outside Sweden and persons who had been treated for cancer before their first operation. After these exclusions, the cohort consisted of 10 785 persons, with a total follow-up of 58 437 person–years. Observed and expected numbers and SIRs (95% CIs) after one year of follow-up were reported. Expected numbers were calculated using national cancer data from the cancer registry. For cancers at all sites combined, the SIR was 0.96 (95% CI, 0.90–1.03); the SIR for lung cancer was 0.8 (95% CI, 0.6–1.0).

A cohort study undertaken in Sweden included persons recorded in the Swedish Inpatient Register with hip replacement between 1965 and 1983 (Nyrén et al., 1995). Persons with a discharge diagnosis of cancer during the same hospitalization or the previous six months, as well as any individual with an erroneous or incomplete national registration number, or registered in any database with invalid codes, were excluded. Record linkage to the Register of Causes-of-Death and the Swedish Cancer Registry was based on the nine-digit national registration number. A total of 14 869 men and 24 285 women were followed up from the date of entry until cancer diagnosis, death, emigration or the end of the observation period (31 December 1989). Overall, 327 922 person–years were included. Expected numbers were calculated using national cancer rates from the cancer registry. Cancers in the first year of follow-up (444 cases and [36 769 person–years]) were excluded from the analysis. For men and women combined, the SIR was 1.03 (95% CI, 1.00–1.06) for cancers at all sites combined. Increased risks were identified for cancers of the kidney (in men and women combined; SIR, 1.3; 95% CI, 1.1–1.5) and prostate (SIR, 1.1; 95% CI, 1.0–1.2) and for melanoma (in men and women combined; SIR, 1.2; 95% CI, 1.0–1.5). Decreased risks were seen for gastric cancer in men and women combined 10–25 years after exposure (SIR, 0.6; 95% CI, 0.4–0.8).

A cohort study performed in Sweden included all individuals registered in the Swedish Knee Arthroplasty Register as having undergone a total knee replacement between 1975 and 1989 (Lewold et al., 1996). Persons who had emigrated from Sweden were excluded. Record linkage with the Swedish Cancer Registry was performed using the national registration number. The final analysis was based on 4260 men (18 134 person–years) and 10 291 women (48 488 person–years). Results were presented separately for osteoarthritis and for rheumatoid arthritis for subgroups at 36 and 60 months latency, for all cancers combined and for 20 primary sites. For cancer at all sites combined, the SIR was 0.8 (95% CI, 0.7–0.9) for patients with rheumatoid arthritis; the corresponding SIR for osteoarthritic patients was 0.86 (0.7–0.9). Although the risk of lymphoma was not elevated in patients with osteoarthritis, an increase of risk was seen in patients with rheumatoid arthritis (relative risk, 1.8; 95% CI, 1.0–2.9). Incidence of colon cancer and rectum cancer was decreased in both patient groups (see Table 32).

A cohort study carried out in Finland included 579 persons given a McKee–Farrar total hip replacement in two hospitals of Helsinki between 1967 and 1973 (Visuri &

Koskenvuo, 1991; Visuri et al., 1996). Results given here are those in the second follow-up of the cohort study (Visuri et al., 1996). Persons with a diagnosis of operative indications other than osteoarthritis were excluded. Cases were ascertained by linkage of the surgical registers with the Central Statistical Office of Finland and the Finnish Cancer Registry. In total, 9092 person–years were accumulated. The cumulative annual incidence was calculated for 15 years of follow-up for all cancers. Expected numbers were calculated using national cancer data from the cancer registry. For cancers at all sites combined, the risk was similar to that in the general population (SIR, 0.95; 95% CI, 0.79–1.13). SIRs for cancers at specific sites were 0.8 (95% CI, 0.4–1.5) for breast, 0.4 (95% CI, 0.2–0.9) for lung, 0.7 (95% CI, 0.2–1.6) for colon, 1.3 (95% CI, 0.5–2.7) for rectum and 2.3 (95% CI, 0.9–4.8) for leukaemia.

A cohort study performed in Helsinki, Finland, included 1585 individuals with osteoarthritis of the hip who underwent primary total hip arthroplasty with polyethylene on metal between 1973 and 1985 at two hospitals in Helsinki (Visuri et al., 1996). Earlier results were presented by Visuri and Koskenvuo (1991). Persons with a diagnosis of hip disease other than osteoarthritis were excluded. The mean follow-up time was 12.5 years, yielding 19 846 patient–years. Observed cases were ascertained by linking the surgical registers with the Finnish Cancer Registry. Expected numbers were calculated using national cancer data from the cancer registry. For cancers at all sites combined, the SIR was 0.8 (95% CI, 0.7–0.9). SIRs for individual cancer sites were 0.8 (95% CI, 0.5–1.3) for breast, 0.5 (95% CI, 0.3–0.7) for lung, 0.8 (95% CI, 0.5–1.4) for colon, 0.9 (95% CI, 0.4–1.6) for rectum and 0.6 (95% CI, 0.2–1.6) for leukaemia.

Paavolainen et al. (1999) reviewed 31 651 patients who had received a metal-on-polyethylene total hip replacement between 1980 and 1995 in Finland. The study overlaps slightly with the study reported by Visuri et al. (1996). Patients suffering from rheumatoid arthritis were excluded. Data sources were the Finnish National Register of Arthroplasties, the Finnish Cancer Registry and the Finnish Population Register Centre. Numbers of cases observed and person–years at risk were calculated for five-year age groups, separately for three periods (1980–85, 1986–90 and 1991–95). Latency data were grouped by time since operation (0–2, 3–9, and ≥ 10 years of follow-up). Accrued follow-up was 199 996 person–years. Cancer incidence was lower than expected overall (SIR, 0.90; 95% CI, 0.87–0.93). There was no excess risk for any individual cancer site. The relative risk for non-Hodgkin lymphoma was slightly decreased (0.9; 95% CI, 0.7–1.1). Latency data were presented overall and for 12 selected cancers or cancer groups; no significant increase or reduction was identified.

A matched cohort study performed in the Seattle area of Washington state (United States) (Gillespie et al., 1996) included 2039 men and women who had undergone a joint replacement of the hip ($n = 1005$) or knee ($n = 1034$) between 1972 and 1984 within Group Health Cooperative. A cohort of 7599 persons without this treatment at the time of enrolment was used for comparison, matched for age and gender. Patients with a diagnosis of lymphoma, leukaemia or other cancer made before the index date were excluded from the study. Follow-up was performed from the date of operation until development of lymphoma or leukaemia, departure from the Cooperative, or the most recent date of file updating. Results were given for lymphoma and leukaemia (ICD-9 codes 200–202.9, 204–208) only. Expected numbers were calculated from the control group. Persons with knee replacement had a relative risk of 0.5 (95% CI, 0.1–1.9; 2 cases) for lymphoma or leukaemia. The relative risk was similar for persons with a hip replacement (relative risk, 0.7; 95% CI, 0.3–1.4; 8 cases). [The Working Group noted there is overlap in this study for both cases and controls with the Group Health Cooperative case–control study reported by Gillespie et al. (1996) (see below).]

A matched cohort study included 2734 men (average age at operation, 65.4 years) and 5015 women (average age at operation, 67.8 years) recorded as having undergone hip or knee replacement for arthritis in Scottish hospitals between 1981 and 1983 (Gillespie et al., 1996). Controls were 10 936 men and 20 060 women from hospital morbidity registers who underwent surgery for reasons unrelated to arthritis or neoplasia, matched for age, gender and date of surgical procedure. Record linkage was performed with the Scottish National Cancer Registry and the Register of Deaths. Persons with a diagnosis of femoral neck fracture at the time of operation or a prior diagnosis of lymphoma or leukaemia were excluded from the study. The median follow-up time was approximately 10.5 years. Results were given for lymphoma and leukaemia (ICD-9 codes 200–202.9, 204–208). The relative risk for lymphoma or leukaemia was 1.1 (95% CI, 0.8–1.5). After controlling for a main diagnosis of rheumatoid arthritis, the relative risk remained essentially unchanged (relative risk, 1.1; 95% CI, 0.8–1.5).

A cohort study in Denmark (Fryzek et al., 1999) investigated the incidence of cancer after insertion of finger or hand joint (858 patients) or temporo-mandibular joint (TMJ) implants (389 patients). A range of different materials had been used for these implants (silicone, Teflon, rubber, polyethylene, ceramics and metals). Patients had been operated between 1977 and 1992 and were followed up until the end of 1995. There were no stated exclusion criteria, but patients with a hospital discharge diagnosis of rheumatoid arthritis (ICD-8 712) were identified and a separate analysis was conducted. Data sources were the Danish Hospital Discharge Register, the Danish Cancer Registry and the Danish Central Population Register. Stratification of the data by implant material was not possible. Accrued follow-up was 7664 person-years for finger/hand arthroplasty and 2365 person-years for TMJ arthroplasty. There was no overall excess of cancer in either implant cohort (finger/hand cohort, SIR, 1.0; 95% CI, 0.8–1.2; TMJ cohort, SIR, 1.1; 95% CI, 0.8–1.7). There was an excess risk for lymphohaematopoietic cancers in the finger/hand arthroplasty cohort (SIR, 2.1; 95% CI, 1.0–3.8). The risk for non-Hodgkin lymphoma was elevated in patients with a clear diagnosis of rheumatoid arthritis (SIR, 5.5; 95% CI, 1.1–16) and for the other patients (SIR 3.1, 95% CI, 0.8–7.9). No latency data were available.

A cohort study performed in Denmark (Olsen et al., 1999) included 22 997 osteo-arthritis patients who had received a hip replacement between 1977 and 1989, and 4771 osteoarthritis patients who had received a knee replacement during the same period. Data sources were the Danish Hospital Discharge Register, the Danish Cancer Registry and the Central Population Register. Exclusions before the study included 971 patients who had died within one year of joint replacement surgery, 2168 patients with a diagnosis of rheumatoid arthritis or other connective tissue disease prior to operation (to avoid confounding by the association between these diseases and malignant lymphomas) and 964 patients who had a prior hospital admission for fracture of the hip, knee or ankle (to avoid a possible confounding effect of tobacco smoking and alcohol abuse). Accrued follow-up was 180 000 person–years for hip replacement and 31 000 person–years for knee replacement. There was no excess of cancer in either the hip replacement cohort (SIR, 0.94; 95% CI, 0.91–0.98) or the knee implant cohort (SIR, 0.97; 95% CI, 0.89–1.06). There was an elevated risk for melanoma (SIR, 1.5; 95% CI, 1.2–1.8) in the hip replacement group. Overall, there was no excess risk of lympho-haematopoietic cancers, the relative risk for the hip replacement cohort being 1.1 (95% CI, 1.0–1.3) and that for the knee replacement cohort being 0.9 (95% CI, 0.6–1.3). The role of time between implantation and diagnosis (up to 16 years) was examined for cancers of the stomach and colon; there was no pattern of risk reduction over time.

(b)   Case–control studies

Morgan and Elcock (1995) performed an analysis of subjects included in a case–control study conducted by Kang *et al.* (1987) in the United States Armed Forces Institute of Pathology between 1975 and 1980. Cases were 217 men diagnosed with soft-tissue sarcoma between 1 January 1975 and 31 December 1980 identified from the records of the institute. Controls were 599 men without a record of soft-tissue sarcoma, matched for age, from the same institute. Data on orthopaedic implants were obtained by telephone interview of cases and controls or their next-of-kin. No adjustment for confounding was described, but analysis was performed controlling for respondent status (case/control or next-of-kin). The odds ratio for soft-tissue sarcoma and all implants was 0.7 (95% CI, 0.3–1.3). [The Working Group noted that the exposure data were self-reported and there was no validation with medical records].

A case–control study (Gillespie *et al.*, 1996) was performed in the Seattle area of Washington state (United States). Cases were 1177 individuals with a diagnosis of lymphoma or leukaemia (ICD-9 codes 200–202.9, 204–208) who were included in the Group Health Cooperative database. Average time between exposure and diagnosis was three years (range, 0–15 years). Controls were 4708 individuals from the same database matched for gender, date of birth and person time. Length of exposure was on average five years (range, 0–16 years in male controls). For cases and controls, information on hip or knee replacement was obtained from the Group Health Cooperative database. Adjustment was made for possible confounding by use of phenylbutazone and by rheumatoid arthritis status. Overall, no elevation in risk was observed (odds ratio, 1.1; 95% CI, 0.6–2.0). [The Working Group noted that there was overlap in this study for both cases and controls with the Group Health Cooperative (see Gillespie *et al.*, 1996, Seattle, Washington study) cohort study reported by the same authors.]

2D. Other Foreign Bodies

2D.1 Metallic foreign bodies

Compilations of the published case reports describing malignant tumours at the site of metallic foreign objects that have entered the body either accidentally or as a result of war are presented in Table 33 (sarcomas, 23 cases), Table 34 (carcinomas, 23 cases) and Table 35 (brain tumours, seven cases). Cases in which the missile was removed immediately after wounding have been excluded. There appears to have been particular attention paid to neoplasms arising after war injuries in Germany (Frey & Knauer, 1949; Dietrich, 1950; Kunze, 1965) and underreporting of cases is considered to be likely. It should be noted that the classification of sarcomas has changed and continues to change, but the older nomenclature cannot be modified reliably to take this evolution into consideration. Lead is likely to represent an important component of many of these foreign bodies. Data on human carcinogenicity of elemental lead and inorganic lead compounds have been evaluated by IARC (1980, 1987c).

The time lapse between the entry of the foreign object and the discovery of a malignant tumour ranged from four to 63 years for sarcomas arising near metallic objects (23 cases), nine of which were more than 20 years; from 5 to 48 years for carcinomas (23 cases), 21 of which were discovered after 10 or more years; from two to 40 years for malignant brain tumours (seven cases), five of which were discovered after 17 or more years.

2D.2 Non-metallic foreign bodies

Table 36 summarizes 10 case reports of cancer at the sites of various foreign objects in the body. The time lapse between the entry of the foreign object and the discovery of a malignant tumour ranged from 12 to 49 years for miscellaneous malignancies at the sites of non-metallic objects.

Table 33. Sarcomas at the site of metallic foreign bodies in war and accidental injuries in men

Reference	Foreign body/ composition	Site	Age at injury	Injury	Histopathology	Interval between injury and development of cancer (years)	Remarks
Krevet (1888)	Bullet	Thoracic wall, axilla	28	War injury, soft-tissue wound	Round-cell sarcoma	15	Chronic sinus, bullet inside tumour
Seydel (1892); Löwenthal (1895)	Bullet	Thigh	21	War injury, compound fracture	Sarcoma (not specified)	21	Chronic sinus, fragment of the bullet inside tumour
Philippsberg (1922)	Shrapnel	Back	25	War injury, soft-tissue wound	Fibrosarcoma (spindle-cell sarcoma)	6	Removal of foreign body 2 years after injury, radiotherapy 3.5 years after injury
Melzner (1927)	Bullet	Thigh	24	War injury, soft-tissue wound	Fibrosarcoma	11	Removal of foreign body 3 years after injury
Kopas (1929)	Shotgun pellets	Testicle	42	Accident, soft-tissue wound	Carcinosarcoma	4	Several pellets inside tumour
Thies (1936)	Shrapnel (numerous lead fragments)	Hand	NR	War injury, compound fracture of metacarpal bone 3	Spindle-cell sarcoma	20	Infection during 1 year after trauma
May (1937)	Shrapnel	Forearm	22	War injury, compound fracture of forearm	Spindle-cell sarcoma	18	

Table 33 (contd)

Reference	Foreign body/ composition	Site	Age at injury	Injury	Histopathology	Interval between injury and development of cancer (years)	Remarks
Keller (1938) [cited in Frey & Knauer, 1949]	Shrapnel	Back	NR	War injury. Fracture of the 3rd lumbar vertebra, paraplegia	Haemangiosarcoma	12	
Scheid (1938)	Shrapnel (numerous fragments)	Leg	20	War injury, compound fracture of left leg and right thigh	Spindle-cell sarcoma	18	
Desjacques (1939)	Shrapnel	Knee	31	War injury, soft-tissue wound	Polymorphic sarcoma	21	Multiple shrapnel injuries
Frey & Knauer (1949)	Bullet	Femur	18	War injury, infraction of the distal femur	Osteosarcoma	7	Foreign body removed 2 months after trauma
Dietrich (1950) [cited in Nolte, 1966]	Shrapnel	Thigh, proximal tibia	NR	Shrapnel injury of tibia	Polymorphic cell sarcoma	16	
Prosinger (1952)	Shrapnel	Humerus	32	War injury, soft-tissue wound	Chondromyxosarcoma	36	Chronic osteomyelitis
Dontenwill & Graf (1953)	Shotgun pellets	Femur and knee	39	Accident, soft-tissue wound	Neurosarcoma	15	
Ebert (1954)	Shrapnel, numerous metal fragments	Femur	44	War injury, soft-tissue wounds	Polymorphic spindle-cell sarcoma	8	Multiple shrapnel wounds

Table 33 (contd)

Reference	Foreign body/composition	Site	Age at injury	Injury	Histopathology	Interval between injury and development of cancer (years)	Remarks
Blümlein (1957)	Shrapnel	Vertebra C2	35	War injury, soft-tissue wounds	Round-cell sarcoma or lymphosarcoma	8	Multiple shrapnel wounds
Kunze (1965)	Shrapnel	Pleural cavity	27	War injury, penetrating thoracic wound	Spindle-cell sarcoma	18	
Nolte (1966)	1) Explosive bullet 2) Wires	Arm	21	War injury, compound fracture of radius	Rhabdomyosarcoma	22	Infection for 6 months. Pseudoarthrosis, reconstruction with tibial graft
Nolte (1966)	Landmine fragments	Thigh	26	War injury, soft-tissue wound	Spindle-cell sarcoma	46	4 metal fragments inside tumour
Hayman & Huygens (1983)	Grenade fragment	Chest wall	21	War injury, soft-tissue wound	Angiosarcoma	63	
Jennings et al. (1988)	Bullet, antimonial lead	Thigh	25	War injury, soft-tissue wound	Angiosarcoma	54	
Lindeman et al. (1990)	Shrapnel	Humerus	21	War injury, compound fracture	Malignant fibrous histiocytoma	44	
Schneider et al. (1997)	Metal fragment 7 mm, lead with 2.5% antimony	Tibia	NR	War injury, compound fracture	Angiosarcoma	46	Chronic osteomyelitis, previous curettage, bone graft

NR, not reported

Table 34. Carcinomas at the site of metallic foreign bodies in war and accidental injuries

Reference	Foreign body/composition	Site	Age at injury/sex	Injury	Histopathology	Interval between injury and development of cancer (years)	Remarks
Trampnau (1922)	Shotgun pellet, 5 mm	Frontal sinus	30/M	Accident, penetrating wound	Adenocarcinoma	25	Pellet inside tumour
Weiss & Krusen (1922)	Pin	Lung	1/F	Pulmonary abscess, foreign body	Squamous-cell carcinoma	36	Autopsy findings, pin inside tumour
Luckow (1933)	Shrapnel 1–2 cm	Lung	43/M	War injury, penetrating wound	Small-cell carcinoma	14	Autopsy findings
Blake (1943)	Metal crucifix 4 × 7 mm	Lung	50/M	Ingurgitation	'Anaplastic' carcinoma	6	
Haslhofer (1950)	Bullet	Lung	22/M	War injury	Squamous-cell carcinoma	34	Autopsy findings, bullet inside tumour
Leicher (1950)	Shrapnel	Parotid gland	35/M	War injury, soft-tissue wound	Adenocarcinoma of the parotid gland	5	Chronic sinus, shrapnel removed 1 year later
Dahlmann (1951)	Shrapnel, 2.6 × 0.5 × 1.3 cm	Lung	32/M	War injury, penetrating thorax wound	Small-cell, undifferentiated carcinoma	32	Autopsy findings shrapnel inside tumour

Table 34 (contd)

Reference	Foreign body/composition	Site	Age at injury/sex	Injury	Histopathology	Interval between injury and development of cancer (years)	Remarks
Fischer-Wasels (1951)	Shrapnel (numerous fragments)	Hip, amputation stump	31/M	War injury	Squamous-cell carcinoma	30	Above knee amputation after trauma, chronic ulceration
Montag & Mondry (1952)	Dum-dum bullet (numerous fragments)	Femur	26/M	War injury compound fracture	Squamous-cell carcinoma	25	Chronic osteomyelitis
Siddons & MacArthur (1952)	Bullet	Lung	23/M	War injury, penetrating thorax wound	Carcinoma (no histology)	34	
Siddons & MacArthur (1952)	Shrapnel ball	Lung	24/M	War injury, penetrating thorax wound	Squamous-cell carcinoma	32	
Birnmeyer (1963)	Shrapnel, several fragments	Frontal sinus	19/M	War injury, penetrating wound	Low differentiated large-cell carcinoma	41	Chronic suppuration
Kunze (1965)	Shrapnel 5 mm	Leg	NR/M	War injury soft-tissue wound	Squamous-cell carcinoma	48	Chronic ulceration

Table 34 (contd)

Reference	Foreign body/ composition	Site	Age at injury/sex	Injury	Histopathology	Interval between injury and development of cancer (years)	Remarks
Kunze (1965)	Shrapnel	Lung	21/M	War injury, penetrating wound	Small-cell lung carcinoma	29	Autopsy findings, shrapnel outside the tumour
Peter (1966)	Shrapnel, 1.8 × 0.7 cm	Lung	38/M	War injury, penetrating wound	Squamous-cell carcinoma	20	Shrapnel inside tumour
Pomplun (1970)	Shrapnel, 97.2% Fe, 1.9% Mn, 0.6% Si, 0.3% C	Lung	39/M	War injury, penetrating wound	Squamous-cell carcinoma	21	Shrapnel inside tumour
Kurpat & Baudrexl (1971)	Shrapnel	Lung	38/M	War injury, penetrating wound	Squamous-cell carcinoma	20	Shrapnel in the vicinity of the tumour
Kurpat & Baudrexl (1971)	Bullet	Lung	33/M	War injury, penetrating wound	Squamous-cell carcinoma	25	Bullet in the vicinity of the tumour
Kurpat & Baudrexl (1971)	Shrapnel 1.2 cm	Lung	21/M	War injury, penetrating wound	Squamous-cell carcinoma	28	Shrapnel in the vicinity of the tumour
Philip (1982)	Steel bullet, lead fragments	Buttock	NR/M	War injury, penetrating pelvic wound	Well differentiated squamous-cell carcinoma	33	Persistent gluteal sinus, autopsy

Table 34 (contd)

Reference	Foreign body/composition	Site	Age at injury/sex	Injury	Histopathology	Interval between injury and development of cancer (years)	Remarks
Stambolis et al. (1982)	Shrapnel 1.2 cm	Lung	28/M	War injury penetrating wound	Small-cell carcinoma with squamous cell carcinoma	36	Autopsy: siderosis around foreign body
Dubeau & Fraser (1984)	Shrapnel 1 mm	Lung	15/M	War injury penetrating wound	Well differentiated papillary adenocarcinoma and undifferentiated large-cell carcinoma	40	Autopsy
Eistert et al. (1989)	Shrapnel	Larynx	20/M	Shrapnel injury of the larynx	Squamous-cell carcinoma	41	Shrapnel inside tumour

NR, not reported

Table 35. Malignant brain tumours at the site of metallic foreign bodies

Reference	Foreign body/composition	Site	Age at injury/sex	Injury	Histopathology	Interval between injury and development of cancer (years)	Remarks
Reinhardt (1928)	Metal fragment 0.3 mm × 1 cm	Brain	36/M	Explosion penetrating wound	Meningeal sarcoma	20	Autopsy findings
Müller (1939)	Shrapnel, numerous fragments	Brain	35/M	War injury, penetrating skull wound	Astrocytoma and glioblastoma multiforme	22	Autopsy findings
Bauer & Frey (1955) [cited in Kunze, 1965]	Shrapnel	Brain	NR		Polymorphic glioblastoma	35	
Dietrich (1958)	Shrapnel	Skull	37/M	War injury, compound fracture	Malignant meningioma	13	
Schmidt & Jaquet (1963)	Darning needle, 0.786 × 24.6 mm, stainless steel	Brain	After birth/M	Murder attempt	Meningioma	40	Autopsy findings
Schäfer (1965)	Shrapnel (multiple shrapnel injuries)	Brain	31/M	War injury, penetrating skull wound	Meningioma	21	Autopsy findings
Schulze & Bingas (1968)	Silver clip	Brain	11/F	Removal of ependymoma	Meningioma	2	Clip inside tumour, recurrence of ependymoma needed 3 operations

NR, not reported

Table 36. Malignant tumours at the site of non-metallic foreign bodies

Reference	Foreign body/composition	Site of implant	Age at implantation/sex	Injury	Histopathology	Interval between injury and development of cancer (years)	Remarks
Hallervorden (1948)	Vegetable matter, bone fragments	Brain	3/F	Fall, open fracture	Oligodendroglioma	39	Autopsy findings
Leicher (1950)	Paraffin injections	Larynx	35/M	Paresis of the vocal cords	Squamous-cell carcinoma	15	
Thompson & Entin (1969)	Lucite spheres (poly(methyl methacrylate))	Pleural cavity	42/F	Pulmonary tuberculosis	Chondrosarcoma	18	
Button (1979)	Pipette glass fragments	Thumb	19/F	Thumb wound	Epithelioid sarcoma	12	
Pennisi (1984)	Paraffin injections	Breast	27/F	Cosmetic augmentation	Intraductal [adeno]-carcinoma	41	Injection in both breasts
Jennings et al. (1988)	Surgical sponge	Abdominal cavity	50/F	Cholelithiasis	Malignant mesothelioma	20	
Jennings et al. (1988)	Bone wax	Leg	34/F	Donor site for bone graft	Angiosarcoma	30	
Maier & Beck (1992)	Paraffin injections	Larynx	32/M	Perforating missile wound, vocal cord lesion	Squamous-cell carcinoma	49	
Ben-Izhak et al. (1992)	Sponge	Colon	55/F	Surgery	Angiosarcoma	25	
Harland et al. (1993)	Lucite spheres (poly(methyl methacrylate))	Lung	21/F	Pulmonary tuberculosis extrapleural pneumonolysis	Squamous-cell carcinoma of the lung	42	

3. STUDIES OF CANCER IN ANIMALS SEEN IN VETERINARY PRACTICE

3.1 Dogs

3.1.1 *Case reports*

Case reports in the veterinary literature describing malignant tumours at the site of metallic implants and miscellaneous non-metallic foreign bodies in dogs are summarized in Table 37. Sarcomas developed after metallic implants or deposition of other foreign bodies. The time lapse from implantation to sarcoma development was reported in 48 individual cases and ranged from one to fifteen years, with an average of approximately six years. The orthopaedic devices included pins, nails, plates and wires or combinations of these materials. Sarcomas developing adjacent to implants were most commonly found in the diaphyses of long bones (approximately 85%) in large breed dogs; about half occurred in the femur. The male:female ratio was 1.8:1. Non-metallic and miscellaneous foreign bodies included a surgical sponge, a pacemaker, glass and a total hip prosthesis. The sarcomas most commonly reported to develop at sites of implantation of foreign objects were osteosarcoma, chondrosarcoma, fibrosarcoma and undifferentiated sarcoma.

3.1.2 *Analytical studies*

Li *et al.* (1993) reported a case–control study that assessed the relationship between metallic implants used to stabilize fractures in dogs and the development of cancer in the canine population. The cases consisted of 222 dogs with tumours of any kind, preceded by fractures and fixation. The controls consisted of 1635 dogs who had a fracture and fixation for fracture without later development of tumours. The analysis considered the type of fixation, i.e., internal (implanted methods of fixation) versus external (casts). Information on the type of internal fixation was not available. In a multivariate analysis (controlling for sex, age, body weight and infection), the odds ratio for internal versus external fixation was 0.6 (95% CI, 0.4–0.8) for bone tumours and 2.2 (95% CI not reported) for soft-tissue tumours. No significant association was found between the type of fixation and the development of bone and soft-tissue tumours. [The Working Group noted that 400 potentially eligible cases and 1315 potentially eligible controls had been excluded from the analysis due to lack of information on the operative procedures.]

3.2 Cats

3.2.1 *Case reports*

Individual case reports of vaccination-site sarcomas in cats are summarized in Table 38.

Table 37. Case reports of sarcomas in dogs associated with metallic implants and miscellaneous foreign bodies

Reference	Device	Implantation age (years)	Site	Diagnostic interval (years)
Fracture-associated fixation				
Banks et al. (1975)	Plate	1	Radius	3.5
	Pin	2	Tibia	6
Harrison et al. (1976)	Pin	1	Humerus	11
	Plate	6	Tibia	5.5
Sinibaldi et al. (1976)	Pin	8	Radius	6
	Pin	4.5	Femur	2.5
	Pin	10	Humerus	1
	Pin	NR	Femur	4
	Pin	NR	Femur	NR
	NR	2	Femur	4
	Plate	0.7	Femur	4
Madewell et al. (1977)	Pin	7	Femur	11
Knecht & Priester (1978)	Splint	NR	Humerus	NR
	Pin	NR	Humerus	NR
	Pin	NR	Humerus	NR
	None	NR	Humerus	NR
	Splint	NR	Femur	NR
	Pin	NR	Femur	NR
	Pin	NR	Femur	NR
	Nail	NR	Femur	NR
	Pin	NR	Femur	NR
	NR	NR	Femur	NR
	Cast	NR	Tibia	NR
	Pin	NR	Tibia	NR
Bennett et al. (1979)	Plate	1	Tibia	12
Brunnberg et al. (1980)	Plate	4	Humerus	4
	Nail	0.7	Tibia	7
	Wire	2	Humerus	7
Van Bree et al. (1980)	Nail	0.7	Humerus	5
Stevenson et al. (1982)	Plate/screw	0.9	Femur	8.5
	Plate/screw	0.5	Femur	6
	Plate/screw	2.5	Tibia	3.5
	Plate/screw	0.8	Tibia	4
	Plate/screw	0.7	Femur	6
	Plate/screw	2.5	Femur	3.8
	Plate/screw	1.2	Radius and ulna	6.8

Table 37 (contd)

Reference	Device	Implantation age (years)	Site	Diagnostic interval (years)
Golubyeva & Mitin (1984)	Pin	6	Humerus	3
Stevenson (1991)	Pin/wire	1	Femur	7
	Plate/screw	4	Tibia	3
	Plate/screw	1	Femur	5
	Pin	< 1	Femur	7
	Plate/screw	< 1	Tibia	8.3
	Plate/screw	NR	Tibia	< 4
	Plate/screw	NR	Tibia	1
	Screw	1	Humerus	10
	Plate/screw	NR	Femur	NR
	Wire	1.5	Femur	6
	Plate/screw	4	Humerus	6
	Lag screw	0.7	Tibia	7
	+ plate	7	Radius and ulna	3
	Plate	1	Carpus	9
	Plate/pins	1.5	Femur	7
	Plate	0.5	Femur	6.5
	Pin/wire	2	Femur	7
	Plate	0.3	Femur	8.5
	NR	3	Humerus	4
	Plate/wire	1	Radius	10
	Plate/pin Plate/screw	1	Femur	15
Non-metallic and miscellaneous foreign bodies				
Pardo et al. (1990)	Sponge	1	Jejunal	6
Rowland et al. (1991)	Pacemaker	15	Subcutaneous	0.7
McCarthy et al. (1996)	Glass	1	Subcutaneous	10
Murphy et al. (1997)	Total hip	2	Femur	7

NR, not reported

Table 38. Case reports of vaccination-site sarcomas in cats

Reference	Tumour site	Lag time (years)	Vaccine	Histological type
Dubielzig et al. (1993)	Thigh	0.3	Rabies	Fibrosarcoma
Esplin & Campbell (1995)	Interscapular	2	FeLV	Fibrosarcoma
Esplin et al. (1996)	Interscapular	0.5	FeLV	Liposarcoma
Rudmann et al. (1996)	Interscapular	1.1	Rabies FeLV	Fibrosarcoma
Sandler et al. (1997)	Flank	Not reported	Rabies	Fibrosarcoma
Briscoe et al. (1998)	Interscapular	1	Rabies	Fibrosarcoma

3.2.2 Case series

A temporal relationship between previous vaccination and subsequent development of sarcomas at vaccination sites in cats has been reported. A 61% increase was noted in the number of fibrosarcomas in feline biopsy accessions from 1987 to 1991 at the University of Pennsylvania School of Veterinary Medicine and corresponded to the introduction of two vaccines for feline leukaemia and rabies containing adjuvant in the late 1980s in the United States. These fibrosarcomas occured primarily at sites of previous vaccination. A 25% increase in fibrosarcomas in cats was reported in a large veterinary diagnostic laboratory in the western United States during the same five-year period. Vaccination-site tumours were sarcomas of various subtypes, fibrosarcoma being the most commonly reported. Vaccination-site sarcomas were differentiated from non-vaccination-site sarcomas by their higher mitotic rate, pleomorphism, presence of inflammation, subcutaneous location and the presence of macrophages that contained foreign material identical to that previously described in post-vaccinal inflammatory site reactions. The substance in the macrophages is thought to be vaccine adjuvant and one study has identified it as containing aluminium in some clinical cases (Hendrick et al., 1992, 1994).

Although most studies have implicated feline leukaemia virus (FeLV) vaccines and rabies vaccines (Hendrick et al., 1992; Kass et al., 1993; Coyne et al., 1997), no single vaccine has been singled out or excluded from suspicion. All FeLV and rabies vaccines used are killed viral products, and most, but not all, contain adjuvants. FeLV and rabies vaccines with both aluminium or non-aluminium adjuvants have been associated with vaccination-site sarcomas (Kass et al., 1993; Hendrick et al., 1994).

Only one study has reported a vaccine other than FeLV or rabies to be associated with vaccination-site sarcoma (Lester et al., 1996). In this study, 18 cases of vaccination site sarcomas were reported in association with the use of a killed panleukopenia vaccine containing adjuvant.

Adjuvants are rarely used with vaccines other than FeLV and rabies. Tumorigenesis is thought to result from a profound inflammatory response to a localized high concentration of adjuvant and vaccine antigen. This hypothesis is supported by the observation that, in some clinical cases, 'transitional' microscopic foci of sarcoma have been found in areas of granulomatous inflammation similar to those observed in sarcomas that develop in the eyes of cats following persistent or previous trauma (Hendrick et al., 1992).

In a series of cases reported by Kass et al. (1993), the median time from previous vaccination to sarcoma development in cats was 340 days, with a range of three months to 3.5 years. The risk for sarcoma development increased with the number of vaccines given at an individual site. The prevalence of vaccine-associated sarcomas has been reported to be between one and 3.6 cases per 10 000 cats for FeLV and rabies vaccine (Coyne et al., 1997) and 13 per 10 000 for a killed panleukopenia vaccine containing adjuvant (Lester et al., 1996).

A summary of the 652 cases reported in five case series is presented in Table 39.

Table 39. Case series of vaccination-site sarcomas in cats

Reference	No. of cases	Site
Hendrick et al. (1992)	222	Interscapular/thigh
Lester et al. (1996)	18	Interscapular
Kass et al. (1993)	185	Interscapular/thigh
Coyne et al. (1997)	158	Interscapular/thigh
Hendrick et al. (1994)	69	Interscapular/thigh

3.2.3 Analytical studies

Kass et al. (1993) performed a retrospective study involving 345 cats with fibrosarcoma diagnosed between January 1991 and May 1992. Cats with fibrosarcomas developing at body locations where vaccines are typically administered ($n = 185$) were compared with controls ($n = 160$) having fibrosarcomas at locations not typically used for vaccination. In cats receiving FeLV vaccination within two years before tumorigenesis, the time between vaccination and tumour development was significantly shorter for tumours developing at sites where vaccines are typically administered than for tumours at other sites. Univariate analysis, adjusting for age, revealed associations between FeLV vaccination (odds ratio, 2.8; 95% CI, 1.5–5.2), rabies vaccination at the interscapular space (odds ratio, 2.1; 95% CI, 1.0–4.3) and rabies vaccination at the femoral region (odds ratio, 1.8; 95% CI, 0.7–5.1) with fibrosarcoma development at the vaccination site within one year of vaccination. The risk of cats developing fibrosarcoma from a single vaccination in the interscapular region was almost 50% higher than in cats not receiving vaccines at that site; the risk in cats with two vaccinations was 127% higher and the risk with three or four vaccinations was approximately 175% higher.

4. STUDIES OF CANCER IN EXPERIMENTAL ANIMALS

4A. Metallic medical and dental materials

4A.1 Metallic chromium
4A.1.1 *Intrapleural administration*

Mouse: A group of 50 male C57BL mice, approximately six weeks of age, received six intrapleural injections of 10 µg per mouse of chromium powder in 0.2 mL of a 2.5% gelatin–saline solution every other week; 32 mice lived for up to 14 months, at which time no tumour was observed (Hueper, 1955a). [The Working Group noted the relatively short period of exposure and the low dose.]

Rat: Groups of 17 female and eight male Osborne-Mendel rats, approximately four months of age, were given six monthly intrapleural injections of 16.8 mg per rat of chromium powder in 50 µL lanolin; 25 male Wistar rats, of approximately the same age, received six weekly intrapleural injections of 0.5 mg per rat of chromium powder suspended in 0.1 mL of a 2.5% gelatin–saline solution. Six Osborne-Mendel rats survived up to 19–24 months and 12 Wistar rats up to 25–30 months. Three female Osborne-Mendel rats developed adenofibromas of the thoracic wall; in addition, one of these rats also had a retroperitoneal haemangioma. Two other rats [group unspecified] had a haemangioma and an angiosarcoma, and another rat [group unspecified] had an intra-abdominal round-cell sarcoma. No Osborne-Mendel control rats were used. Of 12 male Wistar rats receiving gelatin alone, three developed intra-abdominal round-cell sarcoma (Hueper, 1955a).

4A.1.2 *Intramuscular administration*

Rat: A group of 25 male and 25 female weanling Fischer 344 rats received monthly intramuscular injections of 100 mg per rat of chromium powder (99.9% pure) in 0.2 mL tricaprylin. Treatment was continued until definite nodules appeared at the injection site in more than one animal [time unspecified]. The study was terminated at 644 days [survival figures not given]. A single injection-site fibrosarcoma was reported in a male rat. No local tumour was seen in 50 vehicle control rats (Furst, 1971).

4A.1.3 *Intraperitoneal administration*

Mouse: A group of 50 male C57BL mice, approximately six weeks of age, was given weekly intraperitoneal injections for four consecutive weeks of 10 µg per mouse of chromium powder (diameter, >100 µm to colloidal particle size) suspended in 0.2 mL of a 2.5% gelatin–saline solution. Forty mice survived up to 21 months, at which time the experiment was terminated. One mouse developed myeloid leukaemia; no other tumour was noted (Hueper, 1955a). [The Working Group noted the low dose given and the absence of controls.]

Rat: A group of 25 male Wistar rats, 3–4 months of age, was given weekly intraperitoneal injections for six consecutive weeks of 50 µg per rat of chromium powder in 0.1 mL of a 2.5% gelatin–saline solution. One rat developed a scirrhous carcinoma of the caecal submucosa, two rats developed intra-abdominal round-cell sarcomas, one rat had both a sarcoma of the leg of cartilaginous osteoid origin and an insulinoma of the pancreas, and one rat had an insulinoma (Hueper, 1955a). [The Working Group noted that no vehicle control group was reported and that the authors stated that, although round-cell sarcomas also occurred in controls, insulinomas were found only in treated rats.]

4A.1.4 *Intravenous administration*

Mouse: A group of 25 C57BL mice [sex unspecified], approximately eight weeks of age, received six weekly injections into the tail vein of 2.5 µg per mouse of chromium powder (particle size, ≤ 4 µm) in 0.05 mL of a gelatin–saline solution. Six animals lived up to 12 months, but none to 18 months. No tumour was observed (Hueper, 1955a). [The Working Group noted the small number of animals and the low dose.]

Rat: A group of 25 male Wistar rats, approximately seven months of age, was given six weekly injections of 90 µg per rat of chromium powder in 0.18 mL of a 2.5% gelatin–saline solution into the left saphenous vein. Fifteen were still alive at one year and 13 at two years, at which time the study was terminated. Round-cell sarcomas were observed in four rats—three in the ileocaecal region and one in the intrathoracic region. One rat had a haemangioma of the renal medulla and two rats had papillary adenomas of the lungs, one of which showed extensive squamous-cell carcinomatous changes. Use of vehicle-treated controls was not reported. The author stated that, although round-cell sarcomas also occurred in groups of control rats in this series of studies, lung adenomas were found only in treated rats (Hueper, 1955a).

Rabbit: Eight albino rabbits [sex unspecified], approximately six months of age, received six weekly intravenous injections of 25 mg/kg bw of chromium powder in 0.5 mL of a 2.5% gelatin–saline solution into the ear vein. The same course of treatment was given four months later, and three years after the first injection, a third series of injections was given to the three surviving rabbits. Four rabbits given intravenous injections of the vehicle alone served as controls. One of three treated rabbits that survived six months after the last injection developed a tumour of uncertain origin (evidently an immature carcinoma) involving various lymph nodes, but no tumour occurred in controls (Hueper, 1955a).

4A.1.5 *Intrarenal administration*

Rat: Six groups of 20 or 18 female Sprague-Dawley rats (weighing 120–140 g) received an injection of 5 mg of various metallic powders [reagent grade, particle size unspecified] into each pole of the right kidney (total dose, 10 mg per rat). The metallic powders, which included cadmium, chromium, cobalt, gold, lead and nickel, were suspended in 0.05 mL glycerine for injection. A group of 16 females receiving an injection of 0.05 mL glycerine into each pole of the kidney served as negative controls; a further group of 16 females receiving an injection of 5 mg of nickel subsulfide powder into each pole of the right kidney (total dose, 10 mg per rat) served as positive controls. No renal tumour developed within the 12-month period of observation in the six groups of rats that received intrarenal injection of metallic powders, although 1/20 rats treated with metallic nickel powder developed a rhabdomyosarcoma involving the injected kidney and mesentery. No renal tumour was observed in the negative control group, but renal carcinomas were found in 7/20 rats in the positive control group which received nickel subsulfide by intrarenal injection (Jasmin & Riopelle, 1976). [The Working Group noted the short duration and inadequate reporting of the experiment.]

4A1.6 *Intraosseous administration*

Rat: A group of 25 male Wistar rats, approximately five months of age, received an intramedullary injection into the femur of 0.2 mL of a 50% (by weight) suspension of chromium powder (approximately 45 mg) in 20% gelatin–saline and was observed for 24 months; 19 survived over one year. No tumour developed at the injection site. Similarly, a group of 25 male Osborne-Mendel rats, approximately five months of age, received a similar dose of chromium powder in 0.2 mL lanolin injected into the femur and was observed for 24 months; 14 rats survived for one year, and one developed a fibroma at the injection site (Hueper, 1955a).

Rabbit: Two groups of 15–20 rabbits [strain, sex and age unspecified] received an implantation in the femoral cavity of metallic chromium dust or metallic cobalt dust [purity and particle size unspecified]. Physical examination by palpation and X-ray examination at three years after implantation revealed no implantation-site tumour in 11 survivors of the chromium-treated group or six survivors of the cobalt-treated group (Vollmann, 1938). In a follow-up study of survivors [number unspecified] at intervals up to six years after implantation, sarcomas were observed at the implantation site in three chromium-treated rabbits and two cobalt-treated rabbits (Schinz & Uehlinger, 1942). [The Working Group noted the limited reporting.]

4A.2 Metallic cobalt
4A.2.1 *Intramuscular administration*

Rat: A group of 10 male and 10 female hooded rats, 2–3 months of age, received a single intramuscular injection of 28 mg per rat of cobalt metal powder (spectrographically pure with particle sizes of 3.5 µm × 3.5 µm to 17 µm × 12 µm, with large numbers of long narrow particles of the order of 10 µm × 4 µm) in 0.4 mL fowl serum into the thigh; a control group of 10 males and 10 females received fowl serum only. Average survival times were 71 weeks in treated males and 61 weeks in treated females; survival of controls was not specified. During the observation period of up to 122 weeks, 4/10 male and 5/10 female treated rats developed a sarcoma (mostly rhabdomyosarcoma) at the injection site compared with 0/20 controls. A further group of 10 female rats received a single intramuscular injection of 28 mg cobalt metal powder in 0.4 mL fowl serum; others received injections of 28 mg zinc powder (5 rats) or 28 mg tungsten powder (5 rats). Average survival time for cobalt-treated rats was 43 weeks. During the observation period of up to 105 weeks, sarcomas (mostly rhabdomyosarcoma) developed in 8/10 cobalt powder-treated rats; none occurred in the zinc powder- or tungsten powder-treated rats. No other tumour occurred in the cobalt-treated or other rats, except one malignant lymphoma in a zinc-treated rat (Heath, 1954, 1956).

4A.2.2 *Intrarenal administration*

Rat: Six groups of 20 or 18 female Sprague-Dawley rats (weighing 120–140 g) received an injection of 5 mg of various metallic powders [reagent grade, particle size unspecified] into each pole of the right kidney (total dose, 10 mg per rat). The metallic powders, which included cadmium, chromium, cobalt, gold, lead and nickel, were suspended in 0.05 mL glycerine for injection. A group of 16 females receiving an injection of 0.05 mL glycerine into each pole of the kidney served as negative controls; a further group of 16 females receiving an injection of 5 mg nickel subsulfide powder into each pole of the right kidney (total dose, 10 mg per rat) served as positive controls. No renal tumour developed within the 12-month period of observation in the six groups of rats that received intrarenal injection of metallic powders, although 1/20 rats treated with metallic nickel powder developed a rhabdomyosarcoma involving the injected kidney and mesentery. No renal tumour was observed in the negative control group, but renal carcinomas were found in 7/20 rats in the positive control group which received nickel subsulfide by intrarenal injection (Jasmin & Riopelle, 1976). [The Working Group noted the short duration and inadequate reporting of the experiment.]

4A.2.3 *Intrathoracic administration*

Rat: Two groups of 10 female hooded rats, 2–3 months of age, received intrathoracic injections of 28 mg cobalt metal powder (spectrographically pure with particle sizes of 3.5 μm × 3.5 μm to 17 μm × 12 μm, with many long narrow particles of the order of 10 μm × 4 μm) in fowl serum through the right dome of the diaphragm (first group) or through the fourth left intercostal space (second group) and were observed for up to 28 months. Death occurred within three days of the treatment in 6/10 rats injected through the diaphragm and in 2/10 rats injected through the intercostal space. The remaining rats in the first group (diaphragm) survived 11–28 months and those in the second group (intercostal space) survived 7.5–17.5 months. Of the 12 rats that survived the injection, four developed intrathoracic sarcomas (three of mixed origin, including rhabdomyosarcomatous elements, one rhabdomyosarcoma arising in the intercostal muscles). No controls were used (Heath & Daniel, 1962).

4A.2.4 *Intraosseous administration*

Rabbit: Two groups of 15–20 rabbits [strain, sex and age unspecified] received an implantation in the femoral cavity of metallic chromium dust or metallic cobalt dust [purity and particle size unspecified]. Physical examination by palpation and X-ray examination three years after implantation revealed no implantation-site tumour in 11 survivors of the chromium-treated group or six survivors of the cobalt-treated group (Vollmann, 1938). In a follow-up study of survivors [number unspecified] at intervals up to six years after implantation, sarcomas were observed at the implantation site in three chromium-treated rabbits and two cobalt-treated rabbits (Schinz & Uehlinger, 1942). [The Working Group noted the limited reporting.]

4A.3 Metallic nickel

4A.3.1 *Inhalation exposure*

Mouse: A group of 20 female C57BL mice, two months of age, was exposed by inhalation to 15 mg/m^3 metallic nickel powder (> 99% pure nickel; particle diameter, ≤ 4 μm) for 6 h per day on four or five days per week for up to 21 months. All mice had died by the end of the experiment. No lung tumour was observed. No control group was available (Hueper, 1958).

Rat: Groups of 50 male and 50 female Wistar rats and 60 female Bethesda black rats, 2–3 months of age, were exposed by inhalation to 15 mg/m^3 metallic nickel powder (> 99% pure nickel; particle diameter, ≤ 4 μm) for 6 h per day on four or five days per week for 21 months, when the experiment was terminated. Histological examination of the lungs of 50 rats showed numerous multicentric, adenomatoid alveolar lesions and bronchial proliferations that were considered by the author as benign neoplasms. No control group was included in the study (Hueper, 1958).

A group of 60 male and 60 female Bethesda black rats [age unspecified] was exposed by inhalation to metallic nickel powder (98.95% nickel; particle diameter, 1–3 μm) [concentration unspecified] in combination with 20–35 ppm (50–90 mg/m^3) sulfur dioxide as a mucosal irritant; powdered chalk (1:1) was added to the nickel to prevent clumping. Exposure was for 5–6 h per day. Forty-six of 120 rats lived longer than 18 months. No lung tumour was observed, but many rats developed squamous metaplasia and peribronchial adenomatoses (Hueper & Payne, 1962).

Guinea-pig: A group of 32 male and 10 female guinea-pigs (Strain 13), approximately three months of age, was exposed by inhalation to 15 mg/m^3 metallic nickel powder (> 99% nickel; particle diameter, ≤ 4 μm) for 6 h per day on four or five days per week for up to 21 months. Mortality was high; only 23 animals survived to 12 months and all animals had died by 21 months. Almost all animals developed adenomatoid alveolar lesions and terminal bronchiolar proliferations. No such lesion was observed in nine controls. One treated guinea-pig had an anaplastic intra-alveolar carcinoma, and another had an apparent adenocarcinoma metastasis in an adrenal node, although the primary tumour was not identified (Hueper, 1958).

4A.3.2 *Intratracheal administration*

Rat: Two groups of 39 and 32 female Wistar rats, 11 weeks of age, received either 20 or 10 weekly intratracheal instillations, respectively, of 0.3 or 0.9 mg metallic nickel powder [purity unspecified] in 0.3 mL saline (total doses, 6 mg and 9 mg, respectively) and were observed for almost 2.5 years. Lung tumour incidence in the two groups was 10/39 (nine carcinomas, one adenoma) and 8/32 (seven carcinomas, one mixed), respectively; no lung tumour developed in 40 saline-treated controls maintained for up to 124 weeks. Pathological classification of the tumours in the two groups combined revealed one adenoma, four adenocarcinomas, 12 squamous-cell carcinomas and one mixed tumour. Average time to observation of the tumours was 120 weeks, the first tumour being observed after 98 weeks (Pott *et al.*, 1987).

Hamster: A group of 27 male and 31 female Syrian golden hamsters (strain Cpb-ShGa51), 10–12 weeks of age, received 12 intratracheal instillations of 0.8 mg metallic nickel powder (99.9% nickel; mass median aerodynamic diameter, 9 µm) in 0.15 mL saline at two-week intervals (total dose, 9.6 mg). Median lifetime was 111 weeks for males and 100 weeks for females. One lung tumour, an adenocarcinoma, was observed in females that received nickel powder. No lung tumour was observed in males or in vehicle-treated controls (Muhle *et al.*, 1992).

4A.3.3 *Intrapleural administration*

Rat: A group of 25 female Osborne-Mendel rats, six months of age, received five injections of a 12.5% suspension of metallic nickel powder in 0.05 mL lanolin into the right pleural cavity [6.25 mg nickel powder] once a month for five months. A group of 70 rats received injections of lanolin only. The experiment was terminated after 16 months. Four of the 12 nickel-treated rats that were examined developed round-cell and spindle-cell sarcomas at the site of injection; no control animal developed a local tumour (Hueper, 1952).

A group of five male and five female Fischer 344 rats, 14 weeks of age, received injections of 5 mg metallic nickel powder suspended in 0.2 mL saline into the pleura once a month for five months (total dose, 25 mg nickel). Two nickel-treated rats developed mesotheliomas within slightly over 100 days; no tumour occurred in 20 controls (Furst *et al.*, 1973). [The Working Group noted the small number of animals and the limited reporting of the experiment.]

4A.3.4 *Subcutaneous administration*

Rat: A group of five male and five female Wistar rats, 4–6 weeks of age, received subcutaneous implantation of four pellets (approximately 2 mm in diameter) of metallic nickel. [No control group of sham-operated rats was available.] The animals were observed for 27 months. Sarcomas (fibrosarcoma or rhabdomyosarcoma) developed within 7–23 months around the implants in 5/10 rats that received metallic nickel pellets (Mitchell *et al.*, 1960).

4A.3.5 *Intramuscular administration*

Rat: Groups of 25 male and 25 female Fischer 344 rats [age unspecified] received five monthly intramuscular injections of 5 mg metallic nickel powder in 0.2 mL trioctanoin. Fibrosarcomas occurred in 38/50 nickel-treated animals but in none of a group of 25 male and 25 female controls given trioctanoin alone (Furst & Schlauder, 1971).

Groups of 20 or 16 male Fischer 344 rats, 2–3 months old, received a single intramuscular injection of 14 mg metallic nickel powder (99.5% nickel) in 0.3–0.5 mL penicillin G procaine vehicle into the right thigh. The metal was ground to median particle diameter of < 2 µm. Of the 20 rats receiving nickel powder, 13 developed tumours (mainly rhabdomyosarcomas) at the site of injection, with an average latency of 34 weeks. No local tumour developed in 44 controls given penicillin G procaine or in 40 controls given an injection of glycerol (Sunderman, 1984).

Two groups of 10 male Fischer 344 rats, three months of age, received a single intramuscular injection of 3.6 or 14.4 mg per rat of metallic nickel powder in 0.5 mL penicillin G procaine suspension. Surviving rats were killed 24 months after the injection. Sarcomas at the injection site were found in 0/10 and 2/9 nickel-treated rats, respectively, compared with 0/20 vehicle controls (Sunderman & Maenza, 1976). [The Working Group noted the small number of animals.]

Groups of 20 WAG rats [sex and age unspecified] received a single intramuscular injection of 20 mg metallic nickel powder in an oil vehicle [type unspecified]. A group of 56 control rats received 0.3 mL of the vehicle alone. Local sarcomas developed in 17/20 nickel-treated and 0/56 control rats injected with oil (Berry *et al.*, 1984). [The Working Group noted the inadequate reporting.]

A group of 40 male WAG rats, 10–15 weeks of age, received a single intramuscular injection of 20 mg metallic nickel in paraffin oil; 10 of these rats also received intramuscular injections of 50 000 U interferon per rat twice a week beginning in the 10th week after nickel treatment. Rhabdomyosarcomas occurred in 14/30 and 5/10 rats in the two groups, respectively. No local tumour occurred in 60 control rats that received the vehicle (Judde *et al.*, 1987).

Hamster: Furst and Schlauder (1971) studied the local tumour response to metallic nickel powder in Syrian hamsters compared with that in Fischer 344 rats (see above). Groups of 25 male and 25 female hamsters, 3–4 weeks of age, received five monthly intramuscular injections of 5 mg nickel powder in 0.2 mL trioctanoin. Two fibrosarcomas at the injection site occurred in males. No local tumours occurred in 25 male and 25 female controls injected with trioctanoin alone.

4A.3.6 *Intraperitoneal administration*

Rat: In a study reported in an abstract, a group of male and female Fischer rats [number and age unspecified] (weighing 80–100 g) received 16 intraperitoneal injections of 5 mg metallic nickel powder in 0.3 mL corn oil twice per month for eight months. A control group received injections of corn oil only. In the nickel-treated group, 30–50% of rats were reported to develop intraperitoneal tumours (Furst & Cassetta, 1973).

A group of 50 female Wistar rats, 12 weeks of age, received 10 weekly intraperitoneal injections of 7.5 mg metallic nickel powder [purity and particle size unspecified] (total dose, 75 mg nickel). Abdominal tumours (sarcoma, mesothelioma or carcinoma) developed in 46/48 (96%) nickel-treated rats, with an average tumour latency of approximately eight months. Concurrent controls were not reported, but in non-concurrent groups of saline controls, abdominal tumours were found in 0–6% of animals (Pott et al., 1987).

4A.3.7 Intraosseous administration

Rat: In groups of 20 WAG rats [sex and age unspecified], subperiosteal injection of 20 mg metallic nickel powder resulted in local tumours in 11/20 rats; intramedullary injection of 20 mg metallic nickel powder resulted in local tumours in 9/20 rats (Berry et al., 1984). [The Working Group noted the absence of controls and the inadequate reporting of tumour induction.]

4A.3.8 Intrarenal administration

Rat: A group of male Fischer 344 rats, approximately two months of age, received an intrarenal injection of 7 mg metallic nickel powder in 0.1 mL saline solution into each pole of the right kidney (total dose, 14 mg nickel per rat). The study was terminated after two years; the median survival time was 100 weeks compared with 91 weeks in a group of saline-treated controls. Renal tumours occurred in 0/18 rats compared with 0/46 saline-treated controls (Sunderman et al., 1984).

4A.3.9 Intravenous administration

Mouse: A group of 25 male C57BL mice, six weeks of age, received two intravenous injections of 0.05 mL of a 0.005% suspension of metallic nickel powder in 2.5% gelatin into the tail vein (2.5 µg nickel). Nineteen animals survived more than 52 weeks, and six survived over 60 weeks. No tumour was observed. No control group was used (Hueper, 1955b). [The Working Group noted the short period of observation.]

Rat: A group of 25 Wistar rats [sex unspecified], 24 weeks of age, received intravenous injections of 0.5 mL/kg bw (0.1–0.18 mL) of a 0.5% suspension of nickel powder in saline into the saphenous vein once a week for six weeks. Seven rats developed sarcomas in the groin region along the injection route [probably from seepage at the time of treatment]. No control group was used (Hueper, 1955b).

4A.4 Metallic titanium

4A.4.1 Intramuscular administration

Rat: Groups of 15 male and 15 female Sprague-Dawley rats, 20–30 days old, received intramuscular implants of polished rods (1.6 mm in diameter, 8 mm in length) of metallic titanium (> 99% titanium) and were observed for up to two years [survival unspecified]. Two groups of 15 male and 15 female untreated or sham-operated control animals were available. No benign or malignant tumour developed at the implantation site or in the sham-operated control group. The incidences of malignant tumours at distant sites did not differ significantly between control and treated rats (Gaechter et al., 1977).

4A.4.2 Intraosseous administration

Rat: Four groups of 11–15 male and 11–15 female Sprague-Dawley rats, 30–43 days of age, received implants in the femoral bone of metallic titanium as small rods (1.8 mm in diameter, 4 mm in length), as powders (fine, diameter < 28 µm; coarse, diameter 28–44 µm) or as compacted wire (4 × 2.8 mm). A total of 77 rats in three groups of 12–13 male and 13 female untreated or sham-operated controls were available. Average survival in all groups exceeded 21 months; the animals were observed for up to 30 months. No sarcoma at the implantation site was observed in rats that received titanium implants or in two groups of 25 and 26 untreated rats or in a group of 26 sham-treated control rats. Two implant site-associated lymphomas were observed in the groups receiving titanium powder, but none in sham-operated controls (Memoli et al., 1986).

4A.5 Metallic foils

4A.5.1 Subcutaneous administration

Rat: Three groups of Wistar rats [initial number, sex and age unspecified] were given subcutaneous implants of gold, silver or platinum foils as discs (17 mm diameter [thickness unspecified]) and observed for 23 months. The total number of sarcomas at the implantation site was 68/77 (88.3%) for gold foil, 65/84 (77.4%) for silver foil and 39/73 (53.4%) for platinum foil (Nothdurft, 1956). [The Working Group noted that no sham-operated controls were available.]

Five groups of 25 male Wistar rats [age unspecified] were given subcutaneous implants of silver, tin, tantalum, Vitallium or stainless steel foils as discs or squares (1.5 cm; two discs or squares per rat) and observed for > 596 days. Local sarcomas were found in 14/25 (56%) rats with silver foil, 5/21 (24%) rats with steel foil, 2/23 (8.7%) rats with tantalum foil, 0/25 (0%) rats with tin foil and 5/23 (21.7%) rats with Vitallium foil (Oppenheimer et al., 1956). [The Working Group noted that no sham-operated controls were available and that the composition of the stainless steel was not specified.]

4A.5.2 Intraperitoneal administration

Mouse: A group of 43 female Marsh mice, three months of age, received intraperitoneal implants of open-end tin foil cylinders (2 × 4 mm; 151 mm^2 surface area). A control group of 39 female mice was sham-operated. The animals were observed for 18 months. Local sarcomas were found in 8/31 test animals versus 1/23 controls. [The low effective numbers of test and control rats reflect the occurrence of pneumonia.] (Bischoff & Bryson, 1977).

Rat: Groups of 31 male and 29 female Evans rats, five to six weeks of age, received intraperitoneal implants of open-end tin foil cylinders (25 × 8 mm; 628 mm² surface area). Four control groups of 29–31 male and female mice were sham-operated. The animals were observed for 18–24 months. Local sarcomas were found in the four groups of effective animals as follows: experiment 1, males, 10/16; females 8/13 and experiment 2, males 7/8; females 9/12. In controls the corresponding incidences were 0/16, 0/21, 0/8 and 0/14. Histiocytic lymphomas appeared sporadically in all groups of test and control animals (Bischoff & Bryson, 1977).

4A.6 Metal alloys

The results of experimental carcinogenicity studies on metal alloys are tabulated in Table 40. Alloy composition is specified by the chemical symbol of each metal followed by its percentage. Silica, carbon and other elements are not always given.

4A.6.1 *Intratracheal administration*

Hamster: Groups of 50 male and 50 female Syrian golden hamsters, three months of age, received a single intratracheal instillation of 10, 20 or 40 mg metallic nickel powder (particle diameter, 3–8 μm) or powders of nickel-containing alloys (particle diameter, 0.5–2.5 μm; alloy I: Fe39Ni27Cr16; alloy II: Ni67Cr13Fe7) or four intratracheal instillations of 20 mg of each of the substances every six months (total dose, 80 mg). In the groups receiving single instillations of alloy II, the incidences of malignant intrathoracic tumours were reported to be 1, 8 and 12%, respectively, suggesting a dose–response relationship. In the group receiving repeated instillations of alloy II, 10% of animals developed an intrathoracic malignant neoplasm (fibrosarcoma, mesothelioma or rhabdomyosarcoma). Metallic nickel induced comparable numbers and types of intrathoracic neoplasms, but no tumour was observed in animals treated with alloy I or in control animals (Ivankovic *et al.*, 1987, 1988).

A group of 27 male and 31 female Syrian golden hamsters (strain Cpb-ShGa51), 10–12 weeks of age, received 12 intratracheal instillations of 0.8 mg metallic nickel powder (99.9% nickel; mass median aerodynamic diameter, 9 μm) in 0.15 mL saline at two-week intervals (total dose, 9.6 mg). Three additional groups (28–31 animals of each sex per group) were treated with 12 intratracheal instillations of 3 or 9 mg nickel stainless-steel dust (Fe59Cr14Ni7C4Al2Mn1; mass median aerodynamic diameter, 3–5 μm) or 9 mg chromium stainless-steel dust (Fe68Cr13C3Al2; mass median aerodynamic diameter, 3–5 μm). The observation period was 26 months for females and 30 months for males. The median lifespan was 90–111 weeks in the various groups. One lung tumour was observed: an adenocarcinoma in the group that received nickel powder. No lung tumour was observed in vehicle-treated controls or in the groups treated with the stainless-steel powders (Muhle *et al.*, 1992).

Table 40. Studies of cancer in animals given implants of metallic alloy medical and dental materials

Implant material/composition (wt %)	Route/size/amount	Species	Duration of observation	Local tumour outcome No.	Local tumour outcome %	Reference	Comments
Nickel-containing alloys except stainless steels							
Ni67Cr13Fe7	Intratracheal/powder 0.5–2.5 μm/	Hamster				Ivankovic et al. (1987, 1988)	
	10 mg			1/100	1		Single instillation
	20 mg			8/100	8		
	40 mg			12/102	12		
	20 mg × 4			10/100	10		Repeated instillation
Ni27Fe39Cr16	Intratracheal/powder 0.5–2.5 μm/	Hamster				Ivankovic et al. (1987, 1988)	
	10 mg			0/100	0		Single instillation
	20 mg			0/100	0		
	40 mg			0/100	0		
	20 mg × 4			0/100	0		Repeated instillation
Ni60Ga40	Subcutaneous/pellets (~2 mm diameter)/ 4 pellets	Rat	27 months	9/10	90	Mitchell et al. (1960)	
Ni35Co35Cr20Mo10 (MP35N alloy)	Intramuscular/rod (8 × 1.6 mm diameter)/ 1 rod	Rat	2 years	0/30	0	Gaechter et al. (1977)	
Ni35–36Co33Cr20–22Mo9 (MP35N alloy)	Intraosseous/rod (4 × 1.6 mm diameter) powder (<28 μm)/43 g	Rat	30 months	0/26 3/26	0 12	Memoli et al. (1986)	
Ni38Fe62	Intramuscular/particles (<2 μm)/14 mg as Ni	Rat	2 years	0/16	0	Sunderman (1984)	In penicillin G procaine vehicle

Table 40 (contd)

Implant material/composition (wt %)	Route/size/amount	Species	Duration of observation	Local tumour outcome No.	%	Reference	Comments
Nickel-containing alloys except stainless steels (contd)							
Ni50Al50	Intraperitoneal/powder (< 10 μm)/50 mg (as Ni)	Rat	30 months			Pott et al. (1989, 1992)	52% Ni after milling
	3 × 50 mg (as Ni)			8/35	23		
				13/35	37		
Ni32Fe55Cr21Mn1	50 mg (as Ni)			2/33	6.1		29% Ni after milling
	2 × 50 mg (as Ni)			1/36	2.8		
Ni74Cr16Fe7	50 mg (as Ni)			12/35	34		66% Ni after milling
	3 × 50 mg (as Ni)			22/33	66.7		
Ni38Fe62	Intrarenal/powder/ 14 mg (as Ni)	Rat	2 years	1/14	7	Sunderman et al. (1984)	
Ni67Cu30Fe2Mn1	Ear tag	Rat	2 years	14/168	8.3	Waalkes et al. (1987)	Observed in a carcinogenicity study on cadmium compounds
				2/193	1.0		
Cobalt-based alloys							
Vitallium (CoCrMo)	Subcutaneous/pellet (~ 2 mm diameter)/ 4 pellets	Rat	27 months	0/10	0	Mitchell et al. (1960)	
Co67Cr26Mo7Mn1	Intramuscular/particles (0.1–1 μm)/2 mg	Rat	29 months	3/16	18.8	Heath et al. (1971); Swanson et al. (1973)	Obtained by frictional movement of prostheses in Ringer's solution
				4/14	25.0		
				15/50	30.0		

Table 40 (contd)

Implant material/composition (wt %)	Route/size/amount	Species	Duration of observation	Local tumour outcome No.	Local tumour outcome %	Reference	Comments
Cobalt-based alloys (contd)							
Co68Cr28Mo4	Intramuscular/powder (100–250 μm)/28 mg powder (0.5–50 μm)/28 mg	Rat	2 years	0/51	0	Meachim et al. (1982)	
				0/61	0		
Co53Cr19W15Ni10 (wrought Vitallium)	Intramuscular/rod (8 × 1.6 mm diameter)/1 rod	Rat	2 years	0/30	0	Gaechter et al. (1977)	
Co63Cr29Mo6Ni2 (cast Vitallium)	Intramuscular/rod (8 × 1.6 mm diameter)/1 rod	Rat	2 years	0/30	0	Gaechter et al. (1977)	
Co68Cr28Mo4	Intramuscular/powder (0.5–50 μm)/28 mg	Guinea-pig	Lifetime	0/46	0	Meachim et al. (1982)	
Co41Cr18Zr16Si11	Intraosseous/powder (<28 μm)/42 mg	Rat	30 months	1/18	5.6	Memoli et al. (1986)	
Co51Cr20W14Ni10 Fe2Mn2	Wire			3/32	9.4		
Co70Cr25Mo5	Rod (4 × 1.6 mm diameter)			0/25	0		
Co47Cr20W14Ni12	Rod (4 × 1.6 mm diameter)			0/26	0		

Table 40 (contd)

Implant material/composition (wt %)	Route/size/amount	Species	Duration of observation	Local tumour outcome No.	Local tumour outcome %	Reference	Comments
Cobalt-based alloys (contd)							
Co67Cr27Mo6 (F 75 alloy)	Smooth, solid extraosseous half-cylinder (5 mm diameter × 13 mm) on lateral femur	Rat	24 months	14/101	14.0	Bouchard et al. (1996)	Not sintered
	Sintered porous extraosseous half-cylinder (5 mm diameter × 13 mm) on lateral femur	Rat		3/102	3.0		Sintered
	Injection of a suspension of microspheres (50–80 μm diameter) in the dorsal subcutis	Rat		15/103	15.0		
Co59Cr29Mo6Mn1Si1 (F 75-82)	Intra-articular/wear debris (1.5–50 μm)/20 mg	Rat	24 months	0/12	0	Lewis et al. (1995)	In saline vehicle
Titanium-based alloys							
Ti75V8Cr6Mo4Zr4Al3 (RMI alloy)	Intramuscular/rod (8 × 1.6 mm diameter)/ 1 rod	Rat	2 years	0/30	0	Gaechter et al. (1977)	
Ti89Al6V4	As above	Rat	2 years	0/30	0		
Ti89Al6V4 (F 136 alloy)	Intraosseous/half-cylinder (33 mm × 5 mm diameter)	Rat	24 months	23/102	22.5	Bouchard et al. (1996)	Not sintered
Ti89Al6V4 (F 136 alloy)	Intra-articular/wear debris (20–650 μm)/20 mg	Rat	24 months	0/8	0	Lewis et al. (1995)	In 50% glycerol vehicle

Table 40 (contd)

Implant material/composition (wt %)	Route/size/amount	Species	Duration of observation	Local tumour outcome		Reference	Comments
				No.	%		
Stainless steels							
Fe59Cr14Ni7C4Al2Mn1	Intratracheal/dust (3–5 μm)/12 × 3 mg	Hamster	26–30 months	0/63	0	Muhle et al. (1992)	
	(3–5 μm)/12 × 9 mg	Hamster		0/62			
Fe68Cr13C3Al2	(3–5 μm)/12 × 9 mg	Hamster		0/56	0	Muhle et al. (1992)	
Stainless steel[a]	Intramuscular/discs 18-, 12- and 4-mm diameter; 1.5 mm thick	Guinea-pig Rat	> 30 months	0/47 6/59	0 10	Stinson (1964)	
Fe65Cr17Ni14Mo2	Intramuscular/rod (8 × 1.6 mm diameter)/ 1 rod	Rat	2 years	0/40	0	Gaechter et al. (1977)	
Fe65Cr17Ni14 (316L solid)	Intraosseous/rod (4 × 1.6 mm diameter)	Rat	30 months	0/26	0	Memoli et al. (1986)	
Fe68Cr16Ni13 (316L powder)	Powder (< 2 μm)/40 mg			0/52	0		
Fe70 Cr15 Ni12	Intrabronchial/wire (28 gauge, approx. 10 mm long)	Rat (35)	24 months	0/32	0	Autian et al. (1976)	

[a] Metal composition unspecified

4A.6.2 *Intrabronchial administration*

Rat: A group of 35 male Bethesda black rats, approximately three months old, received implants via tracheotomy into the left inferior bronchus of a coiled wire fabricated of surgical-grade stainless steel suture material (Fe70Cr15Ni12, 28 gauge, approximately 1 cm long). Thirty-two of the rats survived for two years; none developed a lung tumour at the implant site. In contrast, three squamous-cell carcinomas were observed after 17–21 months in another group of rats that received intrabronchial implants of a polyether chlorinated polyurethane sheet (1 × 1 × 10 mm) (Autian *et al.*, 1976).

4A.6.3 *Subcutaneous administration*

Rat: Six groups of five male and five female Wistar rats, 4–6 weeks of age, received subcutaneous implants of four pellets (~2 mm diameter) of: (*a*) Vitallium alloy, (*b*) metallic nickel, (*c*) metallic copper, (*d*) Ni60Ga40 alloy, (*e*) metallic silver or (*f*) AgHg dental amalgam. [The percentage compositions of the metal constituents of the Vitallium alloy and the dental amalgam were unclear. No control group of sham-operated rats was available.] The animals were observed for 27 months. Sarcomas (fibrosarcoma or rhabdomyosarcoma) developed around the implants in 5/10 rats that received metallic nickel pellets and in 9/10 rats that received Ni60Ga40 alloy pellets. No local tumour occurred in the other groups of treated rats (Mitchell *et al.*, 1960).

4A.6.4 *Intramuscular administration*

Rat: A group of 59 female rats of the Chester-Beatty strain, three months old, received intramuscular implants of stainless steel discs (18-, 12- and 4-mm diameter, 1.5 mm thick). Each rat received one large (18-mm) disc into the left buttock and one small (4-mm) and one medium (12-mm) disc into the right buttock. Three animals were killed at 6, 12, 18, 24 and 30 months; the remainder were observed for their lifespan. Six rats developed a total of seven sarcomas in juxtaposition to the large discs or medium-sized discs. The minimum latent period was 332 days (Stinson, 1964). [The Working Group noted that no sham-operated controls were available.]

In a series of three experiments, a total of 80 female hooded rats, 7–9 weeks of age, received an intramuscular injection of 28 mg of wear particles (Co67Cr26Mo7Mn1; particle diameter, mostly 0.1–1 µm; obtained following repeated frictional movement in Ringer's solution of artificial hip or knee prostheses) in 0.4 mL horse serum and were observed for up to 29 months [survival not specified]. No control group was reported. Sarcomas developed at the injection site in 3/16, 4/14 and 15/50 rats in three series, respectively. Of the 22 tumours, 10 were rhabdomyosarcomas, 11 were fibrosarcomas and one was an unclassified sarcoma with giant cells. Distant metastases were found in 11/22 tumour-bearing rats (Heath *et al.*, 1971; Swanson *et al.*, 1973).

Groups of female Wistar and hooded Lister rats, weighing 190–310 and 175–220 g, respectively, received intramuscular implants of 28 mg of coarse (100–250 µm diameter; 51 Wistar rats) or medium (0.5–50 µm diameter, 85% 0.5–5 µm; 61 Wistar and 53 hooded rats) particles as dry powder (obtained by grinding Co68Cr28Mo4 alloy) and were observed for life. A sham-operated control group of 50 female Wistar rats was used. Survival at two years was 11/51 Wistar rats receiving the coarse particles, 7/61 Wistar rats receiving the fine particles, 0/53 hooded rats receiving the fine particles and 5/50 Wistar controls. No tumour was noted at the implantation site in rats treated with either type of alloy particles or in sham-operated control animals (Meachim et al., 1982).

[The Working Group noted in comparing these two studies that the particle size was smaller in the studies by Heath et al. and Swanson et al. than either of the dry powders tested by Meachim et al., and that the studies differed in the method of production of the test powders (the former being more relevant to the in-vivo situation), and that in the Heath et al. and Swanson et al. studies, horse serum was used as vehicle.]

Seven groups of 15 or 20 male and 15 or 20 female Sprague-Dawley rats, aged 20–30 days, received intramuscular implants of polished rods (1.6 mm in diameter, 8 mm in length) of one of seven alloys: (a) Fe65Cr17Ni14Mo2 alloy (stainless steel 316L); (b) Co53Cr19W15Ni10 alloy (wrought Vitallium); (c) Co63Cr29Mo6Ni2 alloy (cast Vitallium); (d) Ni35Co35Cr20Mo10 alloy (MP35N alloy); (e) metallic titanium (> 99% titanium), (f) Ti75V8Cr6Mo4Zr4Al3 alloy (RMI alloy) and (g) Ti89Al6V4 alloy. The animals were observed for up to two years [survival unspecified]. Two groups of 15 male and 15 female untreated or sham-operated control animals were available. No benign or malignant tumour developed at the implant site in any of the groups receiving metal implants or in the sham-operated control group. The incidence of malignant tumours at distant sites did not differ significantly between any of the treated and two control groups (Gaechter et al., 1977).

Groups of 20 or 16 male Fischer 344 rats, two to three months old, received a single intramuscular injection of 14 mg metallic nickel powder (99.5% nickel) or 14 mg (as nickel) of Fe62Ni38 alloy in 0.3–0.5 mL penicillin G procaine vehicle into the right thigh. Each compound was ground to a median particle diameter of < 2 μm. Of the 20 rats receiving nickel powder, 13 developed tumours (mainly rhabdomyosarcomas) at the site of injection, with an average latency of 34 weeks. No local tumour developed in the 16 rats given the Fe62Ni38 alloy, in 44 controls given penicillin G procaine or in 40 controls given an injection of glycerol (Sunderman, 1984).

Guinea-pig: A group of 47 female guinea-pigs of the Hartley strain, 4–6 months old, received intramuscular implants of stainless steel discs (18-, 12- and 4-mm diameter, 1.5 mm thick). Each guinea-pig received one large (18-mm) disc into the left gluteal muscle, and one small (4-mm) and one medium (12-mm) disc into the right. Three animals were killed at 6, 12, 18, 24 and 30 months; the remainder were observed for their lifespan. No local tumours developed (Stinson, 1964).

A group of 46 female Dunkin-Hartley guinea-pigs (weighing 550–930 g) received intramuscular implants of 28 mg of a dry powder (particle diameter, 0.5–50 μm, 85% 0.5–5 μm) obtained by grinding Co68Cr28Mo4 alloy. The guinea-pigs were observed for life and 12/46 animals were alive at three years. No control group was available.

No tumour was observed at the implantation site in any guinea-pig; nodular fibroblastic hyperplasia was noted in eight animals (Meachim et al., 1982).

4A.6.5 Intraperitoneal administration

Rat: Groups of female Wistar rats, 18 weeks of age, received single or repeated intraperitoneal injections of one of three nickel-containing alloys (milled to particle size < 10 μm) in 1 mL saline solution once or twice per week. The alloys were (*a*) Ni50Al50 alloy (nickel content 52% after milling), (*b*) Fe55Ni32Cr21Mn1 alloy (nickel content 29% after milling) and (*c*) Ni74Cr16Fe7 alloy (nickel content 66% after milling). All animals were killed 30 months after the first injection. The incidences of local sarcomas and mesotheliomas in the peritoneal cavity are shown in Table 41. A dose–response trend was apparent for metallic nickel and the tumour responses to the nickel alloys increased with the proportion of nickel present and the dose (Pott et al., 1989, 1992).

Table 41. Tumour responses of rats to intraperitoneal injection of nickel and nickel alloys

Compound	Total dose (mg as nickel)	Schedule	Mesotheliomas	Sarcomas	Local tumours
Metallic nickel	6	Single injection	2	3	4/34*
	12	2 × 6 mg	3	2	5/34*
	25	25 × 1 mg	9	6	25/35*
Alloy (66% nickel after milling)	50	Single injection	0	12	12/35*
	150	3 × 50 mg	5	19	22/33*
Alloy (52% nickel after milling)	50	Single injection	1	7	8/35*
	150	3 × 50 mg	3	11	13/35*
Alloy (29% nickel after milling)	50	Single injection	1	1	2/33
	100	2 × 50 mg	0	1	1/36
Saline controls		3 × 1 mL	0	1	1/33
		50 × 1 mL	0	0	0/34

From Pott et al. (1989, 1992)
* $p < 0.05$

4A.6.6 Intrarenal administration

Rat: Groups of male Fischer 344 rats, approximately two months of age, received an intrarenal injection of 7 mg metallic nickel powder or 7 mg (as nickel) Fe62Ni38 alloy in 0.1 or 0.2 mL saline solution into each pole of the right kidney (total dose, 14 mg nickel per rat). The study was terminated after two years; the median survival time was 100 weeks in the two treated groups compared with 91 weeks in a group of saline-treated controls. Renal tumours occurred in 0/18 (nickel-treated) and 1/14 (alloy-treated) rats, compared with 0/46 saline-treated controls. The tumour, a nephroblastoma, was observed at 25 weeks (Sunderman et al., 1984).

4A.6.7 Intraosseous administration

Rat: Groups of 10–17 male and 8–15 female Sprague-Dawley rats (total number, 409), 30–43 days of age, received implants in the femoral bone of various metallic materials as small rods (1.6 mm diameter, 4 mm length), powders (fine, diameter < 28 µm; coarse, diameter 28–44 µm) or porous compacted wire. A total of 77 rats in groups of 12–13 male and 13 female untreated or sham-operated controls was available. Average survival in all groups exceeded 21 months; the animals were observed for up to 30 months. Sarcomas at the implantation site were observed in 1/18 rats given Co41Cr18Zr16Si11 powder, 3/32 rats given Co51Cr20W14Ni10Fe2Mn2 compacted wire and 3/26 rats given Ni35Co33Cr22Mo9Ti1 powder (MP35N alloy). No sarcoma at the implant site was observed in rats that received other metallic implants or in two groups of 25 and 26 untreated rats or in a group of 26 sham-treated control rats. A total of 12 implant site-associated lymphomas was observed sporadically in the test groups, but none in sham-operated controls (Memoli et al., 1986).

Four groups of 52 male and 52 female Sprague-Dawley rats, four weeks of age, were given implants of metal half-cylinders (5 mm in diameter, 13 mm in length) fixed on the left, lateral femur by an intraosseous cylindrical peg (1.5 mm diameter, 3 mm length) (groups 1, 2 and 3) or subcutaneous injections of metal microspheres (50–80 µm diameter, group 4). Group 1 received half-cylinders of Ti89Al6V4 alloy (F 136 alloy); group 2 received half-cylinders of Co67Cr27Mo6 alloy (F 75 alloy); group 3 received half-cylinders of sintered-porous Co67Cr27Mo6 alloy (F 75 alloy); and group 4 received microspheres of Co66Cr28Mo6 (F 75 alloy). No sham-operated or vehicle-injected control groups were available. The experiment was terminated 24 months after implantation [survival data not specified]. Implant-associated tumours were observed in 23/102, 14/101, 3/102 and 15/103 rats of Groups 1, 2, 3 and 4, respectively. The total of 55 implant-associated tumours included 52 malignant tumours (mostly sarcomas) and three benign tumours (lipomas, all in Group 4). Within Groups 1–3, 34/40 of the tumours were associated with loose implants, 3/40 with undetermined implant fixation status and 3/40 with implants fixed to the bone, supporting an association between implant looseness and implant-associated neoplasms ($p < 0.001$) (Bouchard et al., 1996).

4A.6.8 Intra-articular administration

Rat: Two groups of 12 and eight male Fischer 344 rats, 2–4 months old, received an intra-articular injection into the suprapatellar pouch of 20 mg wear-debris powders of either Co59Cr29Mo6Mn1Si1 alloy (F 75-82 alloy; particle dimensions, 1.5–50 µm; suspended in 0.1 mL saline vehicle) or Ti89Al6V4 alloy (F 136-84 alloy; particle dimensions, 20–650 µm; suspended in 0.1 mL 50% glycerol vehicle). Two control groups were available: a negative control group of 11 rats received a similar intra-articular injection of metallic manganese powder (Mn 94%, O 6%; median particle diameter, 1.5 µm;

suspended in 0.1 mL saline vehicle); a positive control group of 12 rats received a similar intra-articular injection of nickel subsulfide powder (median particle diameter, 1.5 µm; suspended in 0.1 mL saline vehicle). The animals were followed up to 24 months after injection. Median survival exceeded 18 months in the test groups and the negative control group, and was 10 months in the positive control group. Tumours (mostly malignant fibrous histiocytomas) developed at the injection site in 10/12 rats in the positive control group. No injection site tumour was observed in either test group or in the negative control group (Lewis *et al.*, 1995).

4A.6.9 *Implantation of ear tags*

Rat: In two studies on the carcinogenicity of cadmium salts, groups of male Wistar rats, six weeks of age, received identification ear-tags made of a Ni67Cu30Fe2Mn1 alloy. In one study, a total of 14/168 rats surviving to two years developed a tumour (mostly osteosarcoma) at the site of ear-tag implantation. In the second study, 2/193 surviving rats developed a tumour (one osteosarcoma, one giant-cell tumour) at the site of ear-tag implantation within two years. The authors implicated nickel in the alloy as the probable causative agent and suggested that local microbial infection might be a contributory factor (Waalkes *et al.*, 1987).

4B. Non-metallic Medical and Dental Materials

4B.1 Polydimethylsiloxanes (silicones)

4B.1.1 *Subcutaneous administration*

Mouse: Three groups of 50 male and female C57BL/6JN mice [age unspecified] received subcutaneous implants of a silicone rubber cube (prepared by heat-curing of linear gum (polysilicone gum) with silica powder and a catalyst (benzoyl peroxide)) (10 mm thickness, 200 mg), a polysilicone gum ball (200 mg) or silica powder (200 mg) into the nape of the neck. All animals were observed for a maximal period of 24 months. No tumour was found at the site of implantation with any sample (Hueper, 1961).

Rat: A group of Wistar rats [sex and age unspecified] was given subcutaneous implants of plain films of Silastic (15 × 15 mm × 0.25 mm). Of the 35 rats that survived at the minimal latent period, 14 animals developed malignant tumours at the implantation site within a latent period of 300–609 days (Oppenheimer *et al.*, 1955).

Five groups of 25–30 male and female Wistar rats, weighing 60 g, received subcutaneous implants of Silastic 250, 450, 675, 2000 or 9711 (4 × 5 × 0.16 mm) and were observed for two years. At 300 days, 112 rats were still alive. Two malignant fibrosarcomas developed at the site of implantation of Silastic 250 and Silastic 2000 at 583 and 562 days, respectively (Russell *et al.*, 1959). [The Working Group noted the small size of the film.]

Three groups of 30 female Bethesda black rats, three months of age, received subcutaneous implants of a Silastic cube (300 mg), a polysilicone gum ball (300 mg) or silica powder [not characterized] (30 mg) into the nape of the neck. All animals were observed for a maximal period of 24 months. The total numbers of tumours at the site of implantation were 10/30 for Silastic, 1/30 for polysilicone gum and 0/30 for silica powder (Hueper, 1961).

A group of 20 male and 20 female Wistar rats [age unspecified] was given subcutaneous implants of silicone film (10 × 20 × < 1 mm); 1/14 males and 2/19 females developed malignant fibrous histiocytomas at the site of implantation during the two-year test period (Maekawa et al., 1984).

A group of male Wistar rats, five weeks of age, was given subcutaneous implants (20 × 10 × 1 mm) of a silicone film of known composition (methylvinylpolysiloxane was mixed with 25% of silica, a small amount of methylhydrogenpolysiloxane as curing agent and platinum catalyst, and rolled out to a 1-mm thick film and cured at 70°C for 3 h). The first tumour at the site of implantation was seen after 24 months, at which time 14 rats survived. Two local malignant fibrous histiocytomas were observed after 24 months (Nakamura et al., 1992).

A group of 50 Sprague-Dawley rats [age and sex unspecified] was given 0.1 mL of Bioplastique by subcutaneous injection. The Bioplastique contained 38% silicone, with particles as small as 5 μm, but mostly in the range 100–150 μm, in a hydrogel carrier. The animals were observed for two years. Thirty-four of the 48 animals examined had developed one or more tumours: breast adenomas (22), pituitary tumours (18), mediastinal hibernomas (2), retroperitoneal liposarcoma (1) and breast adenocarcinoma (1). There was no significant difference in the total number of breast and pituitary tumours between the treated group and a control group housed and fed under the same conditions as the injected animals. Three tumours associated with the injection site were found, all of which were poorly differentiated sarcomas (Dewan et al., 1995).

4B.1.2 *Intraperitoneal administration*

Mouse: A group consisting of 50 male and female C57 BL/6JN mice [age unspecified] received implants of a silicone rubber cube (Silastic, produced by heat curing of linear polydimethylsiloxane gum (polysilicone gum) with silica powder and a catalyst (benzoyl peroxide); 200 mg), a polysilicone gum ball (200 mg) or silica powder (20 mg) into the abdominal cavity and were observed for 24 months. A spindle-cell sarcoma located in the lower abdominal cavity not connected with the Silastic implant was found in one of the 50 mice; one of the mice with a polysilicone gum pellet had a spindle-cell sarcoma in the right lower abdominal cavity and a second mouse in the polysilicone gum group developed a lymphatic leukaemia; among the mice given silica powder, two mice developed malignant lymphomas in the abdominal cavity (Hueper, 1961).

Rat: Three groups of female Bethesda black rats, three months of age, were given implants of a silicone rubber cube (Silastic, produced by heat curing of linear polydimethylsiloxane gum (polysilicone gum) with silica powder and a catalyst (benzoyl peroxide); 300 mg), a polysilicone gum ball (300 mg) or silica powder (25 mg) into the abdominal cavity. All animals were observed for maximal period of 24 months. No tumour was found at the site of implantation with the Silastic, polysilicone gum or silica powder (Hueper, 1961).

4B.1.3 *Intraosseous implantation*

Rat: Cylinders (1.8 mm diameter, 4.0 mm length) of polydimethylsiloxane Silastic were implanted into a drill hole of about 2 mm diameter through the lateral cortex of the left distal femur of a group of 13 male and 13 female Sprague-Dawley rats. No tumour was found at the site of implantation during the 30-month experimental period (Memoli *et al.*, 1986).

4B.2 Polyurethane

4B.2.1 *Subcutaneous and/or intraperitoneal administration*

Rat: Six groups of 30 female Bethesda black rats, three months of age, were given subcutaneous implants into the nape of the neck or into the right side of the abdominal cavity of one of three forms (a disc cut from a sheet, cubes cut from polyurethane foam or a powder derived from the foam by micropulverization, each sample weighing 65 mg) of polyurethane (made from toluene diisocyanate). A group of 30 control rats was given four intraperitoneal injections of saline. Animals were observed for up to 24 months. The discs gave rise to one subcutaneous tumour, the foam caused one subcutaneous and nine abdominal tumours and the powder gave rise to one abdominal tumour. The latency of tumour appearance was 10 months for the foam and 22 months for the disc. Tumours distant from the site of implantation were similar to those seen in controls (see Table 42; Hueper, 1960). [The Working Group noted that the effective numbers of rats were not reported.]

Groups of 30 female Bethesda black rats, three months of age, were given subcutaneous (in the nape of the neck) or intraperitoneal implants of polyurethane sheet,

Table 42. Sites and types of tumours observed in rats with implants of polyurethane

Type of polyurethane	Site of implantation	No. of tumours	
		Local	Distant
Disc	Subcutaneous	1	5
	Intraperitoneal	0	6
Foam	Subcutaneous	1	5
	Intraperitoneal	9	4
Powdered foam	Subcutaneous	0	4
	Intraperitoneal	1	6
Controls		0	4

From Hueper (1960)

foam cubes or powder. The sheet, made by reacting toluene diisocyanate 80/20, adipic acid and diethylene glycol, and containing the flame retardant tris(β-chloroethyl) phosphate, was cut into two discs (3 and 5 mm in diameter). The foam was cut into cubes measuring 25 × 20 × 3 mm; each cube was further subdivided into four pieces for subcutaneous implantation. Powder was obtained by micropulverizing the foam. Each sample weighed 65 mg. A group of 200 female rats served as controls. Polyurethane sheet and foam each produced only one subcutaneous sarcoma; however, intraperitoneal implantation of the foam produced eight adenocarcinomas of the caecum within a latency of 10–19 months. One subcutaneous sarcoma was found following subcutaneous implantation of the powdered form, and one invading adenocarcinoma of the caecum following intraperitoneal implantation. There was no indication of any excess of tumours at distant sites (Hueper, 1961).

Groups of 20 male and 15 female rats Bethesda black rats [age unspecified] were given subcutaneous implants into tissue of the nape of the neck and/or implants into the abdominal cavity (pericaecal or perigastric region) of two polyurethane foams (a linear polyester of adipic acid and diethylene glycol coupled with toluene diisocyanate, old or freshly prepared) and three rigid types of polyurethane. The 65-mg implants varied from 6 × 5 × 2 mm to 25 × 20 × 4 mm in size because of differences in density. Animals were observed for 24 months. Among the 210 rats given intraperitoneal implants of foam, 27 tumours related to the implants were detected (including five stomach sarcomas and 16 adenocarcinomas of the colon). Subcutaneous implants of rigid polyurethane foams resulted in nine sarcomas in 135 rats; the intraperitoneal implant of rigid foam produced two abdominal fibrosarcomas in 135 rats (Hueper, 1964).

Groups of 18 and 10 albino rats [sex and age unspecified] were given subcutaneous implants into the neck region of two polyurethane foams (Etheron, derived from diisocyanate polyethers, and Polyfoam, from toluene diisocyanate; 20 × 20 × 5 mm). Etheron induced two sarcomas in 18 animals that lived for 15–28 months. Polyfoam induced four local sarcomas in 10 animals, the average age at death being 22.5 months. The two foams disappeared almost entirely within two years after implantation (Walter & Chiaramonte, 1965).

Groups of about 30 male Bethesda black rats, three months of age, were given intraperitoneal implants of 17 isocyanate polyurethane samples containing various substituent groups (aromatic, alphatic or ester groups). Thirteen polyurethane samples were implanted as sheets and four as granular material. The sheets were cut into rectangular pieces with no side greater than 3 mm. Thirteen of the polyurethane samples were also implanted into females. Each rat received 1.5 g of test samples. Of the 1015 rats implanted with polyurethane samples, 292/577 males and 248/438 females developed malignant tumours at the implantation site during the 24-month study, about 90% of which were fibrosarcomas. Wide variations in tumour rates were observed among the 17 experimental groups. Local malignant tumours developed in 0/37 sham-operated male controls and 1/37 female controls (Autian et al., 1975). [The Working Group noted that incomplete pathological data were reported.]

A chlorinated poly(ether urethane) (Y-238, prepared from toluene diisocyanate and cured with 4,4'-methylenebis(*ortho*-chloroaniline) (MOCA)), which demonstrated the highest relative tumorigenicity of 17 polyurethane samples tested in the study by Autian *et al.* (1975), was selected for further evaluation. Five groups of 35 male Bethesda black rats, three months of age, were given intraperitoneal implants of discs (3.1 mm in diameter) resulting in doses of 93.8, 187.5, 375, 750 and 1500 mg per rat. The animals were observed for two years. The numbers of local fibrosarcomas observed in the five groups were 0, 1, 2, 8 and 24, respectively, suggesting a dose-related response (Autian *et al.*, 1976).

Five groups of 20 male Wistar rats, six weeks of age, were given subcutaneous implants of five kinds of polyurethane (ether-type) films (15 × 15 × 0.2–0.25 mm) (Biomer, Cardiothane, TM-3 purified, TM-3 unpurified and a tailor-made dicyclohexylmethanediisocyanate-based segmented polyurethane (DCHMDI-SPU)). The first tumour at the site of implantation was seen after 14 months for Biomer, Cardiothane and TM-3 unpurified and after 11 months for TM-3 purified and DCHMDI-SPU. The total incidence of local tumours after 28 months was 4/13 for Biomer, 2/13 for Cardiothane, 1/11 for TM-3 purified, 6/18 for TM-3 unpurified and 3/11 for DCHMDI-SPU, respectively (Imai & Watanabe, 1987).

Four groups of 30 male Wistar rats, five weeks of age, were given subcutaneous implants of three kinds of polyurethane film (containing no additives) of different molecular weight (U-4, 220 000; U-6, 124 000; U-8, 55 600), synthesized from 4,4'-methylenediphenyl diisocyanate, poly(tetramethylene glycol) and 1,4-butanediol with molar ratio of 2: 1: 1, or silicone films (20 × 10 × 1 mm). The rats were observed for one year. As summarized in Table 43, histopathological evaluation showed no relationship

Table 43. Histopathological evaluation in one-year implantation study of polyurethanes of different molecular weight

Implant	No. of animals in rank				Total active incidence (A + B + C)	Capsule thickness (mm)	
	A	B	C	D		Mean	SD
U-4	2	3	9	16	14	0.32	0.12
U-6	0	0	2	28	2	0.32	0.14
U-8	0	1	5	24	6	0.37	0.21
Silicone	0	0	0	27	0	0.30	0.08

Criteria of ranking: A, local tumour was found; B, atypical cell proliferation accompanied by preneoplastic changes was observed at the inner layer of the capsule; C, cell proliferation but no preneoplastic change was observed; D, no cell proliferation was observed
From Nakamura *et al.* (1992)

between molecular weight and active tissue responses, including local malignant fibrous histiocytomas (Nakamura et al., 1992).

Groups of 30 male Wistar rats, five weeks of age, were given subcutaneous implants of polyurethane (U-6), silicone and a 1:1 blend (U-6/silicone films) (20 × 10 × 1 mm) and were held for two years. As shown in Table 44, the polyurethane content governed tissue responses, including tumour formation (Nakamura et al., 1992).

Table 44. Effects of polyurethane content on tissue responses in a two-year study

Implant	No. of animals in rank				Total active incidence (A + B + C)	Capsule thickness (mm)	
	A	B	C	D		Mean	SD
Silicone	2	1	4	21	7	0.27	0.08
U-6/silicone	2	0	9	18	11	0.29	0.10
U-6	11[a,b]	1	10	7	22[c]	0.29	0.11

Criteria of ranking: A, tumour was found; B, atypical cell proliferation accompanied by preneoplastic changes was observed at the inner layer of the capsule; C, cell proliferation but no preneoplastic change was observed; D, no cell proliferation was observed
[a] Significantly different from silicone (χ^2-test, $p < 0.01$)
[b] Trend test (Cochran-Armitage test, $p < 0.01$)
[c] Trend test (Cochran-Armitage test, $p < 0.0001$)
From Nakamura et al. (1992)

Seven groups of 30 male Wistar rats, five weeks of age, were given subcutaneous implants of poly(ether urethane) film (10 × 20 × 1 mm) with smooth or porous (pore size, 20–50 μm) surface morphology, containing different amounts of oligomers, or a silicone film of the same size as control. The poly(ether urethanes) used were: UN (unrefined; molecular weight, 220 000) prepared from 4,4'-methylenediphenyl diisocyanate, poly(tetramethylene glycol) and 1,4-butanediol with molar ratio of 2 : 1 : 1, having oligomer content of 5.6%; UR, refined UN to delete oligomers; and UA, oligomer-added UN, having oligomer content of 11%. Animals were observed for two years. The incidence of local tumours (malignant fibrous histiocytomas) at the site of implantation and the shortest latent period are summarized in Table 45. It was concluded that the amount of oligomers did not affect the local tumour incidence, whereas changing surface morphology from smooth to porous extended the latent period of tumour development and decreased the total incidence of local tumours. There was no increase in the incidence of tumours at sites distant from the implantation site (Nakamura et al., 1995).

Table 45. Injection-site tumours in rats given implants of different polyurethanes

Implant	Surface	Total no. of MFH-bearing animals	Shortest latent period (months)
UR	Smooth	6	12
UR	Porous	7	18
UN	Smooth	8	15
UN	Porous	4	21
UA	Smooth	8	12
UA	Porous	4	21
Silicone	Smooth	3	15

See text for definition of polyurethane types UA, UN and UR
MFH, malignant fibrous histiocytoma
From Nakamura et al. (1995)

4B.2.2 Inhalation and/or intratracheal or intrabronchial administration

Rat: Two groups of 39 and 45 Sprague-Dawley rats [sex and age unspecified] were exposed by inhalation to rigid isocyanate polyurethane foam powder [composition not specified] at concentrations of 3.6 and 20 mg/m^3, respectively, for 6 h per day on five days per week for six weeks. The median particle size was 0.5 μm. One bronchial squamous-cell carcinoma was observed in animals at each dose level after 544 and 349 days, respectively. The median lifespans were 50 and 62 weeks, and the durations of the experiments were 139 and 101 weeks. No tumours were found in 20 untreated rats (Laskin et al., 1972).

Groups of white rats [number, sex and strain unspecified] of different ages (2–3 months or 11–19 months) received intratracheal intubations of 5 mg of powder from an old polyurethane dust (the same product as that used by Laskin et al., 1972) or a freshly prepared polyurethane [composition not specified] suspended in 0.2 mL saline. This dose is the equivalent of inhalation for 8 h per day for 30 days of a concentration between the minimal and maximal levels used in the experiment by Laskin et al. (1972). Pulmonary fibrosis appeared after six months. A sub-pleural adenoma was seen in a rat given the old polymer, and four benign lesions reported to be intrabronchial adenomas were observed 18 months after intubation among 15 young rats given the freshly prepared sample (Stemmer et al., 1975).

Two groups of 35 male Bethesda black rats, three months of age, were given implants via tracheotomy into the left inferior bronchus of a polyether chlorinated polyurethane sheet (Y-238, a polymer formed by reaction of toluene diisocyanate with polyether and cured with MOCA) cut into strips of approximately $1 \times 1 \times 6$ mm (5–8 mg) or $1 \times 1 \times 10$ mm (9–10 mg), through which fine, stainless-steel surgical wire was passed and bent to form two hooks. One squamous-cell carcinoma of the lung was observed after 21.5 months in the first group, in which 31 animals survived one year or more; and three squamous-cell carcinomas of the lung were observed after 17–21 months in the second group, in which 32 animals survived one year or more. No lung tumours were observed in 35 controls given implants of surgical wire alone; 33 animals survived more than one year (Autian et al., 1976).

Groups of 50 male and 50 female Sprague-Dawley rats, eight weeks of age, were exposed by inhalation to a freshly generated rigid polyurethane foam dust (particle diameter, 94% < 5 μm) synthesized from Desmophen FWFA/2 (polyol based on a sucrose-polyether) and Desmodur 44V20 (a polymeric isocyanate based on 4,4′-methylenediphenyl diisocyanate) at a concentration of 8.65 mg/m^3 air for 6 h per day on five days per week for 12 weeks; the experiment was terminated after 140 weeks. There was no difference in tumour incidence in the polyurethane group compared with controls exposed to titanium oxide or to air alone (Thyssen et al., 1978).

Hamster: Two groups of 40 and 50 male Syrian hamsters were exposed by inhalation to respirable dust (0.5–3 μm) generated from rigid polyurethane foam [composition not specified] at concentrations of 3.6 and 20 mg/m^3 in air, respectively, for 6 h per day on five days per week for six weeks. Median survival times were 76 and 87 weeks and the duration of exposure was 139 and 101 weeks, respectively. No lung tumour was reported (Laskin et al., 1972).

4B.3 Poly(methyl methacrylate)

4B.3.1 *Subcutaneous and/or intramuscular administration*

Mouse: A group of 50 Harlan albino Swiss mice [sex unspecified], six weeks of age, was given subcutaneous implants into the lateral abdominal wall of poly(methyl methacrylate) (PMMA) film (10 × 10 × 0.2 mm), prepared by polymerizing commercially obtained monomer liquid (containing 1.0 mg/kg (ppm) hydroquinone) and polymer powder (containing cadmium oxide pigments), similar to that used in making dentures. The first fibrosarcoma at the implantation site was found in mice given PMMA films 257 days after the operation, when 20/50 mice were still alive; four additional fibrosarcomas developed at 405, 438, 454 and 469 days after the implantation. A group of 50 control mice was given subcutaneous implants of cellophane film; one fibrosarcoma at the implantation site was found 400 days after the operation among the seven mice still alive at that time (Laskin et al., 1954).

Two groups of 50 Harlan albino Swiss mice [sex unspecified], six weeks of age, were given subcutaneous implants into the lateral abdominal wall of films (10 × 10 × 0.20–0.25 mm) of cold- or heat-cured polymerized PMMA. An equal number of control mice of the same age, sex and strain were given implants of cellophane film (0.1 mm thick) of identical size. Animals were observed weekly for 420 days. At the end of that time, 22, 13 and 25 mice, respectively, were still alive; one mammary carcinoma, considered to be 'spontaneous', was found near a heat-cured PMMA film implant. The study ended after 575 days, when surviving animals comprised two mice that received heat-cured PMMA film, 10 that received cold-cured PMMA film and five controls. No neoplastic changes at the site of implantation were detected (Kydd & Sreebny, 1960).

Groups of female Swiss albino mice, 7–8 weeks of age, were given subcutaneous implants into the left flank of PMMA films of varying sizes (15 × 15 × 0.5 mm, 12 × 12 × 0.5 mm, 6 × 6 × 0.5 mm or 6 × 12 × 0.5 mm) and observed for 100 weeks. The incidences of sarcomas at the site of implantation were 3/18 (16%), 10/38 (26%), 1/15 (6.6%) and 1/15 (6.6%) (Tomatis, 1966a).

Rat: A group of 25 Wistar rats [sex and age unspecified] was given subcutaneous implants of films of PMMA (15 × 15 mm × 0.14 mm). At the time of appearance of the first tumour, 20/25 rats were still alive; among these, four sarcomas were found at the site of implantation (20%), with latent periods ranging from 581 to 685 days. Of 50 surviving rats given implants of glass coverslips, one developed a fibrosarcoma that appeared 659 days after implantation. Results from an experiment that was still in progress at the time of reporting indicated that 11/25 rats given implants of purified PMMA (instead of commercial grade) developed subcutaneous sarcomas. In this group, the first tumour developed at 447 days (Oppenheimer *et al.*, 1953, 1955).

A group of 153 female Chester Beatty rats, three months of age, were given intramuscular implants of PMMA discs. Each animal received one large disc (18 mm in diameter, 1.5 mm thick) in the left thigh and one medium (12 mm in diameter) and one small (4 mm in diameter) disc in the right thigh. Thirty-four tumours, all spindle-cell sarcomas, were observed in association with the largest discs, with latent periods of 150–807 days; seven animals had metastases to the lungs and/or mesentery. Sarcomas associated with the medium-sized discs were found in 17/142 rats still alive at the minimum latent period (297 days); five animals had metastases to the lungs and mesentery. The 51 sarcomas observed occurred in a total of 46 rats. No tumours were found in association with the smallest discs (Stinson, 1964). [The Working Group noted that the number of animals at risk was not given.]

A group of 34 female Wistar rats, 9–12 weeks of age, was given subcutaneous implants of PMMA (Plexiglas) rings (24 mm in diameter with a hole of 21.5 mm); one fibroblastic sarcoma was detected in one rat after 112 weeks of observation (Zajdela, 1966).

Male Wistar rats weighing 175–200 g [age unspecified] were given implants of PMMA (Surgical Simplex P; cut into discs 18 mm in diameter and 0.14 mm thick) inserted subcutaneously in the abdominal region. One group of 22 rats received the discs bilaterally, and another group of 25 rats received the PMMA disc on one side and a glass disc on the other. Surviving animals were killed after 39 months. Only 22 rats with either bilateral or single PMMA discs were subjected to pathological examination. Two fibrosarcomas were found at the site of implantation of PMMA discs between 349 and 471 days after implantation, but no tumours were associated with the glass discs (Lavorgna *et al.*, 1972).

Guinea-pig: A group of 86 female Hartley guinea-pigs, 4–6 months of age, was given intramuscular implants into the thigh of three PMMA discs (1.5 mm thick) of different diameter (18, 12 and 4 mm). Groups of three animals were killed at six, 12, 18, 24 and 30 months after implantation to examine the tissue reactions around the discs; the remaining guinea-pigs were observed throughout their lifespan. No tumours were detected, even though some animals were still alive 48 months after the implantation (Stinson, 1964). [The Working Group noted that the effective number of animals at risk was not given.]

4B.3.2 *Intraperitoneal administration*

Rat: Two groups of 25 male and 25 female rats [strain unspecified], 3–4 months of age, were given intraperitoneal implants of either glass or PMMA discs (about 20 mm in diameter) and a group of 50 sham-operated animals served as controls. No tumours were found after 21 months in the glass-implanted group (21 survivors at 11 months). In the PMMA-implanted group, 20 rats survived 11 months and two sarcomas were observed around the implant (at 13 and 14 months after implantation), one of which metastasized to the omentum and peritoneal cavity; a third tumour in the peritoneal cavity, found at 20 months, did not arise from the capsule enveloping the disc. One lipoma was observed at 11 months in the 23 sham-operated animals alive at that time (Brunner, 1959).

4B.3.3 *Other experimental systems*

Combined subcutaneous and intraperitoneal implantation: Six groups of 10 male and 10 female rats [strain and age unspecified] were given implants of PMMA discs (17 mm diameter, 1–2 mm thick); each rat received five discs intraperitoneally into the abdominal wall and two subcutaneously under the dorsal skin. The PMMA discs contained 0, 2, 5, 10, 25 and 50% fibrin (to produce increasing roughness of the disc surface). A control group of 30 sham-operated animals was available. The numbers of animals at risk at the time of appearance of the first tumour were 20, 13, 15, 18, 14 and 13, respectively, in the groups given PMMA implants, and 15 in the control group; all animals were killed 17 months after implantation. The numbers of sarcomas were 2 (10%), 5 (38%), 2 (13%), 3 (17%), 4 (29%) and 1 (8%) in the implanted groups. No tumours developed in the sham-operated rats. Overall, 13 intraperitoneal and four subcutaneous tumours were observed; the first tumour appeared after nine months. Tumour development was not related to fibrin concentration (Brunner, 1959).

A group of male and female outbred rats (weighing 100–170 g) [initial number and age unspecified] was given intraperitoneal implants of five discs and subcutaneous implants of two discs of PMMA (16 mm diameter, 0.2–0.4 mm thick). At six months, 13 treated animals and 27 sham-operated controls were still alive; these animals were observed up to 23 months. Of treated animals, one developed a sarcoma near an intraperitoneal implant, one developed a subcutaneous sarcoma (metastasizing to the lung) and two others developed [unspecified] tumours (Klärner, 1962). [The Working Group noted that the time of tumour appearance was not stated.]

Intraosseous implantation: A group of 13 male and 13 female Sprague-Dawley rats, 30–43 days of age, was given an implant of a PMMA bone cement (2 mL, Simplex P) injected into a drill hole about 2 mm in diameter through the lateral cortex of the left distal femur and allowed to polymerize *in vivo*. No tumour was found at the site of injection during the 30-month experimental period (Memoli *et al.*, 1986).

4B.4 Poly(2-hydroxyethyl methacrylate)

4B.4.1 *Subcutaneous administration*

Rat: A group of 15 male Wistar rats, weighing 200 g, was given subcutaneous implants of cross-linked poly(2-hydroxyethyl methacrylate) film (10 × 20 × 0.5 mm) and one animal was killed at three and six months after implantation, for histological examination. The remaining animals were kept until they were moribund, died or developed tumours. Five local tumours [unspecified] were found at the site of implantation in 10 rats that survived for more than 12 months (Imai & Masuhara, 1982).

A group of 20 male and 20 female Wistar rats [age unspecified] was given subcutaneous implants of poly(2-hydroxyethyl methacrylate) film (10 × 20 × < 1 mm); 7/19 males and 9/20 females developed malignant fibrous histiocytomas at the site of implantation during the two-year test period (Maekawa *et al.*, 1984).

Hamster: A group of 11 male hamsters (weighing 120 g) [strain unspecified] was given subcutaneous implants of cross-linked poly(2-hydroxyethyl methacrylate) film (10 × 20 × 0.5 mm) and one animal was killed at three and six months after implantation, for histological examination. The remaining animals were kept until they were moribund, died or developed tumours. Among animals that survived for more than 12 months, no tumours were found at the site of implantation (Imai & Masuhara, 1982).

Guinea-pig: A group of eight male guinea-pigs [age and strain unspecified] was given subcutaneous implants of cross-linked poly(2-hydroxyethyl methacrylate) film (10 × 20 × 0.5 mm) and one animal was killed at three and six months after implantation, for histological examination. The remaining animals were kept until they were moribund, died or developed tumours. Among animals that survived for more than 12 months, no tumours were found at the site of implantation (Imai & Masuhara, 1982).

4B.5 Poly(ethylene terephthalate)

4B.5.1 *Subcutaneous administration*

Rat: Groups of male Wistar rats [initial number and age unspecified] were given subcutaneous implants of discs (15 mm diameter) of a material described as Dacron in various physical forms. The incidence of malignant tumours at the site of implantation is summarized in Table 46 (Oppenheimer *et al.*, 1955).

Table 46. Injection-site tumours in rats given poly(ethylene terephthalate) (Dacron) implants

Material	Thickness (mm)	No. of rats surviving minimal latent period	No. of local tumours (%)	Latent period (days)
Plain film	0.02	41	8 (19.5)	330–693
Perforated film	0.02	42	2 (4.8)	327–651
Textile	0.05	38	0 (0)	–

From Oppenheimer et al. (1955)

4B.6 Polyethylene

4B.6.1 *Subcutaneous administration*

Mouse: A group of albino mice (Paris strain) [initial number, sex and age unspecified] was given subcutaneous implants of a polyethylene film (0.002 mm thick); 3/28 survivors developed local sarcomas (Oppenheimer et al., 1952).

A group of albino (Longacre) mice [initial number, sex and age unspecified] was given subcutaneous implants of a pure, plain polyethylene film (15 mm diameter, 0.02 mm thick); 3/29 survivors developed malignant tumours at the site of implantation (Oppenheimer et al., 1955).

Two groups of 42 male and 45 female or 41 male and 32 female BALB/c An mice, 1–3 months of age, were given subcutaneous implants of commercial polyethylene discs (20 mm diameter, 0.38 mm thick) with either a smooth or roughened surface. The first sarcoma at the site of implantation was seen after 7.5 months, at which time the numbers of survivors in the two groups were 71 and 60 mice. The total number of sarcomas after 13 months was 35/71 in the mice given smooth discs and 7/60 in mice given roughened discs (Bates & Klein, 1966).

Rat: A group of 98 Wistar rats [sex and age unspecified] was given a subcutaneous implant of a commercial polyethylene film (0.002 mm thick); 10/80 survivors developed sarcomas, the first tumour appearing after 392 days. In rats given a polyethylene film without plasticizer, 5/40 developed local sarcomas. No local sarcomas developed in five control rats given implants of surgical cotton (Oppenheimer et al., 1952).

Groups of 25 male and 25 female Wistar or 25 male and 25 female Hisaw rats [age unspecified] were given implants of pure polyethylene film (20 × 15 mm) without plasticizer in the abdominal wall and over the skull; 8/63 developed fibrosarcomas after 434 or more days (two associated with cranial and six with abdominal implants). No such tumours occurred among 28 Hisaw controls subjected to sham operations (Bering et al., 1955).

Groups of Wistar rats [initial number, sex and age unspecified] were given subcutaneous implants of polyethylene film (15 mm diameter) of varying thicknesses and physical state. The incidence of malignant tumours at the site of implantation is summarized in Table 47. The minimal latent period was shorter with the plain films than with the perforated film or the textile (385 and 392 days versus 407 and 497 days, respectively) (Oppenheimer et al., 1955).

Table 47. Injection-site tumours in rats given implants of polyethylene

Type of polyethylene	Thickness (mm)	Effective no. of rats	No. of tumours (%)	Latent period (days)
Plain commercial film	0.05	80	10 (12.5)	392–722
Plain pure film	0.02	55	11 (20)	385–742
Perforated pure film	0.02	41	6 (14.6)	407–784
Textile	0.15	40	1 (2.5)	497
Plain film, high mol. wt	0.07	34	3 (8.8)	352–583
Powder	–	42	0 (0)	–

From Oppenheimer et al. (1955)

A group of 60 male and female Wistar rats (weighing 60 g) received a subcutaneous implant of a sheet of polyethylene measuring 4 × 5 × 0.16 mm and was observed for two years. At 300 days, 51 rats were still alive. No malignant tumour was found at the site of implantation (Russell et al., 1959). [The Working Group noted the small size of the film.]

A group of 90 Wistar rats [sex and age unspecified] was given subcutaneous implants of glass cover-slips (18 mm in diameter) into the left and right flanks. Four months later, in a group of 27 of these rats, polyethylene powder was inserted against the cover-slip on the right and glass powder against that on the left side. Five and six sarcomas developed, respectively, with mean latent periods of 570 and 547 days. In another group of 27 rats, the glass cover-slips were removed after four months and polyethylene powder was implanted into the empty pocket in one side and glass powder into the other; one sarcoma occurred on the side containing polyethylene and none on that containing glass powder. In a third group of 25 rats, the glass cover-slip on the right side was removed after four months and no sarcoma developed, whereas six sarcomas occurred on the left side in which the glass cover-slip was left in place, with a mean latent period of 503 days (Oppenheimer et al., 1961).

A group of 55 albino rats [sex and age unspecified] was given implants of polyethylene film (10 mm diameter) into the left abdominal subcutaneous tissue and of polyethylene mesh (10 mm diameter) on the right side. After 18–24 months, four sarcomas were found at 45 sites at which films had been implanted and one at 52 sites at which mesh had been implanted (Shulman et al., 1963).

Two groups of 20 male CB stock rats, eight weeks of age, were given subcutaneous implants of segments of polyethylene (620 mg) or a gelatin capsule containing 530 mg of the shredded plastic. Two groups of controls were given either a sham operation or empty gelatin capsules. All survivors were killed after 93 weeks. Six sarcomas and one squamous-cell carcinoma developed at the implantation sites in seven rats treated with the solid implants; five sarcomas occurred in rats given the capsules containing shredded polyethylene. No implantation site tumour occurred in sham-operated controls or controls given gelatin capsules (Carter & Roe, 1969).

Groups of male Wistar rats [age unspecified] had high-density polyethylene discs (18 mm diameter, 0.14 mm thick) inserted subcutaneously in the abdominal region. One group of 22 rats received the discs bilaterally and another group of 120 rats received the polyethylene disc on one side and a glass disc on the other. Surviving animals were killed after 39 months. Only 55 rats with either bilateral or a single polyethylene disc were subjected to pathological examination. Five fibrosarcomas were found at the site of implantation of polyethylene discs between 347 and 644 days after implantation, but no local tumours were associated with the glass discs (Lavorgna et al., 1972).

No local sarcomas were reported in a group of 11 male and 21 female Fischer 344 rats given subcutaneous implants of polyethylene powder (particle size, 425–600 µm) and observed for 100–118 weeks (Behling & Spector, 1986).

A group of 12 male Wistar rats, eight weeks of age, was given subcutaneous implants of two porous polyethylene blocks (5 × 10 × 15 mm; average pore size, 400 µm) and two collagen-immobilized porous polyethylene blocks of the same size into the left and right flanks, respectively. All rats were killed one year after implantation. Eleven tumours developed among the 24 sites of implantation with the polyethylene sample, while one tumour developed among the 24 sites of implantation with the collagen-immobilized polyethylene sample (Kinoshita et al., 1993).

A group of 50 male Wistar rats, 11 weeks of age, was given subcutaneous implants of medical grade polyethylene film (20 × 10 × 1 mm); 21/41 survivors developed malignant tumours at the site of implantation during the 24-month experimental period. Most of the tumours were diagnosed as fibrosarcomas, and the minimal latency period was 320 days. No such tumour occurred among 30 controls subjected to sham operations (Nakamura et al., 1994).

Hamster: A group of 50 hamsters [sex and strain unspecified], one month of age, was given subcutaneous implants of polyethylene film (squares of 20 × 20 mm); two survived more than 442 days. Both developed tumours at the site of implantation, which were diagnosed as a malignant mesenchymal tumour and a fibrosarcoma, after 442 and 457 days, respectively (Bering & Handler, 1957). [The Working Group noted the poor survival.]

4B.6.2 *Intraperitoneal administration*

Rat: Four groups of 30 female Bethesda black rats, three months of age, were given intraperitoneal implants of polyethylene cubes (3.5 × 3.5 × 3 mm), discs (12 mm diameter), rolled film (10 × 1.75 cm) or powder (65 mg) and were observed for up to 24 months. Sarcomas associated with the implant were found in 6/25 rats given rolled film, in 0/25 rats given cubes and in 1/22 rats given discs. In rats given polyethylene powder, multicystic foreign-body granulomas of the serosal surface of the liver, kidney, spleen and anterior abdominal wall were observed (Hueper, 1961).

Two groups of 20 and 19 male and female Wistar rats, weighing 55–75 g, were given implants of polyethylene rods (10 × 2 × 2 mm) or powder into the peritoneal cavity, respectively. No local tumours developed; 11 and five rats in the two groups survived up to 800 days (Simmers et al., 1963).

A group of 38 male and 36 female Bethesda black rats, three months of age, was given intraperitoneal implants of particles of polyethylene (> 3 mm diameter, weighing 1.5 g). Within two years, 24 males developed intraperitoneal fibrosarcomas and five other [unspecified] tumours, and 19 females developed intraperitoneal fibrosarcomas and one other [unspecified] tumour. The incidence of local tumours in control male rats was 0/37 and that in female controls was 1/37 (Autian et al., 1975). [The Working Group noted that incomplete pathology data were reported.]

4B.6.3   *Other experimental systems*

Combined subcutaneous and intraperitoneal implantation: A group of 23 BD rats [sex and age unspecified] was given subcutaneous and intraperitoneal implants of polyethylene film; among the 14 rats still alive at the time of appearance of the first tumour (15 months), eight developed subcutaneous sarcomas and one developed an intraperitoneal fibroma (Druckrey & Schmähl, 1954).

Intraosseous implantation: A group of 13 male and 13 female Sprague-Dawley rats [age unspecified] was given implants of ultra-high molecular weight polyethylene cylinders (1.8 mm diameter, 4.0 mm length) placed into a drill hole through the lateral cortex of the left distal femur. No local tumour was found. One case of myeloid leukaemia occurred among the effective number of 24 rats during the 23-month observation period, an incidence similar to that of spontaneously occurring tumours. A similar group of 13 males and 13 females was given implants of 4.8 mg polyethylene in powder form (particle size, 10–383 μm); no local tumour was found (Memoli et al., 1986).

4B.7   Polypropylene

4B.7.1   *Subcutaneous administration*

Rat: A group of 70 E3 rats [sex and age not specified] was given subcutaneous implants of eight polypropylene discs (20 mm diameter, 2 mm thick). The experiment was terminated after 14 months, when 35 animals were still alive. A total of 55 local fibrosarcomas were produced, the first appearing after seven months. In another group of 60 rats, which was given a total of 480 implants, the discs were removed eight months after the implantation. The experiment was terminated at 14 months, when 41 animals were still alive. Two fibrosarcomas were observed at the ninth month, and 32 further local tumours were detected during the following five months (Vollmar & Ott, 1961). [The Working Group noted that no controls were included in these experiments.]

A group of 67 rats [sex, strain and age unspecified] was given a combination of implantation of discs (a total of 536 implants) and X-irradiation (3 × 200 rad, two to three weeks after implantation) which led to reduced survival. When the experiment was terminated after 14 months, a total of 34 local tumours had been found and 18 animals were still alive. After implantation of a total of 560 samples of polypropylene powder to 70 rats, the first local fibrosarcoma was found at 11 months. When the experiment was terminated after 14 months, four rats had developed local sarcomas and 35 were still alive (Vollmar & Ott, 1961). [The Working Group noted that no controls were included in these experiments.]

A group of 20 male Wistar rats, six weeks of age, was given subcutaneous implants of a thin polypropylene film (15 × 15 × 0.1 mm). No local tumour was found among 18 animals that survived for more than 11 months, during a 28-month observation period (Imai & Watanabe, 1987).

A group of 50 Wistar male rats [age unspecified] was given subcutaneous implants of a medical-grade polypropylene film (20 × 10 × 1 mm); 17/50 survivors developed malignant tumours at the site of implantation during the 24-month experimental period. Most of the tumours were diagnosed as malignant fibrous histiocytoma, and the latency period was 512 ± 133 days. One fibroma occurred among 50 sham-operated controls (Nakamura et al., 1997).

4B.8   Polytetrafluoroethylene

4B.8.1   *Subcutaneous administration*

Mouse: A group of 89 random-bred female Swiss mice, 7–9 weeks of age, was given a subcutaneous implant in the left flank of a polytetrafluoroethylene (PTFE) sheet (12 × 12 × 1.2 mm). The first local tumour developed 25 weeks after implantation; a total of 11 (12.5%) fibrosarcomas were found after an average latent period of 54.5 weeks (Tomatis & Shubik, 1963). [The Working Group noted that since the implant was not retained in nine mice and since 70 mice were still alive at the appearance of the first tumour, the effective tumour incidence was 16%.]

Groups of random-bred Swiss mice, 7–9 weeks of age, were given a subcutaneous implant of a PTFE sheet (12 × 12 × 1.2 mm) (89 females and 61 males), a 15-mm diameter PTFE disc (103 females), a Teflon fragment corresponding to one disc [size not specified] (53 females) or a 20-mm diameter PTFE disc (54 females and 50 males). Tumours developed around the implant in 8/89 (10%) and 1/61 (2%), 23/103 (22.7%), 10/53 (21.2%) and 7/54 (15.2%) and 4/50 (8%) mice in the above groups, respectively. No similar tumours were seen in 200 and 100 untreated female and male mice. Of 50 female mice given implanted glass coverslips (12 × 12 × 1.2 mm), six developed sarcomas (13.6%) and of 48 females given implants of fragments of glass corresponding to one sheet, two developed sarcomas (4.3%). The average latent period for gross, palpable tumours was 55 weeks, with two tumours appearing as early as week 25 and nine at 65 weeks after implantation. All neoplasms were fibrosarcomas, and some had angiosarcomatous areas (Tomatis, 1963).

A group of 19 male and 27 female inbred C57BL mice, 7–9 weeks of age, was given subcutaneous implants of PTFE discs (15 mm diameter, 1.2 mm thick). At 50 weeks, 13 males and 13 females were still alive. Among 20 females that retained the implant and were considered to be at risk, four developed local sarcomas at weeks 39, 47, 52 and 58, and four local sarcomas were found in the 15 males considered to be at risk (26%) at weeks 49, 51, 60 and 91. Mice were observed for 90 weeks, at which time only three males and three females were still alive. Tumours always occurred around the discs; one sarcoma tested was found to be transplantable in syngeneic mice. Tumours unrelated to the implant developed in three females and one male. In a control group of 30 male and 33 female mice without implants that were observed for 100 weeks, no subcutaneous sarcoma was found; three females and two males developed spontaneous tumours (Tomatis, 1966b).

A group of 40 male and 40 female random-bred CTM albino mice, eight weeks of age, was given subcutaneous implants into the right flank of PTFE discs (15 mm diameter, 1.2 mm thick) and were observed for lifespan; 18 females and nine males developed sarcomas around the disc, giving a total incidence of 38% of the 69 mice still alive at the time of the appearance of the first tumour. Average ages of tumour-bearing animals at death were 72 and 69 weeks for females and males, respectively. No subcutaneous fibrosarcoma was found in 99 male and 98 female control mice of the same strain observed for lifespan (Tomatis & Parmi, 1971).

Three groups of 38, 38 and 39 female BALB/c, C3Hf/Dp and C57BL/He mice, 6–7 weeks of age, received subcutaneous implants of PTFE discs (15 mm diameter, 1.2 mm thick) in the dorsal area. Fibrosarcomas developed around the discs in 17/38 (44%) BALB/c, 36/38 (94%) C3Hf/Dp and 12/39 (30%) C57BL/He mice, within mean latent periods of 78, 61 and 82 weeks, respectively. All surviving mice were killed at 120 weeks of age. Of the 56 tumours examined histologically, two were rhabdomyosarcomas and the rest were fibrosarcomas (Menard & Della Porta, 1976). [The Working Group noted that the incidence of tumours was calculated on the basis of the number of mice treated initially.]

Rat: Two groups of Wistar rats [initial numbers, sex and age unspecified] were given subcutaneous implants of PTFE discs (15 mm diameter, 0.02 mm thick) in the abdominal wall; in one group, the discs were perforated. The numbers of rats that survived the minimum latent period were 34 and 32 for the groups implanted with plain and perforated discs, respectively. Eight sarcomas (23.5%) were observed in the first group and six sarcomas (18.7%) in the second group (Oppenheimer *et al.*, 1955).

A group of 65 weanling male and female Wistar rats was given single subcutaneous implants of PTFE film (4 × 5 × 0.16 mm) in the abdominal wall; 55 rats were still alive after 300 days and 45 at the time of appearance of the first tumour (659 days). All rats were killed within 800 days. Two subcutaneous sarcomas were found; no tumour was observed in 20 control animals given glass implants of the same size, which survived 300 days and were observed for a similar period of time (Russell *et al.*, 1959). [The Working Group noted the small size of the film.]

A group of 39 male Evans rats [age unspecified] was given subcutaneous implants of PTFE mesh surgical outflow patches (20 × 10 mm). A further 40 rats were given implants of the shredded material, and 41 rats without implants served as controls. The experiment was terminated 19 months later, and no local tumours were observed; at that time, 28 controls and 24 and 23 PTFE-implanted rats were still alive (Bryson & Bischoff, 1969).

A group of 50 Sprague-Dawley rats [age unspecified] was given 0.1 mL of Polytef by subcutaneous injection. The Polytef consisted of 50% PTFE particles of which 90% were < 40 µm in diameter; the remainder of the injection was a glycerol carrier, with a small amount of polysorbate. The animals were observed for two years. Of the 48 injected animals examined, 30 (63%) had one or more tumours: breast adenomas or fibrosarcomas (7/15), pituitary adenomas (18), breast adenocarcinomas (4), lymphoma (1), ovarian tumours (2), uterine carcinoma (1), and a hepatocellular carcinoma (1), respectively, but there was no significant difference in the total number of tumours or in the number of breast and pituitary tumours between the treated group and an untreated control group. No tumours were found in the region of the injection site (Dewan *et al.*, 1995).

4B.8.2 *Intraperitoneal administration*

Rat: Groups of male and female weanling Wistar rats were given intraperitoneal implants of PTFE rods (10 × 2 × 2 mm; 16 rats) or equivalent amounts of PTFE powder (17 rats). After 365 days, 13/16 and 10/17 animals were still alive in the two groups, respectively; after 800 days, 9/16 and 3/17 animals were still alive. Surviving animals were killed 27 months after implantation. No local tumours were found in rats with rod implants, whereas two sarcomas became palpable in the powder-treated animals at 354 and 476 days after implantation. Extraperitoneal tumours included one fibrosarcoma in the inguinal region in a rat with a rod implant and one liposarcoma in the upper part of the leg, one fibrosarcoma in the shoulder and one inguinal fibroadenoma in powder-treated rats. Among 25 untreated controls, one adenoma of the testis and a possible carcinoma in the inguinal region were observed (Simmers *et al.*, 1963).

4B.9 Polyamide (nylon)

4B.9.1 *Subcutaneous administration*

Rat: Groups of male Wistar rats [initial number and age unspecified] were given subcutaneous implants of discs (15 mm diameter) of a material described as nylon in various physical forms. The incidence of malignant tumours at the site of implantation is given in Table 48 (Oppenheimer *et al.*, 1955).

4B.9.2 *Intraperitoneal administration*

Rat: A group of nine BD rats [sex and age unspecified] was given intraperitoneal implants of five films of polycaprolactam (Nylon 6; about 10 mm diameter). Four out of six rats which survived for 360 days had local sarcomas (Druckrey & Schmähl, 1952).

Table 48. Injection-site tumours in rats given polyamide (nylon) implants

Material	Thickness (mm)	No. of rats surviving minimal latent period	No. of local tumours (%)	Latent period (days)
Plain film	0.06	26	7 (27.0)	441–651
Perforated film	0.06	31	2 (6.5)	551–738
Textile	0.08	33	0 (0)	–

From Oppenheimer *et al.* (1955)

4B.10 Poly(glycolic acid)

4B.10.1 *Subcutaneous administration*

Rat: A group of 50 male Wistar rats [age unspecified] was given subcutaneous implants of poly(glycolic acid) film (20 × 10 × 1 mm) that was completely absorbed in the animal body within two months. All animals survived to 24 months, and one developed a fibrosarcoma at the site of implantation with a latency period of 704 days. One fibroma developed among 50 sham-operated controls (Nakamura *et al.*, 1997).

4B.11 Polylactide

4B.11.1 *Subcutaneous administration*

Rat: A group of 50 male Wistar rats, 11 weeks of age, was given subcutaneous implants of purified poly-L-lactide (PLLA) sheets (20 × 20 × 1 mm); 20/41 survivors developed malignant tumours at the site of implantation during the 24-month experimental period. Most of the tumours were diagnosed as fibrosarcomas, and the minimal latency period was 320 days. No such tumour occurred among 30 controls subjected to sham operations. The degradation of PLLA during implantation was slow, the sheets remaining at their initial size at 24 months. However, in a separate group of 15 rats, the average molecular weight of explanted PLLA sheets determined at six-month intervals decreased with time: 253 000 (initial), 49 700 (six months), 45 000 (12 months), 34 800 (18 months) and 21 200 (24 months) (Nakamura *et al.*, 1994).

4B.12 ε-Caprolactone–L-lactide copolymer

4B.12.1 *Subcutaneous administration*

Rat: A group of 50 male Wistar rats, 11 weeks of age, was given subcutaneous implants of ε-caprolactone–L-lactide copolymer sheets (20 × 20 × 1 mm) and observed for two years. Twenty-five local tumours were found at the site of implantation during the experimental period, including 16 fibrosarcomas, seven osteosarcomas, and two malignant fibrous histiocytomas. One fibrosarcoma and one osteosarcoma were found at the site of implantation in a sham-operated control group. The in-vivo degradation of the polymer is discussed in Section 5B.1.2(*d*) of this monograph (Nakamura *et al.*, 1998).

4B.13 Polystyrene and related polymers
4B.13.1 *Subcutaneous administration*

Rat: A group of 30 Wistar rats [sex and age unspecified] was given subcutaneous implants of polystyrene film (15 × 15 mm, 0.01 mm thick). Twenty-seven animals were still alive at the time of appearance of the first tumour, among which seven sarcomas developed at the site of implantation (25.9%) within latent periods ranging from 359 to 556 days (Oppenheimer *et al.*, 1955). The same authors studied the effect of continued presence or removal of the polystyrene implants on tumour formation (Oppenheimer *et al.*, 1958) (see Section 5B.4.2).

Groups of Wistar rats [initial number, sex and age unspecified] were given subcutaneous implants of polystyrene of different physical forms. The incidence of sarcomas observed at the site of implantation is given in Table 49 (Nothdurft, 1956).

Table 49. Injection-site tumours in rats given implants of polystyrene

Form	Effective no. of rats	No. of tumour-bearing rats (%)
Smooth discs (17 mm diameter)	47	37 (78.7)
Perforated discs	51	25 (49.0)
Rods, spheres, fibres	40	15 (37.5)
Powder	Not reported	0 (0)

From Nothdurft (1956)

Groups of 25 Wistar rats from three different sources, 3–4 months of age, were given subcutaneous implants of discs (1.45 cm diameter, 0.026 mm thick) and perforated rings (central hole, 6 mm) of polystyrene. Differences were found in the incidence of local sarcomas (8–48%) according to the source of rats (Wistar E being the most sensitive), but no appreciable difference was found between rings and discs (Rivière *et al.*, 1960).

Polystyrene materials having anionic, cationic and neutral properties were prepared by coprecipitation of two oppositely charged linear polyelectrolytes—a cationic polymer, poly(vinylbenzyltrimethylammonium) chloride, and sodium poly(styrene sulfonate). The anionic material (A) had an excess polyanion content of 0.5 meq/g of dry resin, the cationic material (B) had an excess polycation content of 0.5 meq/g of dry resin, and the neutral material (C) contained equivalent parts of polyanion and polycation. Three groups of 16 male CB Wistar rats, six to eight weeks of age, were given film implants of these materials (A, B and C; 20 × 20 mm) subcutaneously, while a further 16 rats (group D) were not given plastic implants but incisions were made, and these groups of rats were observed for 92 weeks, when only three rats remained alive. Three, nine and one local tumours occurred in groups

A, B, and C, respectively, while no local tumour was found in group D (Carter *et al.*, 1971).

4B.14 Poly(vinyl alcohol)

4B.14.1 *Subcutaneous administration*

Rat: Male Wistar rats [number and age unspecified] were given subcutaneous implants of poly(vinyl alcohol) (Ivalon) sponge of unspecified size into the abdominal wall and were observed for lifespan. Three local sarcomas were found in 34 animals still alive at the appearance of the first local sarcoma at 567 days (Oppenheimer *et al.*, 1955).

A group of 25 Bethesda black rats [sex and age unspecified] was given subcutaneous implants of single doses of 500 mg per animal of poly(vinyl alcohol) powder (molecular weight, 120 000) and was observed for up to two years. No local tumours were seen, but three benign and six malignant tumours at various sites were observed in treated rats, and three benign and 17 malignant tumours were found among 200 controls (Hueper, 1959).

A group of 25 male and female Wistar rats [age unspecified] was given subcutaneous implantations of poly(vinyl alcohol) sponges (4 × 5 × 0.16 mm) into the abdominal tissues; 21 animals survived 300 days. All animals had died or were killed within 800 days. Multiple sections were taken from each implantation site, but no local tumour was detected (Russell *et al.*, 1959).

Groups of 20 Chester Beatty rats [sex unspecified], 70 days of age, were given subcutaneous implants of thick (20 × 20 × 5 mm) and thin (20 × 20 × 2 mm) poly(vinyl alcohol) (Ivalon) sponges into the right flank. Fourteen of the rats with implanted thick sponges lived 10 months or longer and developed local sarcomas, whereas only one of the rats bearing thin sponges had a local sarcoma among 18 rats that lived 12 months or longer (Dukes & Mitchley, 1962).

Groups of male Holtzman rats [number unspecified], 5–6 weeks of age, were given two subcutaneous implants of poly(vinyl alcohol) (Ivalon) sponges (20 mm diameter, 3–4 mm thick). Local sarcomas were found in 9/12 rats (75%) that lived for at least 18 months (only one animal had tumours at both implanted sites) (Dasler & Milliser, 1963).

A group of 39 albino rats [sex and age unspecified] was given subcutaneous implants of poly(vinyl alcohol) (Ivalon) sponges (20 × 20 × 5 mm) into the tissue of the back. Twenty rats were killed at intervals from two days to one year; the remaining 19 were kept until they died or were killed at 29 months. Local tumours developed in three rats (two sarcomas and one fibroma or low-grade fibrosarcoma) (Walter & Chiaramonte, 1965).

The possible role of the thickness of sponge implants was investigated in groups of male Chester Beatty rats, eight weeks of age, that were given subcutaneous implants of poly(vinyl alcohol) (Prosthex) (20 × 20 × 5 mm (2 cm^3) or 33 × 33 × 2 mm (2 cm^3)) into the right flank. Of those given the thicker implant, 9/24 developed local sarcomas, whereas only 1/24 with the thinner implants developed a local sarcoma. In addition, five sarcomas arose in 24 rats with 12.6 × 12.6 × 5 mm (800 mm³) implants, and only 1/24 in animals with 20 × 20 × 2 (800 mm³) implants and 1/24 with 8 × 8 × 5 mm (320 mm³) implants. The incidence of local sarcomas in inbred Woodruff hooded rats given 20 × 20 × 5 mm (2 cm³) implants of Prosthex was similar to that in the Chester Beatty rats (12/24). The experiment lasted 800 days (Roe et al., 1967).

A group of 50 male Wistar rats [age unspecified] was given subcutaneous implants of poly(vinyl alcohol) hydrogel (water content, 80%) film (20 × 10 × 1 mm); 22/50 survivors developed malignant tumours at the site of implantation during the 24-month experimental period. Most of the tumours that developed were diagnosed as malignant fibrous histiocytomas and the latency period was 568 ± 89 days. One fibroma developed among 50 controls subjected to sham operations (Nakamura et al., 1997).

4B.15 Poly(vinyl chloride)

4B.15.1 *Subcutaneous administration*

Rat: A group of 45 Wistar rats [sex and age unspecified] was given subcutaneous implants in the abdominal wall of squares or discs (0.04 mm thick and 15 mm wide) of a commercial poly(vinyl chloride) (PVC) sheet known to contain some additives. At the appearance of the first tumour, 44 animals were still alive. In 17 (38.6%), malignant tumours (fibrosarcomas and one liposarcoma) developed at the site of film implantation, with a latent period of 189–727 days; a similar but perforated film did not produce local tumours in 27 rats at risk. No local tumour was found in a group of 50 rats given a subcutaneous implant of cotton (Oppenheimer et al., 1952, 1955). In a similar group of rats, subcutaneous implants of a pure PVC film (0.03 mm thick) produced four malignant tumours at the implantation site after 533 days (Oppenheimer et al., 1955). [The Working Group noted that the reporting of this experiment was preliminary and that final results were never published.]

Three groups of Wistar rats [initial number, sex and age unspecified] were given subcutaneous implants of a PVC disc (17 mm diameter [thickness unspecified]), perforated discs of the same diameter or a powder form [particle size unspecified] and observed for 23 months. The total number of sarcomas at the site of implantation was 75/95 (79%) surviving rats given unperforated discs and 33/76 (43%) rats given perforated discs, whereas no tumour was found in rats given powder (Nothdurft, 1956).

A group of 35 male and female Wistar rats, weighing 60 g, was given a subcutaneous implant of PVC film (4 × 5 × 0.16 mm) into the abdomen. A group of 25 control rats received an implant of glass of similar size. After 300 days, 30 and 20 animals were still alive in the two groups, respectively; all surviving rats were killed 800 days after implantation. One sarcoma and one fibroma were found after 580 days in the PVC-treated rats, whereas no local tumour developed in the control group (Russell et al., 1959). [The Working Group noted the small size of the film.]

Groups of 20 male and 20 female Wistar rats [age unspecified] were given subcutaneous implants of three kinds of plasticized polyvinyl chloride film from different suppliers (PVC-1, PVC-2 and PVC-3; 10 × 20 × < 1 mm). Tumour incidence at the site of implantation during the two-year test period was 3/17 males and 5/20 females for PVC-1, 5/15 males and 6/20 females for PVC-2 and 8/18 males and 13/20 females for PVC-3. All tumours were diagnosed as malignant fibrous histiocytomas. No local tumours occurred in 12 male and 12 female untreated controls (Maekawa et al., 1984).

4B.15.2 *Other routes of administration*

In 37 male and female albino rats, weighing 120–150 g at the beginning of the study, the right kidney was wrapped in PVC film, following a method developed to induce renal hypertension. Five of 16 rats that survived more than seven months developed sarcomas at the site, four within 7–11.5 months and one after 19 months. Unperforated PVC sheets, 1 mm thick, were implanted near the kidney in 20 other rats; sarcomas developed in 2/5 rats that survived 16–18 months. Perforated PVC sheets were implanted near the kidney in 15 rats; a sarcoma developed in 1/4 rats that survived to 17–18 months after implantation (Kogan & Tugarinova, 1959).

A group of 80 outbred albino rats [sex and age unspecified] was given implants of PVC film [size unspecified] by laparotomy to surround the kidney. The animals were killed at 3, 10, 15, 30, 90, 195, 285, 300 and 380 days after implantation. Of rats that survived 285–375 days, 6/16 developed fibrosarcomas at the site of implantation (Raikhlin & Kogan, 1961).

4B.16 Vinyl chloride–vinyl acetate copolymer

4B.16.1 *Subcutaneous administration*

Mouse: A group of CBA/H-T6 mice including males and females, 1.5–2 months of age, was given subcutaneous implants into each flank of vinyl chloride–vinyl acetate copolymer coverslips (15 × 22 × 0.2 mm). Sarcomas at the site of implantation developed in 65% of the males within 9–12 months and in almost all of the females after 7–12 months. A control group of 80 mice with no implant developed no subcutaneous tumours (Brand et al., 1967a). [The Working Group noted the limited reporting.]

Groups of CBA mice [initial number, sex and age unspecified] were given subcutaneous implants of smooth or roughened films of unplasticized vinyl chloride–vinyl acetate copolymer (15 × 22 × 0.2 mm). When film with a smooth surface was implanted, the first tumour was seen after nine months and the total number of tumour-bearing animals at the site of implantation was 52/53; with the roughened surface, 8/26 mice developed tumours after 16 months (Brand et al., 1975b).

A group of 30 male and 46 female CBA mice, six weeks of age, were given subcutaneous implants of vinyl chloride–vinyl acetate copolymer powder (particle size, 50–100 µm; corresponding by weight to two films of 15 × 22 × 0.2 mm) and were observed until death. No treatment-related tumour was reported; however, one sarcoma found in a female was attributed by the authors to clumping of the powder (Brand et al., 1975c).

Groups of 9–124 male and female mice of 18 strains [age unspecified] were given subcutaneous implants of vinyl chloride–vinyl acetate copolymer films (15 × 22 × 0.2 mm or 7 × 15 × 0.2 mm) to test strain differences in response. The incidence of tumours was 90–100% in CBA/H and CBA/H-T6 female mice, AKR/J males, BALB/cJ and BALB/c Wat females, C57BL/10ScSn females and (C57BL/10ScSc × CBA/H)F$_1$ males and females. No tumour was induced in males of strain I/LnJ or strain SJL/J. The tumour incidence in other strains was intermediate, the males being less sensitive than females, except for AKR mice (Brand et al., 1977).

Further extensive experiments on factors affecting tumour formation after implantation of vinyl chloride–vinyl acetate copolymer films are described in Sections 5B.4.3 and 5B.4.4.

4B.17 Cellophane

4B.17.1 *Subcutaneous administration*

Mouse: Two groups of male albino [Longacre] and C57BL mice [age unspecified] were given subcutaneous implants of a commercial cellophane film (15 mm diameter and 0.04 mm thick); 8/35 and 1/22 survivors developed local sarcomas at the site of implantation within 245–498 and 369 days, respectively (Oppenheimer et al., 1952, 1955).

Rat: A group of 55 male Sherman and/or Wistar rats, 8–10 months of age, was given subcutaneous implants in the abdominal wall of cellophane films (20–30 mm^2). The shortest latent period for development of a local tumour was 471 days, and 42 animals survived beyond this period; among these, 15 (35.7%) developed tumours at the site of implantation (Oppenheimer et al., 1948).

Groups of male Wistar rats [initial number and age unspecified] were given subcutaneous implants of cellophane films (15 mm in diameter) of various qualities and physical states. The incidences of malignant tumours found at the site of implantation and the ranges of latent periods are summarized in Table 50 (Oppenheimer et al., 1955). The same authors studied the effect of continued presence or removal of the cellophane implants on tumour formation (Oppenheimer et al., 1964) (see section 5B.4.2).

A group of 35 male and female Wistar rats (weighing 60 g) [sex unspecified] was given a subcutaneous implant of a square sheet of cellophane film measuring 4 × 5 × 0.16 mm and was observed for two years. At 300 days, 30 rats were still alive. No malignant tumour was found at the site of implantation within two years (Russell et al., 1959). [The Working Group noted the small size of the film.]

Four groups of rats [initial numbers, strain, sex and age unspecified] were given subcutaneous implants of ground cellophane (< 0.1 cm) and a cellophane film of different sizes (10 × 30 mm, 20 × 30 mm and 70 × 25 mm) and were observed for one year. No tumours associated with the implant were found among 144 rats treated with ground cellophane, whereas the incidences of tumours at the implantation site were 6/184 (3.2%), 6/36 (16.6%) and 5/30 (16.6%) for the 10 × 30 mm, 20 × 30 mm and 70 × 25 mm films, respectively. Among the 17 tumours that appeared, nine were

Table 50. Injection-site tumours in rats given cellulose films

Type of cellophane	Thickness (mm)	Effective no. of rats	No. (%) of local tumours	Latent period (days)
A. Commercial sausage casing	0.04	42	15 (35.7)	495–779
B. Type A after extraction with alcohol for 3 days	0.04	44	20 (45.4)	322–665
C. Type B after additional extraction with benzene	0.04	39	18 (46.1)	390–706
D. A special form employed for tissue culture	0.01	19	3 (15.8)	423–521
E. Type D perforated	0.01	22	4 (18.2)	504–594

From Oppenheimer et al. (1955)

polymorphocellular sarcomas, four were spindle-cell sarcomas, one was a fibrosarcoma, one a giant-cell sarcoma and one an osteoblastic tumour (Ol'shevskaya, 1962). [The Working Group noted the short period of observation.]

Groups of 60–290 male rats, weighing 100–120 g, [strain and age unspecified] were given subcutaneous implants of a commercial cellophane film (Cellophane N55; 1 mm thick) of different sizes or 50–100 cut pieces of about 1–2 mm in diameter. The incidence of local tumours is summarized in Table 51. The first tumour appeared 10 months after implantation (Vasiliev et al., 1962).

Table 51. Injection-site tumours in rats given cellulose films

Film size (mm)	No. of rats per group	Effective no. of rats	No. of local tumours	%
Cut pieces	200	180	0	0
10 × 30	290	184	56	30
20 × 30	67	48	29	60
70 × 20[a]	60	24	11	46

[a] Before implantation, each film was folded in half
From Vasiliev et al. (1962)

4B.17.2 *Other experimental systems*

Rat: The left kidney of a group of 55 male Sherman and/or Wistar rats, 8–10 months of age, was wrapped loosely with cellophane film and animals were observed. The shortest time for appearance of a tumour was 362 days from the date of wrapping, and the total number of rats that developed local tumours was 8/23 that survived over 11 months (Oppenheimer et al., 1948).

4B.18 Millipore filters

4B.18.1 *Subcutaneous administration*

Mouse: In a study reported as an abstract, groups of Swiss albino mice [initial numbers, sex and age unspecified] were given subcutaneous implants of Millipore filters [diameter unspecified] of different pore sizes and were observed for 18 months. The total incidence of tumours was 21/35 (60%) for the group given implants of 0.05 µm pore size, 18/34 (53%) for 0.10 µm pore size and 2/39 (5%) for 0.45 µm pore size. One year after implantation of a solid Millipore filter without any pores, tumours were found in 11/33 (33%) animals, while with a solid Plexiglas (poly(methyl methacrylate)) disc and with a Millipore filter of the same diameter with 0.05 µm pores, tumours were found in 14/41 (34.1%) and 18/39 (46.1%) of the animals, respectively (Goldhaber, 1962).

A group of female 93 CBA mice [age unspecified] was given subcutaneous implants of hydrophilic Millipore filter discs (20 mm diameter; eight different pore sizes ranging from 0.025 to 8.0 µm) and the animals were observed until death. The incidence of sarcomas is summarized in Table 52. The latency of the tumours was 7–27 months (Karp *et al.*, 1973).

[The Working Group noted that the exact chemical compositions of the various Millipore filters were not specified.]

Table 52. Tumour incidence in mice given implants of Millipore filters with a range of pore sizes

Pore size (µm)	No. of tumours/no. of implanted animals
0.025	11/11
0.05	6/10
0.10	8/10
0.22	0/9
0.45	0/9
0.45[a]	0/9
0.80	0/9
3.0	0/9
3.0[a]	1/8
8.0	0/9

[a] Millipore filter reinforced with nylon microweb material
From Karp *et al.* (1973)

4B.18.2 *Intraperitoneal administration*

Mouse: A group of male and female BALB/c AnN mice, 4–8 weeks of age, was given intraperitoneal implants of two Millipore filter discs (14 and 17.5 mm diameter) [pore size unspecified]. Four of 30 mice developed sarcomas at the site of implantation (Merwin & Redmon, 1963).

4B.19 Epoxy resins

4B.19.1 *Subcutaneous administration*

Rat: A group of 22 male Wistar rats (weighing 175–200 g) was given subcutaneous implants of an epoxy resin disc (prepared from triglycidyl *para*-aminophenol and a curing agent, nonylphenol and aminoethylpiperazine; 18 mm diameter and 0.14 mm thick) bilaterally on both sides of the abdomen, while another group of 24 rats received the epoxy resin disc and a glass coverslip of the same size on each side of the abdomen. After 39 months, the survivors were killed and examined. None of the effective number of 27 rats developed tumours (Lavorgna *et al.*, 1972).

4B.20 Aluminium oxide ceramics

4B.20.1 *Subcutaneous administration*

Rat: Five groups of male Sprague-Dawley rats, weighing 220 g at the start of treatment, received subcutaneous implants of various forms of an aluminium oxide ceramic (99.6% pure). Group 1 (33 rats) each received eight discs (20 mm diameter, 3 mm thick) implanted subcutaneously; Group 2 (27 rats) each received eight discs of the same size but perforated with 13 1-mm holes; Group 3 (21 rats) each received four porous discs of the same size (pores, 200–400 µm); Group 4 (47 rats) each received aluminium oxide powder [amount and particle size unspecified]; and Group 5 (22 rats) served as sham-operated controls. Sarcomas occurred between nine and 21 months, as shown in Table 53 (Griss *et al.*, 1977).

4B.21 Glass sheet

4B.21.1 *Subcutaneous administration*

In some experiments investigating the carcinogenicity of plastic films by subcutaneous administration, glass sheet was also investigated, often as a control.

Mouse: In Swiss mice, 6/42 effective animals implanted with glass sheet (12 × 12 × 1.2 mm) developed local sarcomas within 90 weeks (Tomatis, 1963). [The Working Group noted that there was no control group of untreated animals.]

Rat: In three experiments using 50 albino, 25 Wistar and 22 Wistar rats given implants of glass discs (18 × 0.2 mm), glass sheets (4 × 5 × 0.16 mm) or glass discs (18 mm diameter, 0.4 mm thick), 0/23, 0/20 and 0/22 surviving rats developed local sarcomas. Observation times were 12–14 months, 300 days and 39 months, respectively (Oppenheimer *et al.*, 1952; Russell *et al.*, 1959; Lavorgna *et al.*, 1972).

Table 53. Injection-site tumours in rats treated with aluminium oxide ceramics

Material	No. of rats	No. of implants	Sarcomas/ no. of animals with sarcoma	Discs with sarcoma (%)
Solid disc	33	264	46/32	17.4
Perforated disc	27	216	55/27	25.4
Porous disc	21	84	16/16	17
Powder	47		0/0	0
Control	22		0/0	0

From Griss et al. (1977)

4B.22 Major factors that affect tumour incidence

4B.22.1 Physical factors

(a) Size (surface area) of the implant

Based upon observations from several studies reported above, it is evident that, following implantation into the tissues of rodents, large films induced more sarcomas than small ones.

Rats that received subcutaneous implants of cellophane films of different sizes developed local tumours (6/184 (3.2%) for 10 × 30 mm film, 6/36 (16.6%) for 20 × 30 mm film and 5/30 (16.6%) for 70 × 25 mm film), while cellophane powder did not produce local tumours (Ol'shevskaya, 1962). Similar results were obtained in another study in rats with cellophane film (56/184 (30%) for 10 × 30 mm film, 29/48 (60%) for 20 × 30 mm film and 11/24 (46%) for doubly folded 70 × 20 mm film), while no local tumour was found for cut pieces (Vasiliev et al., 1962). Following intramuscular implantation of poly(methyl methacrylate) discs of various sizes into rats, the incidences of local tumours were 0/142, 17/142 (12%) and 34/142 (24%) for discs of 4, 12 and 18 mm diameter, respectively (Stinson, 1964). Vinyl chloride–vinyl acetate copolymer films, 7 × 15 or 15 × 22 mm, were implanted subcutaneously into female CBA/H or CBA/H-T6 mice. Local tumour incidences over a 30-month observation period were 63.5 and 95%, respectively (Brand et al., 1973). In another experiment designed to determine dose (surface area)-related tumour incidences, different numbers of polyurethane discs of 3.1 mm in diameter were implanted intraperitoneally into rats to give doses of 93.8, 187.5, 375, 750 and 1500 mg per rat. The local tumour incidences were 0, 1, 2, 8 and 24 for the five groups, respectively (Autian et al., 1976).

(b) Continuity

The following incidences of tumours were found in rats at the site of subcutaneous implantation with plain, perforated and textile films of four polymeric materials of 15 mm diameter: polyester (Dacron): 8/41 (19.5%), 2/42 (4.8%) and 0%, respectively;

polyethylene: 11/55 (20%), 6/41 (14.6%) and 1/40 (2.5%); polyamide (Nylon): 7/26 (27.0%), 2/31 (6.5%) and 0%; and polytetrafluoroethylene: 8/34 (23.5%), 6/32 (18.7%) and no data, respectively; a polyethylene powder of the corresponding weight produced no local tumour (Oppenheimer et al., 1955). Another study of subcutaneous implantation of polyethylene film and mesh into rats gave incidences of 4/45 (8.9%) and 1/52 (1.9%), respectively (Shulman et al., 1963). In the case of polystyrene, the following incidences were observed: 37/47 (78.7%) for smooth discs (17 mm in diameter), 25/51 (49.0%) for perforated discs, 15/40 (37.5%) for rods, spheres, fibres and 0% for powder (Nothdurft, 1956). In contrast, no appreciable difference in tumour incidence was found between the polystyrene discs of 14.5 mm in diameter and rings with a central hole of 6 mm diameter (Rivière et al., 1960).

Following subcutaneous implantation of poly(vinyl chloride) discs of 17 mm diameter into rats, the following incidences of local tumours were observed: 75/95 (79%) for plain film, 33/76 (43%) for perforated film, and 0% for powder, respectively (Nothdurft, 1956). Subcutaneous implantation of 15 × 22 mm films of vinyl chloride–vinyl acetate copolymer into mice induced tumours in almost 100%, while no tumours developed with powdered copolymer of the same weight (Brand et al., 1975b,c). Subcutaneous implantation of rectangular smooth-surfaced poly(vinyl chloride) films (22 × 15 × 0.2 mm) into mice induced local sarcomas in 17/30 (56.6%), whereas the corresponding perforated films with 50–60 holes (0.3 mm wide)/cm^2 induced sarcomas in only 3/29 (10.3%) (Moizhess & Vasiliev, 1989).

A decrease in local tumour incidence was observed on changing the implant from film to powder for other materials: powdered silicone (25 mg) produced no tumours among 30 rats at the subcutaneous implantation site, while 3/30 tumours were produced by a 300 mg Silastic cube (Hueper, 1961).

(c) *Pore size*

The effect of pore size on tumour development after subcutaneous implantation of Millipore filters was studied in mice: during the 18 months of study, the local tumour incidences were 21/35 (60%), 18/34 (52.9%) and 2/39 (5%) for the groups given implants of 0.05, 0.10 and 0.45 μm pore size, respectively (Goldhaber, 1962). In another lifetime study of subcutaneous implantation in mice using Millipore filter discs of 20 mm diameter with eight different pore sizes, tumours did not develop with the filters with pore size larger than 0.22 μm (Karp et al., 1973). Greater pore surface also led to decreasing local tumour incidence following subcutaneous implantation of polyurethane in rats, with a significant delay in the development of the first tumour (Nakamura et al., 1995).

(d) *Surface roughening*

Subcutaneous implantation of polyethylene discs (20 mm diameter) with a smooth surface into rats produced local sarcomas in 35/71 rats compared with 7/60 rats for roughened discs (Bates & Klein, 1966). In CBA mice that received subcutaneous implants of vinyl chloride–vinyl acetate copolymer films (15 × 22 mm) with smooth or rough surfaces. A marked delay in tumour incidence was seen, with 98% of the animals in the smooth-implant group having tumours at the end of their lifetime versus 31% in the rough-implant group (Brand *et al.*, 1975c).

(e) Thickness

Two studies measured the effects of thickness of poly(vinyl alcohol) implants on local tumour incidence. In one, thick (20 × 20 × 5 mm) and thin (20 × 20 × 2 mm) poly(vinyl alcohol) sponges of the same surface area but with different volume induced incidences of 14/20 and 1/18, respectively, of local tumours after subcutaneous implantation into rats (Dukes & Mitchley, 1962). In the other study, poly(vinyl alcohol) implants of the same volume but of different thickness (thus with different surface area) were implanted subcutaneously into rats. Nine of 24 rats developed local sarcomas with the 20 × 20 × 5 mm (2000 mm^3) implants, whereas only 1/24 rats developed a sarcoma with the 33 × 33 × 2 mm (2000 mm^3) implants; the same trend was observed with 12.6 × 12.6 × 5 mm (800 mm^3) and 20 × 20 × 2 (800 mm^3) implants: 5/24 and 1/24 (Roe *et al.*, 1967).

4B.22.2 *Chemical factors*

(a) Composition

Different materials of the same shape and size induced different incidences of local tumour development in the same experimental protocol using the same animal species and strain (see Table 54). Materials included in Table 54 are listed in the order from hydrophilic to hydrophobic and there is no apparent correlation between hydrophilicity/hydrophobicity and tumour development.

Table 54. Subcutaneous implantation studies with various materials in male Wistar rats

Film (10 × 20 × 1 mm)	Tumour incidence (%)	Reference
Poly(vinyl alcohol) hydrogel	22/50 (44)	Nakamura *et al.* (1997)
Poly(2-hydroxyethyl methacrylate)	7/19 (37)	Maekawa *et al.* (1984)
Poly-L-lactide	20/50 (40)	Nakamura *et al.* (1994)
Poly(vinyl chloride)		Oppenheimer *et al.* (1955)
plain film	17/44 (39)	
perforated film	0/27	
Polyurethane	11/30 (37)	Nakamura *et al.* (1992)
Polyethylene	21/50 (42)	Nakamura *et al.* (1994)
Polypropylene	17/50 (34)	Imai & Watanabe (1987)
Silicone	2/30 (6.7)	Nakamura *et al.* (1992)

Tissue responses, including tumour development, to a 1:1 blended film of silicone and polyurethane were intermediate between those of pure silicone and polyurethane of the same shape and size (Nakamura *et al.*, 1992). This suggests that chemical characteristics of the material surface may to some extent determine long-term local tissue effects, including tumorigenesis.

(*b*)   *Effects of purification and leachable oligomers*

Either purification of material by organic solvent extraction or deletion/addition of leachable oligomers from/to the material did not have significant effects on tumour incidence: the incidences with commercial cellophane film, with the same film after alcohol extraction for three days, and after additional extraction with benzene were 15/42 (35.7%), 20/44 (45.4%) and 18/39 (46.1%), respectively (Oppenheimer *et al.*, 1955).

The incidences of tumours with polyurethane TM-3 with and without methanol extraction were 1/11 (9.1%) and 6/18 (33.3%), respectively, but this difference was not statistically significant (Imai & Watanabe, 1987).

Changing the oligomer content in the polyurethane by deletion or addition of oligomers did not lead to a change in the tumour incidence: neat polyurethane produced tumours in 8/30 (26.7%) rats; oligomer-deleted polyurethane in 6/30 (20%) rats; and oligomer-added polyurethane in 8/30 (26.7%) rats (Nakamura *et al.*, 1995).

(*c*)   *Miscellaneous (surface coating, electric charge)*

A marked effect of collagen-immobilization of porous polyethylene blocks in decreasing tumour incidence was found in a one-year subcutaneous implantation study in rats: neat polyethylene produced tumours in 11/24 (45.8%) rats, while collagen-immobilized polyethylene produced tumours in 1/24 (4.2%) rats (Kinoshita *et al.*, 1993).

Polystyrene films having anionic, cationic and neutral electric properties were tested in rats: the tumour incidences were 3/16 (18.8%), 9/16 (56.3%), and 1/16 (6.3%), respectively (Carter *et al.*, 1971).

These studies suggest that surface chemistry may play a more important role in tumorigenesis than bulk chemistry.

4C. Composite Medical and Dental Implants

Rabbit: A total of 40 male and female adult New Zealand White rabbits received subcutaneous implants of eight types of miniature silicone breast prosthesis (21 × 10 mm) into pockets of both flanks. Groups of 10 animals were evaluated at one, six, 12 and 18 months after implantation. The shell of the prostheses was made of polysulfane-based silicone elastomer. This silicone shell was either bare, backed with a piece of perforated silicone, backed with a patch of Dacron mesh or completely covered with polyurethane foam (3 mm thick, pore sizes of approximately

250–800 μm). Four types were silicone gel-filled and another four types were saline-filled. Survivors after one, six, 12, and 18 months were 10, 10, 10 and four, respectively; no local tumour was found in any group (Lilla & Vistnes, 1976).

4D. Other Foreign Bodies

Experimental data on the carcinogenicity of lead and lead compounds were reviewed by IARC (1980, 1987c).

No data on carcinogenic effects of depleted uranium were available to the Working Group.

5. OTHER DATA RELEVANT TO AN EVALUATION OF CARCINOGENICITY AND ITS MECHANISMS

5A. Metallic Medical and Dental Materials

5A.1 Degradation of metallic implants in biological systems

Implanted metallic materials are subject to corrosion, which can result from direct interaction with the surrounding tissue or body fluids or be the consequence of mechanical damage. The resistance of metallic biomaterials to corrosion depends on the presence of a passive, protective film of oxide covering the surface. Titanium, which appears as an active metal in the electromotive series, forms a resistant oxide, which prevents further corrosion. Stainless steel and cobalt alloys form chromium oxide films. The composition of the oxide film has an important influence on biocompatibility. Metallic biomaterials in an aqueous environment represent a system in which active and passive surfaces exist simultaneously in contact with electrolyte (Kelly, 1982). At the surface of the metal oxide film, there is a continuous process of dissolution and reprecipitation, so that the composition of the film can change even though it seems macroscopically stable. Calcium, phosphorus and sulfur have been found to be incorporated into the surface film of titanium bolts surgically implanted into human jaw bone (McQueen *et al.*, 1982). Similarly, calcium and phosphorus have been detected in the oxide film of 316L stainless steel pins and wires that had been implanted during hand surgery and maxillofacial surgery (Sundgren *et al.*, 1985).

5A.1.1 *Mechanisms of degradation*

The principal mechanisms by which surgical alloys corrode are galvanic, crevice and fretting corrosion. These types of degradation involve the release of ions. Galvanic corrosion can occur when two metallic implants of different composition or two regions of the same implant with different electrochemical properties are in contact. For example, during the development of techniques for internal fixation of fractures, plates of one material were occasionally fixed with screws of another material. In modular total hip prostheses, femoral components may have a head made of a cobalt–chromium–molybdenum (CoCrMo) alloy and a stem made of titanium–aluminium–vanadium alloy (Ti 6,4). However, as more corrosion-resistant materials have become used in such mixed metal combinations, the issue of mixed metal galvanic corrosion has become less problematic.

Crevice corrosion can occur in a confined space that is exposed to a chloride solution. Such a space can exist in a gasket-type connection between a metal and a non-metal or between two pieces of metal bolted or clamped together. Crevice corrosion involves an electrochemical reaction which may take six months to two years to develop. Crevice corrosion has been observed in implants in which metals are in contact, such as in some total hip replacement devices, screws and plates used in fracture fixation and some orthodontic appliances (Fontana & Greene, 1978).

Fretting corrosion is a phenomenon of microscopic shear motion between two surfaces. The range of motion is typically less than 100 μm. Fretting corrosion involves continuous disruption of the oxide film and the associated oxidation of exposed metal. In devices that undergo crevice corrosion, fretting corrosion may accelerate the degradation.

Wear is a form of degradation which involves the release of particulate debris. Surface damage due to wear can occur by several mechanisms. On a microscopic scale, contact between two surfaces is not across an entire area, but rather occurs at high points or local asperities. Adhesive wear occurs when asperities of two surfaces adhere to each other, as with local spot welding due to high contact stress. With sliding between the surfaces, portions of one surface are torn off. Abrasive wear involves a harder material ploughing through the surface of a softer one. With ductile materials like metals and some plastics, such ploughing results in a deep furrow with a raised ridge on either side. These ridges may subsequently cause wear of the opposite surface. Three-body wear occurs when free particles in a bearing space abrade the surfaces. They may cause abrasive wear of both, or may become embedded in the softer surface and cause abrasive wear of the counterface. Under suitable conditions, the protective oxide film can be restored following damage (repassivation).

5A.1.2 *In-vitro corrosion of dental alloys*

The expression 'corrosion-resistant' in connection with precious-metal or well passivated base-metal alloys would suggest that there is no corrosion at all. In fact this is not true, as is clear from the fact that patients often claim a metallic taste and mouth burning following metallic restoration in the mouth. The recommended in-vitro test for such corrosion involves immersion of specimens in a solution of 0.1 M lactic acid and 0.1 M sodium chloride (pH 2.2) at 37°C for seven days. The low pH is thought to mimic oral crevice conditions. The total amount of metal(s) released is determined by atomic absorption spectrophotometry (AAS) or mass spectrometry. The corrosion is expressed as μg metal released per cm^2 surface area per day. Typical values are given in Table 55. Because corrosion is exceptionally rapid in the first few days, these measurements are made after a four-day period of conditioning the specimens in a similar test solution. With precious-metal alloys, the ion-specific corrosion rate does not correlate with the amount of alloying elements; the base metals are released at a proportionately higher rate compared with the alloy composition. Beryllium as an alloying element considerably increases the corrosion rate of other metals such as nickel (Kappert *et al.*, 1998; see Table 55).

Table 55. Ion release from preconditioned specimens of various cast alloy types

Alloy type	Composition	Released ions	Amount of release ($\mu g/cm^2$ per day)
High gold	Au 77–87; Pt 9–19; Zn 1–2; In 0.7–1.6	In	1.97–2.88
Low gold	Au 51–57; Pd 31–38; In 8; Ga 1.5	In Ga	0.48–3.84 0.76–3.57
Palladium–copper	Pd 73–78; Cu 8.5–11.5; Ga 7–9; Sn 3–16	Pd Cu Ga	3.65–11.11 6.03–9.98 10.8–21.0
Palladium–silver	Pd 75–77; Ag 6–8; Ga 2–6.5; Au 5–6	Pd Ag Ga	0.1 < 0.1 1.22–2.36
Cobalt-based alloy	Co 63–65; Cr 27–29 Mo 5–7; Mn < 1	Co	0.3
Nickel-based alloy without Be	Ni 65; Cr 22.5; Mo 9.5	Ni	0.07
Nickel-based alloy with 1.5% Be	Ni 76; Cr 13; Mo 3; Be 1.5	Ni Cr Mo Be	101 5.6 2.3 10.3
CPTi (grade 2, cast)	Ti 99	Ti	0.36
NPG	Cu 79.3; Al 17.8; Ni 4.3; Fe 4; Zn 3; Mn 1.6	Cu Al Ni Fe Zn Mn	1226 117 67 45 40 32

From Kappert et al. (1998)
CPTi, commercially pure Ti; NPG, non-precious gold

A similar analysis of various types of alloy used in orthodontics has shown that nickel and chromium were released when these alloys were stored in physiological saline. Soldered stainless steel bows were very susceptible to corrosion. The release of nickel seemed to be related to both the composition of the alloys and the method of manufacture of the appliances, but was not proportional to the nickel content (Grimsdottir et al., 1992).

5A.2 Absorption, distribution and excretion

Implants in soft tissue or bone give rise to exposure in that tissue, and the biological effects depend on the interactions of the tissue with the surface of the implant. Such effects may remain localized to the site of the implant itself, but metal ions or particulate debris released as a result of corrosion or wear may cause effects at distant sites. Oral exposures prevail in the case of dental fillings, while materials released from these may be ingested and give rise to exposure via the gastrointestinal tract.

Published studies of biological effects of implants in surrounding tissue have various limitations; many were based on cases of failed implants, which may have led to additional corrosion and/or wear, hence to stronger effects than would normally be the case. Furthermore, the composition and properties of the implants are often poorly described. In addition, it is not always clear whether the effects observed are due to the implant itself or to material released from it. In terms of their possible carcinogenic hazard, metal ions released systemically can be regarded as metal salts, several of which have been the subject of previous IARC Monographs (IARC, 1990a,b, 1991, 1993a,b). When metal ions are released systemically, accumulation may occur in specific organs. Thus nickel accumulates in the liver, spleen and kidney of mice after administration of high doses of the metal ion (Pereira et al., 1998), vanadium accumulates in the liver, spleen and bone, but titanium is reported to accumulate less (Merritt & Brown, 1995). A complex mixture of ionic species may be formed during corrosion, and a wide range of sizes, shapes and numbers of particles may be produced by wear, but many reports provide very little information on these aspects.

5A.2.1 *Humans*

Doorn *et al.* (1998) described the analysis of metallic particles in tissue from 13 patients with cobalt–chromium–molybdenum metal-on-metal total hip implants for periods ranging from seven months to 25 years. Samples were obtained at either revision or autopsy from different sites around the implant and particles were found in eight patients. There was marked inter- and intra-individual variability in both the number (range, 1–580) and size (range, 6–834 nm, most < 50 nm) of particles. The authors had previously determined volumetric wear in three of these patients (McKellop *et al.*, 1996). They estimated that wear produced 6.7×10^{12}, 4.9×10^{13} and 2.5×10^{14} particles per year in three metal-on-metal prostheses and contrasted these figures with their estimate for polyethylene wear debris of 5×10^{11} particles per year in a metal-on-polyethylene hip implant.

Willert *et al.* (1996) determined metal concentrations in tissue samples from 19 patients with cobalt–chromium metal-on-metal total hip implants for periods of one to 282 months (average, 86). Samples were obtained at revision from various sites around the implant, mainly the joint capsule, and metal particles were found in 15 patients. As far as they were visible in the light microscope, these were irregularly shaped, ranged from 0.5 to 5 μm in size and were most often found in the vicinity of blood vessels. Poly(methyl methacrylate) bone cement particles were found at greater concentrations than metal particles. Both the worn surface and the wear particles undergo repassivation to cobalt(II) hydroxide, chromium(III) oxide, chromium(III) hydroxide and nickel(II) hydroxide. While these cobalt and nickel compounds have solubilities greater than 10^{-4} M at physiological pH, the chromium compounds are essentially insoluble under the same conditions, so that chromium accumulates in local tissues while the other products are eliminated by urinary and faecal excretion. Merritt and Brown (1996) reported that the estimated dissolution of cobalt–chromium alloy is 0.15–0.30 µg/cm² per day, which corresponds to around 11 mg per year for a total hip replacement. This can be increased by corrosion.

Jacobs et al. (1996) determined cobalt and chromium concentrations in serum and chromium concentrations in urine from eight patients with long-term (> 20 years) cobalt–chromium metal-on-metal total hip replacements, six patients with short-term (< 2 years) cobalt–chromium metal-on-metal surface replacement arthroplasties and three controls. Single samples were obtained at average implantation times of 295 (range 266–324) months from the total hip replacements and 12.4 (range 2–19) months from the surface replacements. No details of diet were recorded, nor was this variable controlled. The controls had chromium concentrations in serum and urine of 0.14 ng/mL (2.7 nmol/L) and 0.035 ng/mL (0.66 nmol/L), respectively, and cobalt concentrations in serum were below the detection limit (0.3 ng/mL, 5.2 nmol/L). The mean total 24-h urinary chromium excretion in the controls was 0.071 µg per day (1.37 nmol per day). The mean serum chromium and cobalt concentrations in the total hip replacement patients were nine- and threefold higher respectively, whilst urinary chromium concentrations were 35-fold higher than in the controls. The mean total 24 h urinary chromium excretion was 30-fold higher than in the controls. The mean serum chromium and cobalt concentrations in the subjects with surface replacements were three- and four-fold higher, respectively than in the hip replacement patients, whilst urinary chromium concentrations were four-fold higher. The mean total 24-h urinary chromium excretion was 2.5-fold higher in the surface replacement group than in the hip replacement subjects.

In a study to investigate nickel and chromium concentrations in saliva of patients with different types of fixed dental appliances (containing 8–12% nickel and 17–22% chromium), fresh saliva samples were obtained from each of 47 orthodontic patients before insertion of the appliance and 1–2 days, 1 week and 1 month after treatment. The method of sampling shows the momentary total concentration of soluble nickel and chromium. The saliva concentrations of both metals showed considerable variation, and no significant differences were found in samples taken before and after treatment. The authors note that minor amounts of nickel released from dental fixtures could be important in case of hypersensitivity to nickel or in evoking allergic reactions in the oral mucosa (Kerusuo et al., 1997).

5A.2.2 Experimental systems

Harmand et al. (1994) described the dissolution in culture medium and cellular uptake in an osteoblast cell line of ISO 5832/3 titanium alloy, ISO 5832/1 316L stainless steel and ISO 5832/4 cobalt–chromium alloy (defined in Tables 8–10) over a nine-day period. The presence of the cells had varying effects (increase, decrease or none) on release of metal ions from these metals. Uptake of extracellular ions by the cells was limited to chromium, vanadium, titanium, iron and cobalt, with the highest uptake been observed for chromium.

Gray and Stirling (1950) exposed serum and red blood cell cultures to radioactive chromium (^{51}Cr) with a valency of +3 (^{51}CrCl$_3$) and with a valency of +6 (Na$_2$^{51}CrO$_4$). Almost all of the trivalent chromium remained in the plasma, whereas hexavalent chromium crossed the red cell membrane and was primarily cell-associated. Similar results were obtained with fretting corrosion experiments in cell culture (Merritt et al., 1991). These results imply that the valency of chromium affects its biological activity. It is clear that the biological fate of corrosion products needs to be understood before conclusions can be drawn regarding the relevance of chemical analytical data of tissues and fluids for effects of implant corrosion.

In a study to investigate the effect of anodization on the dissolution of titanium, Sprague-Dawley rats were given anodized or unanodized titanium implants intraperitoneally, in the left paracolic gutter. At days 7, 14 and 28, peritoneal lavages and blood samples were obtained. At day 28 the animals were killed and liver, kidneys, spleen, lung and brain were removed, as well as tissue surrounding the implant. Titanium was not detected in any distant organs or in the lavage fluid. In the capsular tissues surrounding the implants titanium concentrations were higher in animals with unanodized implants than in those with anodized implants, but the difference was not significant. Peritoneal leukocytes showed significantly higher titanium levels in animals from the unanodized implant group, compared with the controls, while titanium levels in leukocytes from animals with anodized implants were not significantly different from the controls. Despite the presence of titanium in leukocytes, only minimal biological responses and histopathological changes were detected. The presence of titanium in the tissue surrounding the implants is probably the result of corrosion. Surface treatment of titanium by anodization reduces passive dissolution (Jorgenson et al., 1999).

To examine the biological transport of released metal ions, Merritt et al. (1984a) injected metal salts (nickel chloride, cobalt chloride, chromium chloride, potassium dichromate) intramuscularly into hamsters. Blood samples were taken at 2, 4, 6, 24, 48 and 96 h after injection. Nickel was found in the blood serum at 2, 4 and 6 h, but the levels dropped rapidly. Levels of nickel in red and white blood cells were low. Cobalt and trivalent chromium were similarly found in serum, but the levels did not drop as rapidly. In contrast, hexavalent chromium from potassium dichromate was found in the red blood cells, confirming the results of Gray and Stirling (1950). Corrosion products generated by fretting corrosion of 316 LVM stainless steel or MP35N plates and screws were suspended in serum and injected intramuscularly into hamsters; chromium was again found in the red blood cells. When serum that had interacted with the metal salts or corrosion products was separated into its components by isoelectric focusing on polyacrylamide gels, almost all of the metal, whatever the source, was detected in the albumin region of the gels, indicating strong albumin binding (Merritt et al., 1984b).

Brown et al. (1988) carried out chemical analysis of urine from Syrian hamsters after intramuscular injection of nickel(ous) chloride, cobalt chloride and potassium dichromate, or after accelerated anodic corrosion both *in vitro* and *in vivo* of stainless steel implants. The amounts of metal injected were 90 µg of nickel, 94 µg of cobalt and 117 µg of chromium in one group of animals, and 5.18 µg of nickel, 5.40 µg of cobalt and 6.91 µg of chromium in the second group. Total daily urine samples were collected during three days. In both dose groups, virtually all of the injected nickel and most of the cobalt were excreted in the first 24 h, whereas less than 50% of the chromium dose was excreted. After accelerated anodic corrosion of stainless steel, nickel excretion was complete within 24 h, while chromium excretion was minimal. Similar studies were performed with rods of a nickel–cobalt–chromium–molybdenum alloy (F 75) with a porous coating. These rods were implanted subcutaneously in Syrian hamsters and subjected to accelerated anodic corrosion *in situ*. Even though the nickel content of F 75 alloy is less than 1%, it was rapidly excreted and detected in the urine, as was the molybdenum. Recovery in urine of cobalt was close to 80%, whereas that of chromium was in the range of 37–67% due to *in vivo* storage and significant binding of chromium to red cells (Brown et al., 1993).

These studies also showed that the corrosion rates of these alloys in 10% serum were much lower those that in saline. The rates *in vivo* were similar to those in serum. Thus, for testing materials for corrosion, the use of proteins in the test solution provides a better simulation of the in-vivo environment (Brown et al., 1988).

The implication of these results is that chemical analysis of body fluids and tissues must be interpreted in light of the mechanism of degradation. If an implant corrodes and releases metal ions, nickel and cobalt will be transported and excreted, while chromium may be cell-bound, either in local tissues or in organs such as the lung, kidney, liver and spleen. Thus tissue levels may be different from that of the alloy composition. Also, if there is significant wear and particulate debris in the tissues, chemical analysis of the tissue will indicate a composition different from that of the alloy.

5A.3   Tissue responses and other expressions of toxicity

5A.3.1   *Humans*

   (a)   *Inflammatory and immunological responses*

No relevant systematic studies of tissue responses in orthopaedic implant patients have been reported, although some reviews of case reports have tried to link the occurrence of tumours to carcinogenic mechanisms. In a review of nine cases of implantation site tumours following knee arthroplasty, and in a wider-ranging review of the use of metallic implants, it was suggested that carcinogenicity could result from the release of carcinogenic corrosion products (Jacobs & Oloff, 1985; Wapner, 1991).

A case series of 20 failed hip replacements (two Charnley (metal (TiAlV)-on-polyethylene) and 18 McKee-Farrar (metal-on-metal)) revealed mild to severe acute inflammatory response (characterized by the predominant occurrence of polymorphonuclear leukocytes) in all 12 cases that failed due to infection. The remaining eight cases failed due to loosening. Chronic inflammation was seen in all but one of the 12 infected cases (predominantly lymphocytes and plasma cells). Acrylic debris from the cement was found in all cases extracellularly and in three also intracellularly; one patient from this group and one other patient showed polyethylene debris (Charosky et al., 1973).

A case was reported of aseptic aggressive granulomatosis seven years after knee arthroplasty. Both titanium- and polyethylene-containing fragments were observed around the prosthesis, some titanium being found within macrophages or giant cells (Tigges et al., 1994).

None of the pathological changes noted in clinical reports are suggestive of precancerous states.

When a material is implanted, it is recognized as a foreign body and macrophages adhere to the surface of the material (Tang et al., 1993; Mrksich & Whitesides, 1996). Large amounts of macrophages and polyethylene debris are observed in tissues around aseptically loosened hip arthroplasty (Dorr et al., 1990; Wroblewski, 1997). Macrophages generate active oxygen species by themselves without being active in phagocytosis, but the production of active oxygen is much higher during this process (Johnston & Kitagawa, 1985; Edwards et al., 1988). The primary oxygen radical (O_2^-) is converted by superoxide dismutase to hydrogen peroxide, which penetrates the metal surface to which the macrophage has adhered. In the case of a titanium implant, hydrogen peroxide reacts with the surface oxide film of titanium, which results in the formation of a stable $TiOOH(H_2O)_n$ complex. This TiOOH matrix traps the superoxide radical so that no or very small amounts of free hydroxyl radicals are formed. Apart from titanium, other biocompatible metals such as zirconium and aluminium also show low hydroxyl radical production (Tengvall et al., 1989).

(b)   Oral contact lichenoid reactions

Contact lichenoid reactions topographically related to dental restorations display various clinical characteristics, ranging from asymptomatic papular, reticular and plaque type lesions to symptomatic atrophic and reticular lesions (Holmstrup, 1991). Contact lesions present with similar clinical characteristics as oral lichen planus. These two types of lesion can be discriminated only by the degree to which the oral mucosa is involved (Bolewska et al., 1990a,b). By definition, contact lesions are limited to areas of frequent contact with dental restorations, whereas oral lichen planus also involves other regions of the oral mucosa. In a study of the effect of replacement of dental amalgam with gold or metal–ceramic crowns on oral lichenoid reactions, Bratel et al. (1996) found that the lesions showed considerable improvement in 95% of the patients. This effect was parallelled by a disappearance of symptoms, in contrast to patients with persisting contact lesions (5%), who did not report any significant improvement. The healing response was not found to correlate with age, gender, smoking habits, subjective dryness of the mouth or current medication. The healing effect in patients who received gold crowns was superior compared with that of patients receiving metal–ceramic crowns. Similar contact lesions have been seen in the topographical relationship to dental composite restorations (Lind, 1988) and palladium-based crowns (Downey, 1989).

The etiology of these lesions remains uncertain. An immunological mechanism is involved in some cases, whereas others seem to be related to irritative or cumulative insult-type reactions. Microbial factors such as viral or fungal infections may also contribute to the clinical appearance. It is unclear whether oral lichen planus is a multivariant group of etiologically diverse diseases or a disease entity characterized by a type IV hypersensitivity reaction to an antigen in the junction zone between epithelium and connective tissue. The premalignant potential of oral lichenoid lesions requires regular follow-up at three- to six-month intervals (for reviews, see Scully *et al.*, 1998; Holmstrup, 1999).

(*c*) *Allergic reactions*

In questionnaire surveys about side-effects associated with dental materials, the prevalence was estimated to be 1:300 in periodontics and 1:2600 in pedodontics. None of these reactions was related to dental casting alloys. In prosthodontics, the prevalence was calculated to be about 1:400, and about 27% were related to base-metal alloys for removable partial dentures (cobalt, chromium, nickel) and to precious-metal-based alloys for porcelain-fused-to-metal restorations. The complaints consisted of intra-oral reactions (such as redness, swelling and pain of the oral mucosa and lips), oral/gingival lichenoid reactions and a few instances of systemic allergic reactions. In orthodontics, the prevalence was 1:100, and most reactions (85%) were related to metal parts of the extra-oral anchorage devices (Hensten-Pettersen, 1992).

Even though the extensive use of base-metal alloys has been of major concern to the dental profession, relatively few case reports of allergic reactions substantiate this concern. Allergy to gold-based dental restorations has been more commonly reported. Palladium-based alloys have been associated with several cases of stomatitis and oral lichenoid reactions. Palladium allergy seems to occur mainly in patients who are highly sensitive to nickel. All casting alloys, except titanium, seem to have a potential for eliciting adverse reactions in individual hypersensitive patients. Induction of tolerance may be a possible benefit of the use of intra-orally placed alloys. In non-sensitized individuals, oral antigenic contacts to nickel and chromium may induce tolerance rather than sensitization (Hensten-Pettersen, 1992).

Both local and systemic reactions may sometimes occur following implantation of metallic devices (Rostoker *et al.*, 1986; Wilkinson, 1989; Guyuron & Lasa, 1992). Metal allergy has been suggested as a predisposing factor for infection of periprosthetic tissues (Hierholzer & Hierholzer, 1984). However, the majority of individuals—even the majority of sensitized individuals—seem to tolerate low levels of allergens in the tissues without adverse effect. Induction of immunological tolerance may be a potential benefit.

The mechanisms by which local cutaneous and systemic reactions are induced by nickel in orthopaedic implants remain obscure and the development of such reactions is unpredictable. Some reactions appear to be type I in nature. In others, there is good evidence of type IV hypersensitivity. In some patients, however, type I, III (Arthus) and IV reactions seem to coexist (Wilkinson, 1989). The reaction patterns elicited by other metals seem to be similar to those induced by nickel.

5A.3.2 *Experimental systems*
 (*a*) *Animal studies*

The chemical carcinogenicity of metal compounds (such as that of chromium, nickel, cobalt and arsenic) is believed to be dependent largely on their oxidation state and solubility, with oxidative DNA damage or interference with DNA repair having been postulated as likely mechanisms (Hartwig *et al.*, 1996). Additional mechanisms of metal carcinogenesis include epigenetic changes, chromatin condensation or altered patterns of gene methylation (Costa, 1997; Salnikow *et al.*, 1997). However, very few experimental studies have provided information on tissue responses to metallic implants that is of relevance to carcinogenicity.

A series of five 18–24-month studies of tumour incidence following implantation of tin revealed unusual non-neoplastic pathology, but only in tumour-bearing groups. The studies were carried out in female Marsh mice and male and female Evans rats given intraperitoneal tin implants (open-end cylinders, 12 × 4 mm in mice, 25 × 8 mm in rats). In addition to tumours (an increase was seen in local sarcomas with metastases, but not in spontaneous lymphoid tumours in rats), atypical mesothelial hyperplasia, adenomatous hyperplasia and osseous metaplasia were noted. Chronic inflammatory responses were also common. These included focal histiocytic aggregation, multinucleate giant cells, granulomata, fibrohyalinized capsular tissue, necrosis, fibrocellular fat, lack of capsule, hyalinized sclerosis and cysts (Bischoff & Bryson, 1977).

Male WAB rats, 20 weeks of age, were given implants of either Walker 256 carcinoma cells (as 5-mg solid tumour fragments) or syngeneic neonatal thymus tissue. These tissues were placed in the centre of platinum–silicone elastomer loops, which had been implanted earlier. Control animals received tissues without implants. Colchicine was used to facilitate the assessment of cell proliferation. Rats with thymus grafts were killed after three weeks and those with tumour grafts after up to six days. Group sizes were not reported. Historical data indicated 100% tumour growth at six days in 1500 controls, whereas tumour growth was inhibited in 200/230 rats with implants. Marked reductions in cell density and mitotic rate were seen, in comparison with controls, at two, three, four and six days after tumour implantation, the cell density being lowest close to the implant. Unlike in controls, proliferation of tumour cells in the vicinity of implants was concentrated into foci of intense activity. In contrast, proliferation of thymus tissue was unaffected by the presence of the platinum–silicone implant. The authors ruled out restriction of the blood supply as a reason for the observed effects and suggested that the selective inhibition of tumour cell proliferation may be a result of an alteration of the electrochemical environment by the implant (Hinsull et al., 1979). [The Working Group found it difficult to interpret these data.]

(b) Cytotoxicity of metal ions

The cytotoxicity of metal ions has been investigated systematically in L-929 fibroblasts (Takeda et al., 1989; Schedle et al., 1995; Yamamoto et al., 1998) and 3T3 fibroblasts (Wataha et al., 1991; Yamamoto et al., 1998). The rank orders of cytotoxicity that were found are: Cr > Co > V > Fe > Mn > Cu > Ni >> Mo (Takeda et al., 1989); $Cd^{2+} > Ag^+ > Zn^{2+} > Cu^{2+} > Ga^{3+} > Au^{3+} > Ni^{2+} > Pd^{2+} > In^{3+}$ (Wataha et al., 1991), $Ag^+ > Pt^{4+} > Co^{2+} > In^{3+} > Ga^{3+} > Au^{3+} > Cu^{2+} > Ni^{2+} > Zn^{2+} > Pd^{2+} > Mo^{5+} > Sn^{2+} > Cr^{2+}$ (Schedle et al., 1995); $Cd^{2+} > In^{3+} > V^{3+} > Be^{2+} > Sb^{3+} > Ag^+ > Hg^{2+} > Cr^{6+} > Co^{2+} > Bi^{3+} > Ir^{4+} > Cr^{3+} > Hg^+ > Cu^{2+} > Rh^{3+} > Tl^{3+} > Sn^{2+} > Ga^{3+} > Pb^{2+} > Cu^+ > Mn^{2+} > Tl^+ > Ni^{2+} > Zn^{2+} > Y^{3+} > W^{6+} > Fe^{3+} > Pd^{2+} > Fe^{2+} > Ti^{4+} > Hf^{4+} > Ru^{3+} > Sr^{2+} > Sn^{4+} > Ba^{2+} > Cs^+ > Nb^{5+} > Ta^{5+} > Zr^{4+} > Al^{3+} > Mo^{5+} > Rb^+ > Li^+$ (data for 3T3 cells; Yamamoto et al., 1998). The concentrations that reduced [^{3}H]thymidine incorporation to 50% of the control ranged between 0.4 and > 435 µmol/L (Wataha et al., 1991) and between 0.017 mmol/L and > 1 mmol/L (Schedle et al., 1995). Yamamoto et al. (1998) calculated the IC_{50} values (50% of cell growth inhibition), which ranged from 1.36×10^{-6} to 1.42×10^{-2} (mol L^{-1}). For both cell types studied, the ions of chromium, cadmium, vanadium, silver and cobalt were generally the more cytotoxic. Sun et al. (1997) tested the effects of Al^{3+}, Co^{2+}, Cr^{3+}, Ni^{2+}, Ti^{4+} and V^{3+} on osteoblast-like cell metabolism and differentiation. DNA synthesis, succinate dehydrogenase and alkaline phosphatase activities, culture calcification and osteocalcin and osteopontin gene expression were investigated in ROS 17/2.8 cells. It was shown that metal ions can alter osteoblast behaviour at subtoxic concentrations, but do not affect the expression of all genes similarly. Granchi et al. (1998) showed that large amounts of nickel and cobalt extracted from the metal powders induced necrosis in vitro in mononuclear cells from human peripheral blood and high concentrations of chromium or limited amounts of nickel and cobalt caused cell death by apoptosis. The cytotoxicity of metal ions extracted from commercial gold alloys, silver alloys and nickel–chromium alloys was tested on L929 mouse fibroblasts (Schmalz et al., 1998a). The TC_{50} values were slightly lower in corresponding salt solutions than in extracts. Nickel and cobalt ions upregulated the expression of adhesion molecules as well as of the cytokines interleukin (IL)-6 and -8 in human endothelial cell cultures, as do proinflammatory mediators (Wagner et al., 1998). Silver, mercury and, to a lesser extent, gold ions induced direct toxicity (histamine release, ultrastructural signs of necrosis) and platinum ions induced cell death through induction of apoptosis in the human mast cell line HMC-1 (Schedle et al., 1998a). Extracts from titanium–nickel alloy (50:50) were not cytotoxic in vitro, not allergenic in vivo in guinea-pig, nor genotoxic in vitro in Salmonella typhimurium for gene mutation or in V79 cells for chromosomal aberrations (Wever et al., 1997). Extracts from cobalt–chromium orthopaedic alloys caused inhibitory effects on cell viability, on alkaline phosphatase activity and, to a lower extent, on protein production in all rat, rabbit and human bone-marrow cell cultures tested, the human cells being most sensitive to exposure to metal ions (Tomás et al., 1997). Ions associated with the titanium–chromium–vanadium alloy Ti 6,4 inhibited the normal differentiation of rat bone-marrow stromal cells to mature osteoblasts *in vitro* (Thompson & Puleo, 1996).

(c) *Cytotoxicity of metallic materials*

Cobalt–chromium alloy was toxic to macrophages *in vitro*, as reflected by release of tumour necrosis factor (TNF) α, prostaglandin E2 and the enzyme lactate dehydrogenase (Horowitz et al., 1998). Test specimens fabricated from copper, cobalt, zinc, indium, nickel and precious-metal cast alloys reduced cell viability by 10–80% (copper being the most active) in a three-dimensional cell-culture system consisting of human fibroblasts and keratinocytes (Schmalz et al., 1998b). Nickel–titanium (Nitinol) did not induce cytotoxic effects in human osteoblasts and fibroblasts *in vitro* (Ryhänen et al., 1997).

(d) *Effects of metal ions and metallic materials on cytokine levels and histamine release*

Effects of dental amalgam and heavy metal cations on cytokine production by peripheral blood mononuclear cells were investigated *in vitro* (Schedle et al., 1998b). Fresh amalgam specimens and salt solutions containing Cu^{2+} and Hg^{2+} induced a decrease in interferon-γ and IL-10 levels, whereas fresh amalgam specimens and Hg^{2+} caused an increase in TNF-α levels. Amalgam specimens preincubated in cell-culture medium for six weeks did not cause any effects. Ag^+, Au^{3+} and Hg^{2+} induced rapid histamine release from human tissue mast cells *in vitro* (Schedle et al., 1998a). Exposure of macrophages cocultured with osteoblasts to cobalt–chromium alloy led to significant release of TNF-α and prostaglandin E2, but no significant IL-6 or IL-1β production (Horowitz et al., 1998).

5A.4 Genetic and related effects

5A.4.1 *Humans*

Case et al. (1996) studied chromosomal aberrations in blood and bone marrow in 71 patients (mean age 73 years) with hip ($n = 69$) or knee ($n = 2$) replacements who required revision surgery because of worn prostheses, and in 30 control patients (mean age 70.3 years) having primary arthroplasty. Bone marrow was taken at the site of the worn prostheses in the case of revision surgery or at the site of the newly inserted prostheses in the case of primary arthroplasty. Bone marrow from the ipsilateral iliac crest and peripheral blood samples were also taken from all patients for metaphase analysis. The frequency of chromosomal aberrations (mean ± SD) in marrow taken from the femur at primary arthroplasty (5.8 ± 4.3 aberrant cells per 100 cells) was not different from that found in the iliac crest marrow taken from revision cases (4.6 ± 3.3 aberrant cells per 100 cells). However, there was a significant increase in the frequency of chromosomal aberrations (mean ± SD; aberrant cells per 100 cells) in the cells taken from the femoral marrow adjacent to a worn prosthesis (11.4 ± 10.2, $n = 16$, ≤ 10 years after primary arthroplasty; 12.7 ± 10.8, $n = 9$, > 10 years) compared with the frequency in the iliac crest marrow from the same patients (3.3 ± 2.7, $n = 11$, ≤ 10 years; 5.6 ± 2.0, $n = 10$, > 10 years) or with femoral marrow from patients at primary arthroplasty (see above). Nine out of 27 femoral marrow samples from revision cases had higher chromosomal aberration frequencies (17–40 aberrations/100 cells) than any of the control femoral bone marrow (1–15 aberrations/100 cells) or iliac crest marrow samples from revision cases (0–15 aberrations/100 cells). Chromosomal aberration frequencies were only slightly higher in patients requiring revision more than 10 years after primary arthroplasty. Two patients with a long duration of arthroplasty (18 and 20 years) showed clonal expansion of B or T cells which was associated in one case with a high level of chromosomal aberrations in the femur (26/100 cells) compared with ipsilateral iliac crest (6/100 cells). The authors cautioned that the results should be seen as preliminary due to the low patient numbers. They discounted concomitant disease and X-rays as predisposing factors, leaving wear debris as a potential causative agent.

5A.4.2 *Experimental systems*

Very few mutagenicity studies have been performed with metallic medical and dental materials. The evaluation of the mutagenic potential is normally based on either the results of tests with extracts or on knowledge of the mutagenic potential of the individual metallic components of the biomaterial.

(a)   Genotoxic activity of metals and metal compounds

Data on the genotoxicity and mutagenicity of some of the metals used in implants have been compiled in previous IARC Monographs and are summarized here.

Chromium[VI] compounds of various solubilities in water were consistently active in numerous studies covering a wide range of tests for genetic and related effects (IARC, 1990a).

The chromium[III] compounds tested were generally not genotoxic in numerous studies and only weak effects were observed in some tests (IARC, 1990a).

Soluble nickel compounds were generally active in the human and animal cells in which they were tested *in vitro* (IARC, 1990b).

Cobalt[II] compounds induced DNA damage, mutations, sister chromatid exchanges and aneuploidy in mammalian cells. Some cobalt[III] complexes with heterocyclic ligands were also active in these assays (IARC, 1991).

Chromosomal aberrations and aneuploidy were observed in mammalian cells *in vitro* and in rodents *in vivo* after treatment with cadmium chloride. DNA strand breaks, mutations, chromosomal damage and cell transformation have been observed after exposure of mammalian cells to cadmium compounds *in vitro* (IARC, 1993b).

DNA damage, sister chromatid exchanges, chromosomal aberrations and aneuploidy (spindle disturbances) have been induced by mercury compounds in mammalian cells *in vitro*. Weak positive genotoxic effects were observed with mercuric chloride in rodents *in vivo* (IARC, 1993a).

Beryllium salts are not mutagenic in most bacterial systems but they induced sister chromatid exchanges and possible chromosomal aberrations in mammalian cells *in vitro*. Beryllium chloride induced gene mutation and chromosomal aberrations in mammalian cells *in vitro* (IARC, 1993c).

(b) Tests using extracts

Extracts for testing are generally prepared by adding the biomaterial to water, saline or cell-culture medium for a few hours or days at 37°C. The corrosion that occurs under these conditions has generally not been compared with the corrosion that is observed *in vivo*. Also, an analysis of leachable material is often not made, so there is no assurance that any such substances have indeed been extracted from the biomaterial. Reference to the mutagenicity of individual metallic components can be misleading, because the ionic species tested may be different from those generated by leaching.

Tests on extracts are often performed for regulatory compliance, and results are not usually published in the open literature. [The Working Group noted that many genotoxicity tests carried out for such purposes are not adequate to identify all mutagenic hazards and they may not address all relevant mutagenic end-points or optimize exposure to the test system.]

Assad *et al.* (1998) studied single-strand DNA breakage in interphase and metaphase human lymphocytes *in vitro* using an in-situ end-labelling method with electron microscopy. Twenty-four-hour extracts of particles of a nickel–titanium alloy (diameter 250–500 µm) were prepared using complete RPMI medium at 37°C. The lymphocytes were exposed to the extracts for 72 h. The results were compared with those obtained with extracts of commercially pure titanium or 316 L stainless steel particles. No determination of the quantity of each metal extracted by the medium was performed. DNA strand breaks were significantly increased in metaphase chromatin with extracts of 316 L stainless steel. Extracts of the nickel–titanium alloy or of pure titanium did not show an effect. However, no information on the metallic species from stainless steel producing the effect was provided. No effect on chromatin in interphase nuclei was observed with any of the extracts.

Wever *et al.* (1997) tested a nickel–titanium alloy (50% nickel) and compared the results with those obtained with stainless steel containing 13–15% nickel. Both alloys were extracted in aqueous 0.9% sodium chloride for 72 h at 37°C. No determination of the metal content of the extracts was performed. Extracts were tested with and without metabolic activation for mutagenic activity in four strains of *Salmonella typhimurium* (TA1535, TA1537, TA98 and TA100) and for induction of chromosomal aberrations in Chinese hamster ovary (CHO) cells. The two alloys gave negative results in both tests.

The potential to induce neoplastic transformation in C3H T½ fibroblasts was tested for eight metals (cobalt, chromium, nickel, iron, molybdenum, aluminium, vanadium and titanium) and their alloys (stainless steel, chromium alloy, titanium–aluminium–

vanadium alloy). The cells were exposed to solutions of the metal salts or to metal or alloy particles (particle size ≤ 5 µm). Cell transformation was observed with soluble forms of cobalt, chromium, nickel and molybdenum, although in some cases only at cytotoxic concentrations. Vanadium, iron, aluminium and titanium salts did not induce cell transformation. The particulate metals and alloys failed to induce cell transformation, although large differences in toxicity were noted (Doran *et al.*, 1998).

5A.5 Mechanisms of carcinogenic action

Surgical alloys and metallic medical devices are insoluble in physiological media, but are subject to corrosion and wear. Corrosion can result in the release of soluble ions. Information with respect to the potential carcinogenic hazard of such ions is available in previous IARC Monographs. However, it is difficult to evaluate whether the metal salts play any significant role in the possible carcinogenic effects observed with implants, because there is a striking lack of data on the actual amounts of ions released into the surrounding tissue and on the nature of the ionic species involved. It is possible that irritation of the surrounding tissue by the implant itself, presumably occurring at the boundary between the metal surface and the tissue, can provoke responses that lead to disturbances of normal cellular function. In addition, inflammatory reactions observed at the site of implants may enhance oxidative processes, inducing cellular damage and regenerative cell proliferation. Particulate debris generated by wear may induce similar reactions in the surrounding tissue or at more distant sites. One single study has reported an enhanced frequency of chromosomal aberrations in cells adjacent to a loose or worn prosthesis (hip or knee replacement) in elderly patients (Case *et al.*, 1996).

5B. Non-metallic Medical and Dental Materials

Of the many components of non-metallic medical and dental materials, only a few are discussed here, which are those for which some data are available.

5B.1 Degradation, distribution, metabolism and excretion
5B.1.1 *Humans*
(a) Degradation of polyurethane foam

Following early studies on degradation of polyurethane foam in implants in humans, it was widely suggested that the foam either broke up or disappeared. However, Szycher and Siciliano (1991) considered that the apparent fragmentation was observed because of ingrowth of tissue into the foam structure and preparation of histological sections cut through the three-dimensional matrix of the foam. It is however clear that degradation of the foam *in vivo* can lead to loss of at least 30% over nine years.

The urine of a female patient was analysed following implantation of Même® polyurethane-covered breast implants. The implants were replaced at a revision operation during which partial absorption of the foam was observed and scar tissue was removed. Urine, collected at several times over a three-month period after implantation, was analysed by gas chromatography/mass spectrometry (GC/MS) of heptafluorobutyryl derivatives following extraction with toluene and cleavage of acetyl conjugates of 2,4-diaminotoluene in urine by boiling in 6 M hydrochloric acid for 1 h. Scar tissue was extracted and hydrolysed in a similar manner. No free 2,4- or 2,6-diaminotoluene was detected in either urine or scar tissue. In acid-hydrolysed scar tissue, total 2,4-diaminotoluene levels were 27.22 µg/g and total 2,6-diaminotoluene levels were 6.02 µg/g. In acid-hydrolysed urine, total 2,4-diaminotoluene levels ranged from 0.27 to 1.69 µg/L and total 2,6-diaminotoluene from 0.11 to 0.61 µg/L. These levels appeared to be related to creatinine clearance values. The authors recognized that the acid hydrolysis of urine could potentially cleave polyurethane oligomers as well as the expected acetyldiaminotoluene metabolites, but doubted whether such oligomers would be readily absorbed and circulated. They suggested that cleavage to toluene diisocyanates with subsequent conversion to diaminotoluenes and acetylation of diaminotoluenes was more likely to occur. In the case of oligomer cleavage, the urinary ratio of 2,4-diaminotoluene to 2,6-diaminotoluene should be the same as in the polymer i.e., 4:1, but would not necessarily be so in the event of in-situ breakdown, due to possible steric effects at enzyme active sites. The observed ratio was 2.4:1, which supports the acetylaminotoluene pathway (Chan et al., 1991a).

The urine of a second female patient was analysed following implantation of Même® polyurethane-covered breast implants. Urine was collected at several times over a seven-month period after implantation and a control sample was obtained before implantation. Extraction, conjugate cleavage and analysis were performed as described above; however, the method was modified by addition of methylenediphenyldiamine as an internal standard before extraction. The first sample, collected 21 days after implantation, and all subsequent samples collected over a seven-month period, contained both free and acid-hydrolysable 2,4-diaminotoluene and 2,6-diaminotoluene. The free 2,4- and 2,6-diaminotoluene levels were 0.47 to 0.92 µg/L and 0.13 to 0.34 µg/L, respectively, equivalent to 4.8–9.0% and 3.1–6.5% of the total, respectively. The total 2,4- and 2,6-diaminotoluene levels were 5.2–18.1 µg/L and 2.0–8.5 µg/L, respectively. The levels appeared to be related to creatinine clearance values. The concentrations in urine were relatively consistent at all time points, possibly reflecting steady-state kinetics. The acetyl metabolite was not measured directly, but the ratio of 2,4-diaminotoluene to 2,6-diaminotoluene was again less than in the polymer (Chan et al., 1991b).

The fibrous capsule and polyurethane foam recovered following explantation of breast implants were studied to characterize the biodegradation of polyurethane foam in vivo. Seventy-five freshly retrieved polyurethane-coated breast implants and surrounding capsule from 47 patients were analysed. The reasons for removal were capsular contracture (48%), infection or exposure of prosthesis (13%) or other (39%). Tissue from several sites around the surface of the implants was digested in a collagenase solution until either foam was recovered or all the tissue was digested. Additional samples were fixed in 10% formalin and were examined histologically. Visibly intact foam was recovered from only 48% of the prostheses after enzymatic digestion of capsular tissue. There was a progressive decline in the recovery of visibly intact foam with increasing time since implantation. Scanning electron microscopy showed fractures and fissures in the foam structure and thinning of the polyurethane struts from 49 ± 1.5 μm in control (unimplanted) foam to 30 ± 3.1, 32 ± 3.1 and 41.2 ± 2.3 μm in those removed due to contracture, infection or other reasons, respectively. In all but two of the samples without visibly intact foam, residual polyurethane foam was observed in the capsule by light microscopy. Histological examination revealed scalloping and fracturing of the foam. Overall, there was convincing evidence that the foam had degraded *in vivo*. It was not possible to quantify the rate of degradation accurately, but capsular contracture, infection and time appeared to have an effect on polyurethane biodegradation in the human body (Sinclair et al., 1993).

A case–control study was conducted among 129 women, of whom 66 had polyurethane foam-coated breast implants and 63 were age- and race-matched controls with an age range of 23 to 62 years. Women who had known contact with either polyurethane such as contraceptive sponges or other polyurethane-coated implants were excluded from the study. Serum and urine samples were collected from fasted participants on two mornings with a 10 ± 3-day interval. Special handling procedures and storage in citrate buffer tubes were required due to the instability of diaminotoluene in biological matrices. Samples extracted with toluene at pH 7–8 and derivatized with pentafluoropropionic anhydride were analysed by GC/MS with negative chemical ionization. The limits of quantification in urine and serum were 10 pg/mL for diaminotoluene and 100 pg/mL for N-acetyldiaminotoluene. The limits of detection for diaminotoluene in serum and urine were 2 and 3 pg/mL, respectively, and for N-acetyldiaminotoluene 20 and 30 pg/mL, respectively. Patients completed a survey as part of the study. Their demographic data combined with the results of this survey indicated that the subjects were a representative sample of the implant population. There was no detectable 2,4-diaminotoluene, 2,6-diaminotoluene or N-acetyldiaminotoluene in sera of either patients or controls at either visit. Unpublished data quoted in the report showed that diaminotoluene is rapidly acetylated in human blood *in vitro*, with a half-life of 15–20 min. The clearance of diaminotoluene in animal studies is rapid, so that the lack of detectable diaminotoluene in serum is not surprising. Quantifiable or detectable levels of diaminotoluene were found in the urine of 48 patients; no quantifiable levels of diaminotoluene were seen in controls, although seven had trace levels of diaminotoluene at one of the two sampling times. There were decreased urinary diaminotoluene levels with increasing time since implantation. After five years, few urine samples had quantifiable levels of diaminotoluene. The urinary data, after normalization for both urinary creatinine and number of implants, were fitted to a concentration versus time curve, the best fit being a one-compartment exponential model. An estimated 'half-life' of 24 months was obtained for biodegradation of polyurethane foam, which is consistent with a recent report of extensive degradation within three years (Sinclair et al., 1993). The estimated half-life suggests that two-thirds of the foam would be degraded within three years

(Hester et al., 1997). [The Working Group noted that the fitting of the data to regression curves involved a variety of common pharmacokinetic assumptions regarding average values assigned to duplicates around the limit of detection, implying that the accuracy of the 'half-life' should be treated with caution.]

In an inhalation study, two male volunteers were exposed to toluene diisocyanate (TDI; isomeric composition 30% 2,4-TDI, 70% 2,6-TDI), in concentrations of 25, 50 and 75 µg/m^3 in air for four hours. Blood and urine were obtained from the subjects at regular intervals after exposure. The samples of plasma and urine were hydrolysed and 2,4- and 2,6-diaminotoluene were determined by capillary gas chromatography. A biphasic elimination of the diaminotoluenes from plasma was observed, with half-time values of 2–5 h (rapid phase) and > 6 days (slow phase). The slowly eliminated fraction may represent protein conjugates of the diaminotoluenes. About 80% of the compounds were excreted in urine within 6 h after the end of the exposure period (Brorson et al., 1991).

Potential exposures to 2,4-diaminotoluene arising from polyurethane-coated breast implants have been calculated using a series of assumptions and a range of possible exposures. The polyurethane used in the manufacture of breast implants is a poly(ester urethane) manufactured from polyethylene glycol adipate (PEGA) and toluene diisocyanate. The amount of foam in two breast implants is approximately 2–3 g. PEGA is not a molecule with a discrete chain length but rather a mixture of various chain lengths, and when used in the foam has an average molecular weight of 1500 Da (Amin et al., 1993). The ratio of 2,4-diaminotoluene to 2,6-diaminotoluene in the foam is 4:1 and it is assumed that these isomers are equally susceptible to cleavage, so that 80% of the total diaminotoluene would be 2,4-diaminotoluene (see, e.g., Chan et al., 1991b).

The potential annual exposures to diaminotoluenes as a result of implant degradation were calculated based on the 0.8% annual degradation *in vitro* estimated by Benoit (1993), the 30% degradation over nine years reported by Szycher and Siciliano (1991) (assumed to be 3.5% per year) and the total disintegration previously described within seven years (assumed to be 16% per year). It was assumed that the rate of degradation was linear and unaffected by the degree of degradation. The total amount of diaminotoluene in 2–3 g of foam (present in two breast implants) formed from PEGA with an average molecular weight of 1500 Da is 218–328 mg, of which 80% is 2,4-diaminotoluene (175–262 mg). This indicates the range of maximal possible exposure to 2,4-diaminotoluene arising from breast implants.

The potential annual exposure to 2,4-diaminotoluene calculated on the basis of the 0.8% annual degradation (Benoit, 1993) is 1.4–2.1 mg, whereas that based on the 3.5% degradation per year (Szycher & Siciliano, 1991) is 6.1–9.2 mg, and that based on a 16% annual degradation (see above) is 28–41.4 mg.

(b)   Wear of dental composites

Quantification of the chemicals and particles released by chemical dissolution and abrasion of dental composites is complicated. In studies among patients who had received dental restorations, Dickinson et al. (1990) reported a 14- or 26-μm mean annual wear of dental composites (with or without the use of a low-viscosity surface-penetrating sealant), and Freilich et al. (1992) reported wear of 45–175 μm after three years, for different composite materials. In a review, different studies were reported to find 7–10 μm mean annual wear (Leinfelder, 1988), while Rasmusson and Lundin (1995) investigated six different composite resin materials and found wear after five years in the range 120–300 μm.

5B.1.2 *Experimental systems*
    (*a*) *Polyurethane-coated breast implants*

The release of diaminotoluene from polyurethane foam requires cleavage of two adjacent urethane bonds. Whilst such cleavage has been reported for the poly(ester urethane) foam coating of breast implants, it has not been observed with poly(ether urethanes).

    (*i*) *Toxicokinetics*

A physiologically based pharmacokinetic model for the assessment of carcinogenic risk following degradation of poly(ester urethane) foam from breast implants comprised five compartments: two exiting compartments (kidney and gastrointestinal tract), slowly perfused tissues, richly perfused tissues and a metabolizing tissue (liver). Rats were treated with 2,4-diaminotoluene by intravenous (0.52 mg/kg bw) or subcutaneous injection (0.44 mg/kg bw), or they received a subcutaneous implant of ^{14}C-labelled foam (dose comparable to 80 mg/kg) synthesized from [^{14}C]toluene diisocyanate. The experimental data obtained were fitted to the model. The model assumed a zero-order foam degradation rate constant of 88 ng 2,4-diaminotoluene/g foam per day. 2,4-Diaminotoluene was assumed to be the only degradation product, with a single active metabolite. Almost all of the 2,4-diaminotoluene produced from breakdown of polyurethane foam was assumed to be bound to plasma protein, as was indicated by the experiment with the intravenously exposed rats. The model parameters were optimized with the rat data, and the model was subsequently used to estimate degradation kinetics from an implant by substituting human parameters. A risk estimate was derived based on the plasma levels (Luu *et al.*, 1998). [The Working Group noted that the model is limited by the same lack of data on local 2,4-diaminotoluene concentrations at the site of foam degradation that bedevils much of the other published data.]

The toxicokinetics of 2,4-diaminotoluene have been studied in rats and mice after intraperitoneal administration and in rats, rabbits and guinea-pigs after oral administration. The majority of the dose (90%) was excreted in urine after both oral and intraperitoneal administration, except for one study with intraperitoneal administration where 22% of the dose was excreted in faeces between 6 and 16 h after administration. Peak tissue levels were observed at one hour after intraperitoneal administration. The metabolites included mono- and diacetylated amines, a number of unidentified hydroxylated metabolites and products of methyl group oxidation. Little unchanged

2,4-diaminotoluene was excreted after oral administration (Waring & Pheasant, 1976; Grantham et al., 1979).

Further toxicokinetic data indicated that acetyl and other acid-labile conjugates are the main metabolites of diaminotoluene in Fischer 344 rats. The monoacetyl derivative was shown to be almost exclusively 4-acetyldiaminotoluene following administration of either diaminotoluene or toluene diisocyanate. Other metabolites included the diacetyl derivative, ring hydroxylation products and both the methyl-oxidized metabolite and its acetylated product. Elimination appeared to be biphasic, with half-time values of 2–5 h for the rapid phase and greater than six days for the slow phase (Bartels et al., 1993).

The distribution of inhaled [^{14}C]toluene diisocyanate in rats was studied over a range of concentrations. Radioactivity was detectable in all the organs studied, but predominantly in trachea, stomach, oesophagus and lung. Virtually all of the radioactivity in plasma was bound to the > 10 kDa fraction, while 41% of the radioactivity in the stomach contents was recovered in this fraction. The results suggest that conjugation is the predominant metabolic pathway of toluene diisocyanate in the rat (Kennedy et al., 1994).

Route-dependent differences were investigated in the metabolism of 2,4-[^{14}C]-toluene diisocyanate following oral administration (60 mg/kg) and inhalation exposure (2 ppm, 4 h) of Fischer 344 rats (oral exposure was about 15-fold higher). After oral administration, the majority of the radioactivity was excreted within 48 h, with 81% in faeces and 8% in urine; the tissues and the carcass contained 4% of the dose. In contrast, after inhalation, 47% was found in faeces and 15% in urine, while tissues and the carcass contained 34% of the administered dose. A significant portion of the carcass radioactivity was associated with gastrointestinal contents. Mono- and diacetylated diaminotoluene were detected in urine after oral administration and inhalation exposure, but free 2,4-diaminotoluene was seen only after oral administration. The results suggest different metabolic routes for oral administration and inhalational exposure to 2,4-toluene diisocyanate: after oral administration, 2,4-diaminotoluene is formed, which is readily absorbed; after inhalation, the diisocyanate is conjugated and only small amounts of acetylated 2,4-diaminotoluene are formed (Timchalk et al., 1994).

(b) Other polyurethane implants

Pacemaker leads are prone to two principal degradation mechanisms, metal-catalysed oxidative degradation and environmental stress cracking. There is little release of degradation products, but this degradation modifies the polymer chain, affecting its mechanical properties and leading to failure of its insulation properties. McCarthy et al. (1997) reviewed polyurethanes commonly used in this application. They studied degradation of sheets of Pellethane™, Tecoflex™ and Biomer® 18 months after subcutaneous implantation into sheep. By scanning electron microscopy, the surface of Biomer showed uniform pitting and superficial fissuring (< 2.0 μm depth) whilst Pellethane and Tecoflex surfaces showed severe local embrittlement with fissures up to 40 µm deep. The chemical changes were localized oxidation of the soft segment and hydrolysis of urethane bonds joining the rigid and flexible segments in the polymer structure. There was also localized hydrolysis of urethane bonds within the aliphatic rigid segment of Tecoflex.

The performance and biostability of a poly(ester urethane) arterial prosthesis was investigated *in vitro* and *in vivo*. The material was exposed *in vitro* to either buffer or buffered collagenase and pancreatin solutions for up to 100 days at 37°C. There was an apparent decrease in molecular weight following exposure to the enzyme solutions and a decrease in the concentration of carbonate groups at the surface. This arose from enzyme-catalysed hydrolysis of surface carbonate groups in the soft segment of the polymer, but the enzymes were unable to reach the more hydrolytically susceptible urethane groups in the hard segment (Zhang *et al.*, 1994a).

The in-vivo study involved implantation of a thoraco-abdominal bypass in dogs for one or 12 months. At one month, the implant appeared similar to unimplanted prostheses, with a few broken microfibres, but at 12 months the inner surface showed more pronounced degradation, with broken, cracked and fissured microfibres, while the external surface remained similar to that of unimplanted prostheses. This was accompanied by an increase in surface carbonate group and a decrease in urethane group concentrations, especially on the luminal side. This indicates a rearrangement in the microstructure of the polymer (Zhang *et al.*, 1994b).

(c) *Polydimethylsiloxanes (silicones)*

Silicone polymers contain different sizes of silicone ranging from small amounts of the monomers (low-molecular-weight silicones) to a variety of sizes of polymers (with molecular weights from 7000 upwards; average 30 000).

Silicone polymer is a large cross-linked hydrophobic molecule that is insoluble in water. In various studies the toxicity of the low-molecular-weight precursors of polymeric silicones has been investigated. The patterns of absorption, distribution, metabolism and excretion of these short-chain linear and cyclic siloxanes are related to their size, solubility and lipophilicity.

A sensitive method was developed to analyse low-molecular-weight silicones by use of gas chromatography coupled with atomic emission detection (GC/AED) or with mass spectrometry (GC/MS). Mouse liver homogenate was incubated with silicone oil for 24 h at 25°C, and the extraction efficiency was determined with the above-mentioned methods for each of the components of the oil. Recoveries of 96–98 % were obtained (Kala *et al.*, 1997).

The diffusion of low-molecular-weight silicones and platinum – a catalyst used in the preparation of silicone gels – from intact implants into surrounding medium was determined by GC/AED and GC/MS (Kala *et al.*, 1997). In lipid-rich medium, leakage of silicones was most prominent, reaching rates of 10 mg/day per 250-g implant at 37°C. Platinum levels in silicone implant gels were determined to be

175 μg per 250-g implant. Platinum diffused from the intact implant into lipid-rich medium at a rate of 20–25 μg/day/250-g implant (Lykissa et al., 1997).

The toxicity of decamethylcyclopentasiloxane (D_5), used as an intermediate in the production of silicone polymers, was tested in a three-month nose-only inhalation experiment with Fischer 344 rats. The dose range was 0–224 ppm, given for 6 h per day on five days per week. At the high dose, an increase was noted in the serum levels of γ-glutamyltranspeptidase in both sexes, and of lactate dehydrogenase in females. Absolute and relative weights of the liver were increased in both sexes at the end of the exposure period, but this effect was resolved after a one-month recovery period. Focal macrophage accumulation and interstitial inflammation were noted in lungs of male and female rats after exposure to the highest dose. These effects appeared not to be entirely reversible after the recovery period (Burns-Naas et al., 1998).

With increasing molecular weight, the solubility and oral absorption of the siloxanes decrease, reaching essentially zero for molecules containing eight or more siloxy units. Half-lives of short-chain siloxanes were reported to be of the order of hours or days. Metabolic demethylation of short-chain silicone precursors does occur, but in no case has the loss of more than two methyl groups been shown, and there is no evidence for demethylation of silicone polymer. Metabolism of siloxanes to silicates has not been demonstrated (Lykissa et al., 1997; Kala et al., 1997).

A series of studies have used nuclear (^1H and ^{29}Si) magnetic resonance (NMR) and ^1H localized spectroscopy to assess the migration and biodegradation of silicone in rats that had received silicone gel-filled implants. There was no evidence for the presence of silicone in the liver until up to six months after implantation. On the basis of ^{29}Si-NMR data obtained nine and twelve months after implantation, it was concluded that migration of silicone to the liver and formation of new silicon-containing compounds (probably silica gel and high coordinated silicon complexes) had occurred. Only limited quantification of silicone metabolism was given and no identification was provided of the chemical structure of the products formed. The authors did not report the use of reference standards for spectroscopic analysis (Garrido et al., 1993; Pfleiderer et al., 1993a,b; Garrido & Ackerman, 1996). The findings could not be confirmed by others, and a number of technical shortcomings in the methodology have been pointed out (Dorne et al., 1995; Macdonald et al., 1995; Taylor & Kennan, 1996).

[The Working Group noted that the available data did not provide convincing evidence that degradation of silicones occurred.]

(d) Degradable polymers

Flat plates of ε-caprolactone–L-lactide copolymer [50:50 (w/w), molecular weight 162 kDa; 20 × 10 × 1 mm in size] were implanted subcutaneously into 50 male Wistar rats. The copolymer was synthesized by bulk ring-opening polymerization of the two components at 190°C for 5 h followed by precipitation from a dichloromethane solution in methanol and drying under reduced pressure. The positive control implant was a 1-mm thick plate of medical-grade polyethylene prepared to identical dimensions on the same machine with no additional chemicals used during processing. Encapsulation of the copolymer implants had occurred by one month, but degradation had also started. The molecular weight decreased to 36% of the initial value within one month, and to 31% by six months. Macroscopically, the implants retained their initial shape up to six months, at which time the surfaces were roughened but no tissue in-growth was observed. After six months, it was not possible to separate the implant from surrounding tissue. By 12 months, the plates had broken into several pieces and by 18 months they had degraded into small fragments with diameter between 10 and 200 µm. The tissue reaction around the fragments became more marked as degradation proceeded, but remained confined within the tissue capsule. By 24 months, fragments were being resorbed and capsules averaged $10 \times 5 \times 0.5$ mm in size with the broken fragments located in a $3 \times 2 \times 1$ mm volume in the centre of the capsule (Nakamura et al., 1998).

The same group (Nakamura et al., 1994) had earlier compared tumorigenicity of plates of poly-L-lactide and medical-grade polyethylene with identical dimensions in a similarly designed study. The viscosity-average molecular weight decreased from 25.3×10^4 initially to 4.97×10^4 at six months, 4.50×10^4 (18% of original) at 12 months and to 2.12×10^4 (8% of original) at 24 months. However, the plates still retained their initial size of $20 \times 10 \times 1$ mm at 24 months although white spots had begun to appear within six months and scanning electron microscopy at 24 months revealed holes with diameters of several micrometres. Clear areas of poly-L-lactide were homogeneous, whereas the white spots had developed a porous structure.

A similar study of plates of polyglycolic acid showed complete absorption within two months (Nakamura et al., 1997).

The synthetic α-polyesters are synthesized from α-hydroxy acids such as glycolic and L-lactic acid. As the D-isomer of lactic acid is not easily metabolized by humans, only the L-isomer is used in biomedical applications. Suitable polymers are obtained by ring-opening polymerization of the cyclic diesters, i.e. the lactide and glycolide. The mechanical properties and the degradation characteristics of biodegradable implants of these materials depend on a number of factors, such as polymer synthesis and purification, the structure of the polymer chains, and the shape, surface roughness and pore size of the implant. Various methods to control the porosity of the polymer have been developed. The degradation rate of synthetic α-polyester implants may vary from a few weeks to over a year and can be modulated by appropriate polymer selection and control of manufacturing conditions. The degradation rate during the early stages of bone healing is of particular importance, because the implant material should be stable enough to act as a substrate for bone-forming cells. Furthermore, an active growth-inducing effect of the implant on bone cells can be achieved by inclusion of growth factors in the implant formulation (Coombes & Meikle, 1994).

(e) *Substances released from dental composites*

After storage of a well-cured composite specimen for one year in water, analysis by high-performance liquid chromatography (HPLC) showed that several substances had been released. However, none of the chromatographic peaks represented an organic substance known to be present in the polymer, except for possible traces of triethyleneglycol dimethacrylate (Ruyter, 1995).

Methacrylic acid is released from all resin systems. Di- and monomethacrylates hydrolyse to methacrylic acid and the alcohol component at neutral pH catalysed by an unspecific esterase (hydrolase) and by enzymes in the saliva. The rate constants of enzymatic hydrolysis of various (di)methacrylates increase in the following order: 2-hydroxypropyl methacrylate (HPMA) < 2,2-bis[4-(2-hydroxy-3-methacryloyloxypropoxy)phenyl]propane (bisphenol A diglycidylether methacrylate; bis-GMA) < lauryl methacrylate (LAMA) < decyl methacrylate (DECMA) < triethyleneglycol dimethacrylate (TEGDMA) < 1,6-bis-(methacryloyloxy-2-ethoxycarbonylamino)-2,4,4-trimethylhexane (UEDMA) < diethyleneglycol dimethacrylate (DEGDMA). Esterase added to aqueous slurries of various powders made of polymerized bis-GMA/TEGDMA mixtures liberated methacrylic acid, presumably resulting from degradation of dimethacrylates bonded only in the matrix by one end of the molecule. It has been proposed that hydrolases in saliva increase the wear rate of composite resin fillings. The hydrolytic activity of saliva is believed to depend on the activity of esterases or hydrolases released from various types of microorganisms, and repeated measurements from various collections of saliva from the same person showed some variation (Munksgaard & Freund, 1990).

The results described above are consistent with previous assumptions that hydrolases from bacteria in the mouth contribute to a breakdown of the substances contained in fixed and removable dentures, such as methyl methacrylate (Engelhardt & Grün, 1972).

Formaldehyde release from dental composite resins immersed in water for 72 h at 37°C ranged from 0.05 to 0.5 µg/cm^2 for different materials. The highest releases were observed with chemically activated materials with inhibition layers, and in one visible-light-activated material. Both grinding and polyester coating of the specimens reduced the release of formaldehyde. Only small or insignificant differences in release of formaldehyde were observed between ground specimens and specimens coated with a polyester film. The release of formaldehyde decreased with time, but it was still detectable after 115 days of immersion in water. The highest quantities of formaldehyde were released by specimens with thicker inhibition layers. As the half-life of formaldehyde is approximately 1.5 minutes, formaldehyde released from dental materials prepared according to technical standards will not reach local concentrations of toxicological relevance. However, the observed concentrations of formaldehyde may be sufficient to elicit allergic reactions (Øysæd et al., 1988).

Bisphenol A and bisphenol A dimethacrylate are monomers of certain dental sealants. A sealant based on bis-GMA showed oestrogenic properties in human MCF7 breast cancer cells by inducing cell proliferation and progesterone receptor expression. In contrast, three resin-based dental composites did not induce proliferation of MCF7 cells. Saliva samples were obtained from 18 patients during 1-h periods before and after they had received applications of 50 mg of the bis-GMA sealant on their molars. Bisphenol A (90–931 μg) was identified in all post-treatment saliva samples, and its methacrylate derivative in 3 out of 18 samples. Samples containing the highest amounts of bisphenol A and bisphenol A dimethacrylate stimulated MCF7 cell growth (Olea *et al.*, 1996).

5B.2 Tissue responses and other expressions of toxicity
5B.2.1 *Humans*
(a) *Polydimethylsiloxanes (silicones)*

Much attention has been paid to assessment of the long-term effects of implanted silicones, mainly following their use for breast augmentation. Only limited data are available on the effects of silicones used for other applications, although several complications following implantation of silicone elastomer prostheses have been reported. In a case series of 94 patients with 'Swanson' silicone elastomer implants, mainly finger joints, followed up for a mean of 116 months, an intact osseous bed was detected radiographically in only 41% of patients, with osteolysis or distant bone cysts evident in the remainder. The extent of these effects was correlated with the duration of implant. Histology of 11 revisions revealed silicone particles and an aggressive histiocytic response, with foreign-body giant cells (Wanivenhaus *et al.*, 1991).

In a case series of 422 augmentation rhinoplasty patients with silicone nasal implants over 10 years, the few late complications were predominantly aesthetic (Deva *et al.*, 1998).

A case was reported of deterioration of a silicone elastomer toe implant leading to an intense foreign-body granulomatous reaction. The implant was fragmented five years after implantation and a surrounding mass with multicystic changes was present. This was diagnosed as a florid granulomatous reaction that presented as a tumour-like condition, possibly subsequent to avascular necrosis of the first metatarsal head (Ognibene & Theodoulou, 1991).

Another case, classified as 'silastic synovitis' in the great toe was reported following implantation with a polyamide (Dacron)-coated silicone elastomer prosthesis eight years earlier (Glod & Frykberg, 1990) and a further case of cystic osteolysis and detritic synovitis was reported two years after placement of a silicone elastomer implant in the wrist. A granulomatous inflammatory response, with foreign-body particles, was noted, involving histiocytes and giant cells with numerous filopodia that resembled osteoclasts by electron microscopy. A histiocytic reaction to silicone particles was postulated as the cause of osteolysis (Ekfors *et al.*, 1984). These studies suggest that normal foreign-body reactions operate in response to silicone elastomer and reveal no specific preneoplastic changes.

Further data have come from studies on silicone breast implants and the tissue response to these implants. A series was reported of 15 resected breast implant capsules, removed from 11 post-mastectomy and four breast augmentation patients. Of these, seven capsules showed a capsule–implant interface lined by a single layer of epithelial cells. Implantation time for these was 36–240 months (median, 60; mean, 100); three were textured and four were smooth-surface implants. The layer of epithelioid cells showed characteristics of true synovial cells, with an occasional multinucleated cell and normal-appearing mitotic figures. Immunoreactivity of synovial cells for macrophage lineage suggested they were of histiocytic origin. The metaplastic synovial cell response was similar to that reported in bone or soft tissues in contact with other materials. The presence of silicone in the capsules was demonstrated. Of the eight other capsules, six were entirely acellular fibro-collagenous membranes of variable thickness. The other two were acellular membranes with diffuse microcalcification. Implantation times were not given. The authors suggested that synovial metaplasia was an adaptive response to silicone gel leakage and prosthesis movement (del Rosario et al., 1995). Although seen in this limited study in association with both smooth- and textured-surface implants, synovial metaplasia has been reported particularly in association with textured implants (Bleiweiss & Copeland, 1995).

Explanted capsular tissue was also studied in a series of 86 cases: 50 silicone gel-filled (46 smooth-surface, four textured), 12 double lumen (one textured), 14 saline-filled (all textured; four tissue expanders), nine poly(ester urethane)-coated and one injected silicone. Capsule pathology was described in some detail and was typical of a chronic inflammatory response. Calcification was seen in 11 capsules, all associated with the presence of implant stabilization patch material and with smooth-surface implants, 10 of them gel-filled. Vacuoles presumed to contain silicone were seen in macrophages in 68 cases. The presence of silicone was confirmed by infrared spectroscopy in 55/76 cases and by Raman microspectroscopy in 15 cases. Vacuolated macrophages formed sheet-like aggregates and were associated with multinucleated giant cells. Synovial metaplasia, with formation of a pseudoepithelium, occasionally with micropapillary structures, was noted in 38 cases, irrespective of filling type but more frequently with textured surfaces. Seven of these were examined immunohistochemically and showed a histiocytic phenotype, staining positive for CD68(KP-1) or lysozyme in six of seven cases (Luke et al., 1997).

A further description of capsule pathology was derived from a series of 71 explantations of silicone gel breast implants and a review of data on the pathological response to silicone leakage. Granuloma formation was associated mainly with extravasation of gel or with silicone injection, giant cells and foam cells being associated with the former. Phagocytosis of silicones in the lymph nodes by multinucleated giant cells was also described. Synovial metaplasia was characterized as changes in the innermost layer of fibroblastic cells surrounding the implant, resembling normal joint synovium. A layer, one to seven cells thick, of large, mostly polygonal epithelioid cells of various sizes was seen. Both phagocytic and secretory cells were noted, together with a prominent reticulin network; marked staining was observed for eosin and Alcian blue and, immunohistochemically, for vimentin (Beekman et al., 1997; van Diest et al., 1998).

In the case series of 86 patients described above (Luke et al., 1997), the presence of talc in tissue surrounding breast implants, presumably arising from the use of surgeons' gloves, could be a significant confounding factor with many implant types. Talc was identified in 42 cases (intracellular) and 14 cases (extracellular), a total of 65% of cases, irrespective of filling type. The identity of talc was confirmed by scanning electron microscopy/energy dispersive X-ray analysis of peaks for O, Mg and Si and by comparison of infrared spectra. Cells containing talc were identified immunohistochemically as macrophages. The significance of this finding in promoting peri-implant fibrosis, a common complication in silicone breast implants, remains to be determined.

[The Working Group noted that the inflammatory and metaplastic changes observed in these studies with breast implants are consistent with a foreign-body reaction and revealed no specific preneoplastic changes.]

(b)   Polyurethane-coated breast implants

In a series of 86 cases (described above) (Luke et al., 1997), the cellular response was found to be more prominent with the nine polyurethane-coated implants than with uncoated silicone shells. The reaction featured vacuolated macrophages, a chronic granulomatous inflammation and multinucleated giant cells, some with asteroid bodies. Two different chemical species of polyurethane were identified by infrared spectroscopy.

Two cases of haematoma were reported, six months and three years after implantation of polyurethane-coated breast implants. The authors suggested that the etiology was related to a highly vascular inflammatory response to the polyurethane coating (Wang et al., 1998).

(c)   Polytetrafluoroethylene implants

Granulomatous responses were noted in a case series of eight cancer patients in whom polytetrafluoroethylene paste (Teflon 50% w/w in glycerine, Mentor) had been injected into the larynx to restore the voice. A further three cases involving the use of the same product for this purpose have also been reported. Chronic inflammatory foreign-body responses were seen, with fibrosis and encapsulation or granuloma formation, but there was no evidence of metaplasia or neoplasia (Stone & Arnold, 1967; Harris & Hawk, 1969; Wenig et al., 1990).

(d)   Joint replacements, polyethylene and bone cement

With cemented joints, which make up the majority of joint implants, bone and surrounding tissues are exposed to acrylic substances that cure *in situ* in an exothermic reaction (a temperature rise of up to 17°C has been reported by Reckling & Dillon (1977)). This inevitably gives rise to release of monomers or additives into surrounding tissue. Wear of articulating surfaces leads to release of particles of varying size, shape, surface characteristics and composition. These circumstances, and the physical stresses related to the load placed on the implant during use, imply that there is a particularly demanding biological environment. Due to concern over the long-term performance of joint replacement prostheses, numerous studies have examined the tissue response to these implants, with special emphasis on determining mechanisms of necrosis, bone resorption or other factors leading to joint failure. Few of these studies have specific relevance to carcinogenicity but they do illustrate the pathological processes that occur in response to the various materials that are used in orthopaedic joint replacement surgery.

The sort of response commonly seen is typified by a series of 23 bone specimens obtained after one month to seven years of exposure to acrylic cement (four specimens were retrieved at five to seven years after implantation). The topographic anatomy of the sites of new and old bone, of fibrocartilage and of fibrous tissue at the cement–bone interface was described. From the distribution of these tissues, an attempt was made to interpret how the load of body weight is transmitted from the cement to the shaft of the femur. Fibrocartilagenous layers produced in response to mechanical pressure were noted, with occasional points of direct contact between cement and bone. Ossification was noted in the vicinity of underlying bone and a foreign-body giant-cell response was seen on the surface of fibrous tissue in direct contact with cement. The latter response appeared to be most prominent at two to five years (Charnley, 1970).

The histological and immunohistochemical characteristics of tissue surrounding the acetabular component were reviewed in a case series of 11 hip revision patients. The fibrous and inflammatory responses were assessed quantitatively. Cathepsin-G activity, associated with monocyte or macrophage-like and fibroblast-like cells, was higher in periprosthetic tissue than in control tissue from synovial capsule or pseudo-synovial fluid. The authors suggested that cathepsin-G, which is known to interact with TNF-α and other enzymes, has a role in the loosening of the prosthesis (Takagi et al., 1995).

Information on allergies or hypersensitivity reactions to non-metallic constituents of orthopaedic devices is scarce. The sensitivity of 25 patients undergoing orthopaedic surgery was studied by collecting venous blood at short intervals during the surgery and measuring serum concentrations of total haemolytic complement and of components 3 and 4. Eleven patients received total hip arthroplasty (no cement used), while two groups of seven patients were treated for hemi-arthroplasty with and without the use of methyl methacrylate cement, respectively. Neither the surgery nor the use of the cement induced activation of the complement (Monteny et al., 1978).

(e) *Dental materials*

In general, dental materials have acceptable biocompatibility for clinical use in patients. Methyl methacrylate monomer and mercury have in a few instances of high occupational exposure led to classical, dose-dependent toxicological problems. With these exceptions, the amounts of individual chemicals to which professionals and patients are exposed do not seem sufficient to cause manifest, systemic toxic effects.

Localized effects of dental materials such as those related topographically to oral lichenoid lesions may have a premalignant potential. These lesions require adequate diagnosis and systematic clinical follow-up (Holmstrup, 1999).

(i) *Irritant contact dermatitis*

This acute toxic reaction is a dermal inflammatory response to primary irritants. It is a result of physical or chemical action due, for instance, to trauma, ionizing radiation, heat, bases, acids or other reactive chemicals. Depending on the concentration and exposure time, the reaction can vary from erythema to necrosis. The substances may exert a direct cytotoxic effect on the cells in the superficial skin or mucosa, most often corresponding exactly with the site of application. In the oral cavity the boundaries of the inflamed area may be more diffuse. This type of reaction is seen when, e.g., phosphoric acid enamel etchant or bonding agents are inadvertently spilled on the mucosa or skin and remain there for some time (Jacobsen *et al.*, 1991).

Cumulative insult dermatitis can develop following repeated contact with low doses of primary irritants over extended time periods and is caused by a gradual deterioration of the natural barriers. Such exposure conditions are mainly seen in occupational settings. The changes in skin or mucosa are localized to the area of contact with the offending agent and they do not spread to other sites. The diagnosis of cumulative insult dermatitis or mucositis cannot be made on the basis of epicutaneous patch testing or other investigations, but is made by exclusion of other possibilities, based on the case history, the clinical appearance of the lesion and negative patch tests. One example is the 'three-finger syndrome' with a clear positive topographical relationship between the skin changes and contact with dental materials in persons who have negative patch tests to the constituents of the relevant dental materials. This type of reaction is often seen on the first three fingers of the left hand, in right-handed persons. These three fingers are exposed to spray from bonding resins when used to reflect the patients' lips during treatment and may also have been in contact with the remnants of spills on the outside of squeeze-bottles containing the liquid monomers (see, e.g., Munksgaard, 1992).

Gloves used for prevention of microbial contamination do not protect from exposure to monomers in dental materials. The monomers penetrate vinyl and latex gloves within a few minutes, and may therefore be in contact with the skin for an extended time period (Munksgaard, 1992).

Paraesthesia related to contact with dental resins has been observed in a few instances. Dental technicians and orthopaedic surgeons may have dermatitis associated with the use of methyl methacrylate monomer, often in the form of marked dryness and fissuring of the skin. A unique feature is a paraesthesia of the fingertips in the form of a burning sensation, tingling and slight numbness. This type of paraesthesia was observed in two orthodontists who had become sensitized to the monomer in orthodontic bonding materials (Fisher, 1982). This might be due to a direct neurotoxic effect of the methyl methacrylate monomer (Seppäläinen & Rajaniemi, 1984).

Biopsies from a dental laboratory technician who had been preparing dental prostheses for more than 30 years have shown direct pathological effects of methyl methacrylate on nerve fibres, resulting in a sensorimotor peripheral neuropathy (Donaghy et al., 1991).

(ii) *Allergic contact dermatitis*

Although allergic reactions are basically different from toxic reactions, their clinical manifestations are often similar or even identical. Most components of dental materials are of low molecular weight. By acting as haptens and combining with body proteins, they may form complete antigens capable of inducing sensitization of immunocompetent cells. The risk of sensitization varies, depending on the type and concentration of the substance and the type and condition of the contacting tissues. The actual contact site with the allergen is usually the first place where clinical symptoms develop. However, contact-sensitized individuals may develop a number of symptoms when exposed to the allergen systemically, either orally or by inhalation, infusion or transcutaneous or transmucosal absorption.

The problems related to systemic allergic contact dermatitis are complex and not completely understood (see, e.g., Nakada et al. (1997) for a discussion of allergic reactions to gold chloride, mercuric chloride and metallic mercury). Allergic reactions to any component of dental materials may occur in patients and in dental professionals handling the materials. More than 130 common allergens have been identified among the various dental materials available today (Kanerva et al., 1995).

(iii) *Anaphylactoid reactions*

Anaphylactoid reactions in children have been reported following the placement of fissure sealants, which are based on the same ingredients as composite materials (Hällström, 1993). An anaphylactoid reaction developed in a four-year-old child after contact with a dental surgeon's latex gloves (Rasmussen, 1997).

(iv) *Photo-related reactions*

Phototoxic or photoallergic reactions have not been documented in the context of oral medicine, but may well represent a new occupational problem as a result of the extensive use of powerful light units in the curing of dental resin-based materials. Substances of dental interest which may have phototoxic properties are sulfonamides (present in some cavity liners), phenothiazines, griseofulvin and some tetracyclines. Examples of photoallergic compounds of interest in the context of dental treatment are eugenol, chlorhexidine, derivatives of *para*-aminobenzoic acid, eosin (a colorant in some lipsticks), sulfonamides and phenothiazines. A generalized, intensely erythematous eruption of the face and submental area in a dental hygienist was traced to a combination of long-term trimethoprim medication and exposure to stray light from a laboratory photocuring unit (Hudson, 1987). The possibilities of photo-related reactions should be taken into account in evaluating dermatoses in dental personnel and patients.

(v) *Contact urticaria*

There have been many reports of patients with urticarial reactions to dental materials. Contact urticaria is a wheal and flare response elicited by the application of various compounds to intact skin. One case of persistent generalized urticaria was traced to a resin-based orthodontic bonding agent (Tinkelman & Tinkelman, 1979). Another case also presented traits of an anaphylactoid reaction (Hallström, 1993).

Immunological contact urticaria is an immunoglobin E-mediated reaction, entailing histamine release from mast cells. It may be localized or widespread and is sometimes associated with features of anaphylaxis. Such reactions have been observed after contact with surgical latex gloves, where both the powder and the latex may contain substances capable of eliciting urticarial reactions (Wrangsjö et al., 1988).

Non-immunological contact urticaria is clinically indistinguishable from the other variety, and occurs without previous sensitization in most exposed persons. The reaction remains localized and does not spread to become generalized urticaria, nor does it cause systemic symptoms. Its pathogenetic mechanism is not clearly understood. This type of contact urticaria may be elicited by a number of compounds, notably benzoic acid, which occurs naturally in many fruits, is added as a preservative (E 210) in salad dressings and other processed foods and is formed as a degradation product of benzoyl peroxide, used as an initiator in dental composites and denture base resins (Koda et al., 1990).

(vi) *Other types of hypersensitivity: hyperreactivity and intolerance reactions*

These types of 'other hypersensitivity reaction' have been studied considerably less than those mentioned above. A fairly large proportion of hypersensitivity problems must still be ascribed to the 'nonallergic type with unknown cause', since there is limited information about which cells and mediators are involved (SOU, 1989).

Hyperreactivity is associated with vasomotoric reactions of the airways and eyes. Vasomotoric rhinitis/conjunctivitis simulates a chronic allergic condition, but may be due to a direct influence on the peripheral nerve endings in the mucosal linings. Reactions may be elicited by certain perfumes, including eugenol, volatile monomers, fumes from soldering fluxes containing colophony and other irritants.

Intolerance reactions may simulate allergic reactions, but are not mediated by the immune system. These reactions are associated with insufficient levels of enzymes that normally metabolize substances such as fructose, sucrose, acetylsalicylic acid, ethanol and benzoic acid. Whether the small amounts of benzoic acid liberated from dental resins (Koda et al., 1990) may contribute to such problems is not known.

(vii) *Local and systemic effects*

Acid etching and adhesive agents

The reactions of the dental pulp to acid etching in combination with different bonding procedures before implantation of composite restorations have been studied in human teeth *in vivo*. The experimental restorations were placed in intact premolars of 11–15-year-old children. The teeth were scheduled for extraction for orthodontic reasons, which took place four months after the treatments. Acid etching of the dentin appeared to increase the penetration of a low-viscosity resin into the dentinal tubules, thus enhancing the adverse effects of this resin, unless the dentin had been protected during the etching procedure. A glycidyl methacrylate-based dental adhesive did not cause pulpal reactions. The effects in the dental pulp, e.g., inflammatory reactions and growth-reduction of odontoblasts, could only partly be explained by a direct toxic effect of the material tested. Other factors, such as tooth position and marginal leakage resulting in bacterial in-growth also contributed to the inflammatory reaction (Qvist et al., 1989).

In a similar study in premolars in children, histological observation of dental pulp revealed that a glutaraldehyde-based dentinal adhesive caused slight to severe responses, changes in odontoblastic layers and inhibition of dentinogenesis after periods of up to 120 days (Elbaum *et al.*, 1991).

The dental pulp of eight permanent premolars and molars was protected during dental restoration by direct capping with a glutaraldehyde-containing dentin adhesive. All eight teeth examined remained vital and without symptoms during an initial observation period of up to six months after treatment (Heitmann & Unterbrink, 1995).

A review on the biocompatibility of dental bonding agents reported that some agents seem to be irritant to pulpal tissue, and recommended pulpal protection, preferably in the form of spot lining in the deepest part of the cavity (Al-Dawood & Wennberg, 1993).

Composite filling materials

The inherent polymerization shrinkage of composite resins may allow bacterial leakage and give rise to pulpal reactions. Pulp tissue was investigated from exfoliated primary teeth in which shallow class II composite restorations without bonding resin had been placed eight months to more than six years earlier. Histological examination revealed no pulpal inflammation in 5/16 teeth, moderate to severe inflammation in 4/16 teeth, and pulpal necrosis in 7/16 teeth. These pulpal effects paralleled the extent of bacterial penetration into the pulp (Varpio *et al.*, 1990).

In a review of the pulpal response to composite restorations, it was confirmed that the toxicity of the materials used was of less concern than bacterial invasion into the dentinal tubules (Barnett, 1992).

From a summary of clinical reports on dental composites, it appeared that pulp inflammation has not been adequately documented in clinical trials, most studies using sensitivity responses as a measure of biological compatibility. However, sensitivity does not seem to have any correlation with pulpal inflammation, which is caused by mechanical, thermal, chemical and bacterial insults (Bayne, 1992).

A comparable occurrence of post-treatment sensitivity was observed between teeth restored with composite filling materials (25%) and those with dental amalgam (21%).

A quarter of the patients accounted for 60% of complaints, leading the authors to suggest that three factors might contribute to the increased sensitivity: the material, the operating procedure and the pain threshold of the patient. In no case was sensitivity reported after six months (Borgmeijer et al., 1991). In another study with a five-year observation period, only one out of 176 restorations was replaced due to increased sensitivity (Rasmusson & Lundin, 1995).

On the basis of surveys among Scandinavian dentists, it can be estimated that adverse reactions of patients to composite materials occur at frequencies of 1:1000 after prosthodontic treatment and 1:10 000 after paedodontic treatment (Hensten-Pettersen & Jacobsen, 1991).

In a recording by 137 dentists over a 10-day period of side-effects of dental materials in clinical practice, no acute reactions were reported from 2400 composite restorations (Kallus & Mjör, 1991).

Lichenoid reactions related to composite restorations were observed in a study of 17 patients, eight of whom received dental composites to replace amalgam restorations that were topographically related to earlier lichenoid lesions. In addition, lichenoid reactions were seen in nine patients with no previous history of such reactions. Total remission in four cases and partial remission in five patients were observed after the composite material had been replaced with gold inlays or porcelain fused to gold crowns (Lind, 1988).

In a study on experimental gingivitis, no difference in the development of plaque and gingivitis was observed on intact enamel and composite fillings during a seven-day period (van Dijken et al., 1987).

Dust particles generated from composite materials during grinding and finishing composite restorations were examined. About 60–80% of the particles trapped on filters were respirable (size 0.5–5.0 μm) and were composed of 70–100% silica. Dust generated from composites containing crystalline silica as a filter was suggested to have potential to cause silicosis, whereas dust generated from composites containing amorphous silica was not expected to have the same potential (Collard et al., 1989, 1991).

5B.2.2 *Experimental systems*
  (a) *Inflammatory, hyperplastic and metaplastic responses*
    (i) *Polydimethylsiloxanes (silicones)*

The inflammatory response to silicones is well characterized and is predominantly lymphocytic, with macrophage involvement and cytokine production; the outcome is normally fibrotic with occasional granuloma (sometimes termed siliconoma) formation. Animal studies have shown that silicones are not significantly immunotoxic but some can act as adjuvants under experimental conditions; however, their ability to elicit specific antibody responses or cell-mediated immunity is limited. Silicones can be found in tissues following implantation of gel or liquid, in deposits ranging from large intercellular or cytoplasmic droplets to microscopic particles within macrophages. Transport of silicones via the lymphatic system has been demonstrated (Rees et al., 1970; Tinkler et al., 1993; Gott & Tinkler, 1994; Shanklin & Smalley, 1995; Marcus, 1996).

With the exception of those investigating foreign-body carcinogenesis or using silicones as control materials, few studies have looked into relevant tissue responses arising from the presence of silicone materials. One study examined the reaction to various components of silicone breast implants in rats. Discs (3/8 × 0.02 inch (9.5 × 0.5 mm)) of various silicone gel breast implant component materials (elastomer shell, xylene-extracted shell, silicone extract (coated onto an implant shell), silica-free silicone) were implanted subcutaneously into groups of three Lew/SsN rats (two discs per rat). Fumed silica (approximately 1 mL) and the liquid silicone oil and viscous gel (1 mL) were injected subcutaneously. Histological examination at 7, 14, 28, 56 and 90 days showed the progression of the inflammatory and fibrotic response and the differences between the materials. The degrees of fibrous capsule formation and migration of silicone were dependent on molecular weight. The response also varied with the degree of compliance of the material, which coincided with fumed silica content. Free-fumed silica induced an intense early response, with fibroblasts, pericytes, macrophages and some surrounding mast cells. Exudate was seen between the capsule and the material together with some neovascularization. Later, cell destruction and the absence of a fibrous capsule were evident, with fibroblasts, lymphocytes and macrophages but no multinucleated giant cells. The authors concluded that there was an immunological component to the response with the silicone extract, based on the strong multinucleated giant-cell response; however, the reported results did not indicate such a response with fumed silica. No other cellular response was noted and there were thus no indications of pre-carcinogenic mechanisms; however, the number of animals and the duration of the study were inadequate to allow firm conclusions to be drawn (Picha & Goldstein, 1991).

(ii) *Polyurethanes*

Highly stable poly(ether urethanes) are now used in most implant applications (e.g., in vascular grafts). However, most investigations into the effects of implanted polyurethanes have concentrated either on estimating the risk arising from degradation of the poly(ester urethane) foam coating in certain breast implants or on assessing the ability of this material to initiate foreign-body carcinogenesis (see Section 5B.1). One study has investigated the response to the poly(ester urethane) used as a breast implant coating material. Four poly(ester urethane) foam discs (6 mm diameter × 3 mm; soaked in ethanol and rinsed) were implanted into pockets between the mammary fat pad and muscle of groups of 25 female $B6D2F_1$ mice. Controls received sham surgery. Mice were killed at 10 time points between one day and 47 weeks for limited histopathological examination and, at four weeks, for electron microscopy. The inflammatory response observed involved macrophages and giant cells, leading to fibrosis. Phagocytosis of polyurethane particles was noted from week 4 and the implants had virtually disappeared by week 47. No inflammatory or other changes that might indicate a predisposition to carcinogenicity were observed (Devor et al., 1993).

A group of 132 female Swiss albino mice were given sub-mammary implants of poly(ether urethane) foam discs (5 mm diameter × 2 mm) and observed for one year. The relatively large pore size used in the foam (40–45 interconnecting pores per inch (16–18 per cm)) was associated with ingrowth of fatty and loose connective tissue, with a small amount of dense collagenous tissue (Dunaif et al., 1963).

(iii) *Polyethylene*

Because of its widespread use in orthopaedic joint implants and the associated clinical damage due to the effects of wear particles, ultra-high-molecular-weight polyethylene has been investigated in many experimental studies on the biological effects of wear debris. These studies give insight into inflammatory processes and their mediators and into the mechanism of necrosis or osteolysis associated with prosthesis loosening. However, the relevance of such studies to carcinogenicity is limited and they are not discussed here.

Male and female Fischer 344 rats were given subcutaneous implants of 65 mg particles (size range, 425–600 μm) of polysulfone (29 rats) or polyethylene (32 rats) dispersed in 0.5 mL saline. Fibrous capsule tissue from around the implants was examined to determine the proportion of particle surface associated with the various inflammatory cell types. Rats were given the implants at 16 weeks and were killed at 100–118 weeks. A group of 26 controls received sham operations. There was no discernible difference between the two polymers in terms of the macroscopic, microscopic or quantitatively measured response. Almost half of the particle surface was covered by macrophages, while giant cells and fibrous tissue each covered about 20%. In a zone around each type of polymer particle, comparable numbers of giant cells were found (see Table 56). Surface texture influenced the adherent cell type: rough particles were predominantly covered by giant cells, whereas smooth particles were more often associated with macrophages or fibroblasts. This finding reached statistical significance, on the basis of a [presumably subjective] assessment of roughness at × 100 magnification. Cell morphology was described from a transmission electron

Table 56. Surface coverage of polysulfone and polyethylene particles by different cell types

Material	Mean particle surface covered by cell type (%)			No. of giant cells
	Macrophage	Giant cell	Fibrous tissue	
Polysulfone	49	21	17	2
Polyethylene	47	18	23	3

Adapted from Behling and Spector (1986)

microscopy study. No differences were found in the ultrastructure of the cells surrounding the polyethylene and polysulfone particles. Numerous cell processes in interfacial macrophages, evidence of phagocytic activity, amorphous extracellular material close to the polymer surface and occasional collagenous material but no fibroblasts at the material surface were observed (Behling & Spector, 1986).

(iv) *Polytetrafluoroethylene*

Groups of 50 Sprague-Dawley rats received 0.1-mL subcutaneous injections of particulate plastics, namely 50% polytetrafluoroethylene in glycerine (90% of the particles were smaller than 40 µm) or a 38% silicone elastomer in hydrogel carrier (most particles were 100–150 µm in size, but some were 5 µm). Controls were untreated. Injection sites and major organs were examined histologically after two years. A normal chronic inflammatory response was seen but no inflammatory infiltrate in the tissue adjacent to the injection site (Dewan et al., 1995a).

The presence of polytetrafluoroethylene beads in the urinary bladder resulted in accelerated cell turnover in a rat model in which the bladder was transplanted into muscle to avoid problems associated with implantation into the bladder (heterotopically transplanted bladder system). Fischer 344 rats in which urinary bladders from syngeneic rats had been transplanted into the gluteal muscle were used, four weeks after the transplantation. Two 6-mm diameter beads of polytetrafluoroethylene were placed in the bladder lumen. One group of 25 rats received the beads and one group of 25 rats had a sham operation. Bladders were filled with saline containing gentamicin after the operation. One week later, groups of rats received either 0.5 mL rat urine or 0.5 mL saline weekly in their transplanted bladder. Histological and autoradiographic ([^{3}H]thymidine incorporation) examination took place one, three or six weeks after bead implantation. Moderate foci of simple epithelial hyperplasia (4–7 cell layers) were seen at all intervals. Foci of inverted or exophytic nodular or papillary hyperplasia were seen occasionally at week 3, with frequent mild acute inflammation and loose fibrosis. At week 6, fibrosis and acute or chronic inflammation were present in the lamina propria beneath hyperplastic foci and multifocal nodular or papillary hyperplasia (up to eight cell layers) was evident. The changes were more severe than those seen in concurrent studies with formalin solution. A significant ($p < 0.01$) increase in [^{3}H]thymidine incorporation was seen in comparison with sham-operated controls, which had occasional mild fibrosis in the lamina propria but no hyperplasia. The hyperplastic response was enhanced in the presence of urine, which had been found, in previous studies, to contain tumour-promoting substance(s) (Homma & Oyasu, 1986).

(v) *Acrylic substances (IARC, 1979b, 1986, 1994b)*

Evidence that a biological response to an implant may be more dependent on toxic components leaching from implanted materials than on the properties of the bulk material itself was obtained in a study investigating the effects of subcutaneous implantation of three acrylic denture base resins in guinea-pigs. A specified auto-polymerized pour resin, a heat-polymerized resin and a specified auto-polymerized dough resin were polymerized in 10 mm × 1.5 mm polyethylene tubes one to four days before implantation. They were not sterilized. A total of 20 female guinea-pigs that had served as controls in a maximization test and had been given Freund's complete adjuvant (FCA) received one implant per animal through a 5-mm incision in the back. Two groups of seven animals were observed for 14 or 30 days and one group of six animals was observed for 90 days. A further group of seven implanted animals that had not previously received FCA was observed for 30 days but no difference from the FCA-treated group was detected. An inflammatory response with a fibrous capsule was observed, which decreased with time. The apparent resolution of inflammation at 90 days was most pronounced with the heat-polymerized resin (reaching statistical significance) and least pronounced with the dough polymer. A reduction in width of the capsule was noted. The authors speculated that the gradation in severity of response was partially linked to the irritant properties of residual methyl methacrylate monomer, which was 3% in the dough (which elicited the greatest response) and the pour resin and 1% in the heat-polymerized resin (which was the best tolerated). Other residual chemicals were also suggested as having a role in mediating the response. A link between inflammation and release kinetics of residues or breakdown products was postulated (Kallus, 1984).

(vi) *Ceramics, hydroxylapatite*

Implants of porous and dense hydroxylapatite ($Ca_{10}(PO_4)_6(OH)_2$; pore sizes 100 μm and 3 μm, respectively) were placed in the ears of groups of Wistar rats. Each ear had two implants, either both porous or both dense, inserted into a hole in the bony wall of the middle ear. A total of 116 dense and 120 porous implants were studied in normal ears, and 70 of each in infected ears. Infection was induced three weeks before analysis by intratympanic injection of a *Staphylococcus aureus* suspension in saline. Histopathological examination and electron microscopy up to one year after implantation revealed a fibrotic and epithelial response in the vicinity of the implants, most pronounced in the first month after implantation (assessed by [^{3}H]thymidine incorporation). Covering of the implant was due not only to cell proliferation but also to cell migration over the implant area. The reaction stabilized after three months. There was a granular layer between the bone and the implant, except where inflammatory cells were present. Pores were initially filled with exudate and fibrous tissue, followed by bony infiltration, the greater pore size being associated with a greater amount of infiltration. In the infected ears, the presence of the hydroxylapatite did not affect the inflammatory reactions (oedema, vasodilatation, osteoresorption followed by bone deposition), nor did infection influence the reactions on or in the implant. No other cellular response was noted (Grote *et al.*, 1986).

Inflammatory changes were noted following the implantation of glass–ceramic materials into rabbit ear bones for up to two years. Inflammation subsided within two months of implantation. Mucous membrane and bone overgrowth of bioactive glass–ceramic was noted. Lysis of the implant as part of bone remodelling (with giant cell infiltration) was seen at one to two years. No changes suggesting a predisposition to neoplasia were evident from this remodelling process (Reck, 1984).

(vii) *Dental composites*

Cell culture studies

The available cell culture techniques are useful as screening tests to compare potential toxicity of dental materials and their components, but not as usage tests, e.g., to predict pulp reactions.

In an in-vitro test system for assessment of the toxicity of dentine bonding agents after penetration through 100-µm or 50-µm slices of dentin (dentin barrier test), three such agents were found to be highly cytotoxic for cultured hamster fibroblasts, in the absence of adequate lining (Meryon & Brook, 1989). In a similar study with human pulpal fibroblasts, cytotoxic effects of bonding materials were also shown following diffusion through dentin. In some cases, such effects were seen even after seven days (Bouillaguet *et al.*, 1998).

In a study with freshly extracted or cryo-preserved teeth, simulated pulpal pressure appeared to increase the toxicity of dental bonding agents towards mouse L-929 fibroblasts (Camps *et al.*, 1997).

The cytotoxicity of various bonding agents was further demonstrated on the basis of growth of mouse L-cells on microscope slides coated with these materials (Schaller *et al.*, 1985).

It has been reported that the toxicity of bonding materials for in-vitro cultured L-929 cells diminished after a few days' pre-incubation of the specimens in culture medium at 37°C, and had disappeared after six weeks of incubation. The authors conclude that bonding agents are unlikely to induce chronic toxicity and that the benefits of preventing microleakage after dental restorations far exceed the potential risk of cytotoxic effects from these materials (Schedle *et al.*, 1999).

A resin-based dental filling material containing bis-GMA and TEGMA produced toxic reactions in cultured BALB/c 3T3 cells, which could be eliminated by extraction of leachable components into suitable organic solvents, such as ethanol, chloroform and toluene. The primary active component was identified as unreacted bis-GMA (Rathbun *et al.*, 1991).

In an in-vitro test system with human HEp-2 cells, the cytotoxicity of light-cured dental composites was shown to decrease with increasing curing time (Puza *et al.*, 1990). Comparable results were found with various dental resin materials tested on human gingival fibroblast cultures (Caughman *et al.*, 1991). Similarly, extracts obtained from composite resins cured by either visible or ultraviolet light showed strong toxicity towards human HeLa cells or mouse L-929 fibroblasts in the early stages of extraction, but the effects diminished rapidly and were no longer detectable after six weeks of extraction (Nakamura *et al.*, 1985; Schedle *et al.*, 1994).

Various types of composite resin were reported to show slight cytotoxicity for an appreciable time after setting (Schedle et al., 1999), in sharp contrast to the marked toxicity of the resin monomer itself (Nakamura et al., 1985).

Animal studies

The pulpal effects of acid etching in deep cavities have been studied in monkeys. Inflammatory responses and odontoblast displacement were seen three days after etching of cavities with 1% citric acid, but the effects were less severe after 59 days and could be largely suppressed in teeth treated with a liner containing calcium hydroxide after acid application (McInnes-Ledoux et al., 1985).

The pulpal effects of citric acid on surgically exposed root dentin have also been studied in cats. After 21 days, the frequency of adverse pulpal responses to surgery and citric acid treatment is significantly greater than to surgery alone (Ryan et al., 1984).

The pulpal effects of bonding agents have been studied in teeth of ferrets and monkeys filled with composite materials, complicating evaluation of the effects of bonding *per se*. The adverse effects of bonding were reported to be less pronounced in the canine teeth of ferrets than effects of the composite filling material and could be almost eliminated with a calcium hydroxide lining (Plant et al., 1986). In similar studies in monkeys, more pulpal reaction was observed in teeth with composite fillings than in those where a bonding and a composite filling had been placed. The presence of bacteria in the cavities has been suggested to cause some of the effects seen in teeth without bonding agents. With increasing observation time, the degree of pulp inflammation tends to decrease markedly (Hörsted-Bindslev, 1987; Harnirattisai & Hosoda, 1991). Other studies in monkeys have revealed more irritation dentin formation—a sign of initial damage to odontoblasts—in teeth lined with dental adhesives before placement of resin-bonded inlays than in teeth where no adhesives were used (Inokoshi et al., 1995).

A comparison was made of the periodontal effects of silver amalgam and composite restorations placed on the roots of incisor teeth which had been extracted from monkeys and were replanted within an hour after the treatment. Whereas the amalgam produced a localized inflammation that subsided with the formation of a fibrous capsule, the composite resin restorations caused a chronic inflammatory response in the periodontal membrane (Nasjleti et al., 1983).

Implantation studies with dental composites have shown persistent inflammation at the implant site after periods of up to three months in rats (Wennberg et al., 1983; Steinbrunner et al., 1991), ferrets (Grieve et al., 1991) and monkeys (Hörsted et al., 1986). As bacterial contamination was found in dentinal tubules below the fillings in all these studies, it is difficult to assess which of the effects can be attributed to the composite materials.

New cohesive bonding systems prevent postoperative hypersensitivity and completely seal the tooth–restoration interface, preventing bacterial infection of the underlying substrate and ultimately reducing recurrent caries beneath the hybridized restoration (Cox et al., 1995).

(viii) *Components of dental composites*

The toxicity of materials used in dental composites is summarized in Table 57.

The potential toxicity of the components of resin composites and/or bonding agents has been studied with cell culture techniques. The inhibitory effects of 11 components of resin composites on DNA synthesis, total protein content and protein synthesis of BALB/c 3T3 fibroblasts were investigated. Ethoxylated bisphenol A dimethacrylate was the most toxic compound tested (LC_{50} between 1 and 10 μmol/L). The LC_{50} values for seven other components, namely, bis-GMA, urethane dimethacrylate (UDMA), TEGDMA, 1,6-hexanediol dimethacrylate, glycidyl methacrylate, bisphenol A and bisphenol A diglycidyl ether ranged between 10 and 100 μmol/L, while the LC_{50} values of N,N-dihydroxyethyl-p-toluidine, camphorquinone and N,N-dimethylaminoethyl methacrylate were above 100 μmol/L. The authors noted that the concentrations to which cells and tissues are actually exposed *in vivo* are not known (Hanks *et al.*, 1991).

The toxic interactions of various methacrylic esters used as dentin bonding agents in mouse BALB/c 3T3 fibroblasts *in vitro* were tested by measuring cell survival with the dimethylthiazolium-diphenyl-tetrazolium-bromide (MTT) test. Toxicity of the single compounds increased in the order 2-hydroxyethyl methacrylate<<<TEGDMA<UDMA<bis-GMA. Cytotoxicity also increased with incubation time (Ratanasathien *et al.*, 1995).

The rank order of cytotoxicity (ED_{50} values) of composite resin components tested in BALB/c 3T3 fibroblasts was reported to be bis-GMA (0.12 mmol/L) > 2,6-di-t-butyl-4-methylphenol (0.16 mmol/L) > triphenyl antimony (0.51 mmol/L) > camphoric anhydride (1.75 mmol/L) > 2-hydroxy-4-methoxybenzophenone (3.54 mmol/L) > dimethyl-p-toluidine (3.6 mmol/L) (Lehmann *et al.*, 1993).

The cytotoxicity of UDMA in human KB cells was investigated by means of flow cytometric analysis of cellular DNA content. Depending on the concentration of the oligomer, UDMA functions in both a cytostatic (at 10 and 25 μmol/L) and cytotoxic (at 50 μmol/L) manner (Nassiri *et al.*, 1994).

The resin components UDMA, bis-GMA, TEGDMA, bisphenol A, glycidyl methacrylate and N,N-dihydroxyethyl-p-toluidine were reported to evoke either immunosuppressive or immunostimulatory activities on the mitogen-driven proliferation *in vitro* of purified T-lymphocytes, activated by accessory cells from the dental pulp, and spleen cells of the rat (Jontell *et al.*, 1995).

The components of resin composites are hazardous in so far as all show significant toxicity in direct contact with fibroblasts. However, these components have different cytotoxic potencies and the risk to dental pulp depends upon the quantities which permeate the dentin and accumulate in the pulp (see also Wataha *et al.*, 1994).

Blood lipid peroxidation and haemolysis were observed upon irradiation of cultured dog erythrocytes overlaid with a solution of photoinitiators used for light-cured composites. These effects were concentration-dependent (Fujisawa *et al.*, 1986).

Table 57. Acute and chronic toxicity of materials used in the composition of dental resins

Compound	In-vitro toxicity	In-vivo toxicity	Mutagenicity/genotoxicity	References
Methacrylic acid	Day 10 rat embryos in culture: positive indices of teratogenicity and cell death at 1.2–2.1 mM	Corrosive to eye and skin	In vitro: DNA-binding: positive S. typhimurium: negative In vivo: no data	Rogers et al., 1986 Greim et al., 1995
Bisphenol A-glycidyl methacrylate	ID_{50} growth inhibition test: 3T3 mouse fibroblasts: 120 μM Gingiva fibroblasts: 80 μM Growth inhibition of human gingival carcinoma cells: ID_{10} = 10 μg/mL; no-effect conc. 0.6 μg/ml Inhibition of DNA synthesis in BALB/c 3T3 cells: ID_{50} = 13 μM	Irritating	Negative in Salmonella umu test No increase in chromosomal aberrations in occupationally exposed workers	Lehmann et al., 1993 Leyhausen et al., 1995 Hanks et al., 1991 Mitelman et al., 1980 Imai et al., 1988
Bisphenol-A dimethacrylate	Oestrogenic activity in MCF7 cells (1/10 000 of oestradiol)	No data	No data	Olea et al., 1996
Ethoxylated bisphenol-A dimethacrylate	Inhibition of DNA synthesis in BALB/c 3T3 cells: ID_{50} = 3.3 μM	No data	No data	Hanks et al., 1991
Triethylene glycol dimethacrylate	Inhibition of DNA synthesis in BALB/c 3T3 cells: ID_{50} = 70 μM Growth inhibition of rat osteoblasts: IC_{50} = 700 μM Stimulation of mitogen-driven T-lymphocyte proliferation	No data	S. typhimurium negative, 5 strains, ± S9 (up to 10 000 μg/plate) Positive in V79/HPRT gene mutation assay and in micronucleus assay in V79B cells	Suda & Kawase, 1991 Jontell et al., 1995 Hanks et al., 1991 Schweikl et al., 1998 Schweikl & Schmalz, 1999
Ethylene glycol dimethacrylate	Moderate reaction with cellular glutathione (EC_{50} = 1.3 mM)	No data	No data	McCarthy et al., 1994
Diethylene glycol dimethacrylate	No data	No data	S. typhimurium negative, 5 strains, ± S9, 40–2500 μg/plate	Waegemaekers & Bensink, 1984
Tetraethylene glycol dimethacrylate	Reduced survival of mouse lymphoma L5178 cells at 350–525 μg/mL	No data	Positive in mouse lymphoma L5178 tk-locus mutation assay, micro-nucleus test and chromosomal aberration test in L5178 cells, at 350–525 μg/mL	Dearfield et al., 1989

Table 57 (contd)

Compound	In-vitro toxicity	In-vivo toxicity	Mutagenicity/genotoxicity	References
Urethane dimethacrylate	Growth inhibition of human gingival carcinoma cells: $ID_{10} = 9$ µg/mL; no-effect conc. 0.6 µg/mL; Inhibition of DNA synthesis in BALB/c 3T3 cells: $ID_{50} = 11$ µM Stimulation of mitogen-driven T-lymphocyte proliferation	No data	No data	Imai et al., 1988 Hanks et al., 1991 Jontell et al., 1995
1,4-Butanediol dimethacrylate	No data	No data	S. typhimurium negative, 5 strains, ± S9, 40–2500 µg/plate	Waegemaekers & Bensink, 1984
1,6-Hexanediol dimethacrylate	No data	No data	S. typhimurium negative, 4 strains, ± S9, 40–2500 µg/plate	Waegemaekers & Bensink, 1984
2-Hydroxyethyl methacrylate	Growth inhibition of human gingival carcinoma cells: $ID_{10} = 250$ µg/mL; no-effect conc. 30 µg/mL Human gingival cells, inhibition of cell growth rate to 24% of control	No data	S. typhimurium negative, 4 strains, ± S9, 40–2500 µg/plate	Imai et al., 1988, 1992 Waegemaekers & Bensink, 1984
Methyl methacrylate	Growth inhibition of human gingival carcinoma cells: $ID_{10} = 1000$ µg/mL; no-effect conc. 100 µg/mL	Release from poly(methyl methacrylate) orally from palatal appliances in humans, local concentration: 180 µg/mL; release rate 29 µg in the first hour (non-toxic) Dermatitis, eczema and sensitization can be adverse reactions in dentists and dental technicians Allergic sensitization also observed in dental patients	S. typhimurium negative, 5 strains ± S9, 40–10 000 µg/plate Positive in mouse lymphoma L5178 tk-locus mutation assay, micronucleus and chromosomal aberration assay in L5178 cells, and in induction of chromosomal aberrations in rat bone marrow in vivo	Imai et al., 1988 Waegemaekers & Bensink, 1984 Baker et al., 1988 IARC, 1994b Fisher, 1982 Seppäläinen & Rajaniemi, 1984 Donaghy et al., 1991
Benzoyl peroxide	Induction of DNA strand breakage in mouse keratinocytes	Skin tumour promoter in mice	S. typhimurium negative, 7 strains ± S9	Hartley et al., 1987 IARC, 1999b

Table 57 (contd)

Compound	In-vitro toxicity	In-vivo toxicity	Mutagenicity/genotoxicity	References
Bisphenol A	Oestrogenic activity in MCF7 cells (1/10 000 of oestradiol). Inhibition of DNA synthesis in BALB/c 3T3 cells: $ID_{50} = 30\ \mu M$	No developmental toxicity at maternal toxic (rats) or lethal (mice) dose levels	*In vivo* DNA-adduct formation in livers of male rats	Olea *et al.*, 1996 Hanks *et al.*, 1991 Morrissey *et al.*, 1987 Atkinson & Roy, 1995
2-Hydroxy-4-methoxy-benzophenone	No data	Common ingredient of sunscreens and tanning agents; may cause contact dermatitis in sensitive individuals. No irritation or inflammation in human pulpa. Depigmentation of the skin in occupationally exposed persons. No irritation in the rabbit eye.	*S. typhimurium* negative, 5 strains ± S9 *In vitro*: *S. typhimurium* weakly positive with S9 Induction of sister chromatid exchange and chromosomal aberrations *In vivo*: no genotoxicity in mice Positive in mouse lymphoma test at 22–52 μg/mL	Bonin *et al.*, 1982 National Technical Program, 1992 Stanley *et al.*, 1979
Camphorquinone	Inhibition of DNA synthesis in HeLa cells in the cytotoxic range	No data	*S. typhimurium* negative, TA 100 ± S9, up to 25 μmol/plate *S. typhimurium* negative, in 5 strains ± S9 up to 10 μmol/plate	Leyhausen *et al.*, 1995 Dorado *et al.*, 1992 Cameron, 1993
p-Methoxyphenol	No data	Depigmentation of the skin of occupationally exposed workers. Dietary admin. in mice at 0.1%, slight growth depression; in rabbits at 10% little or no growth depression; in dogs fed 6 g/day, no deleterious effects. Undiluted application (> 1 day) on rabbit eye or skin causes damage and necrosis	*S. typhimurium* negative, 5 strains, ± S9	Chivers, 1972 Clayton & Clayton, 1993

Table 57 (contd)

Compound	In-vitro toxicity	In-vivo toxicity	Mutagenicity/genotoxicity	References
N,N-Dimethyl-p-toluidine	No data	No data	S. typhimurium negative, 3 strains ± S9 S. typhimurium positive, 1 strain ± S9 Positive in mouse lymphoma test and in micronucleus test in V79 cells Induction of DNA breakage in vivo in mouse and rat liver	Taningher et al., 1993 Cameron, 1993

ID_{50} or IC_{50} = concentration inhibiting the effect by 50%; S9 = liver homogenate preparations for metabolic activation
(Modified from Schedle et al., 1999)

The metabolism of camphorquinone (used as a composite initiator) was studied in rabbits following oral administration of 500–800 mg of the compound. Although 40% of the dose was excreted as the glucuronide in urine, camphorquinone did not possess any pharmacological activity (Robertson & Hussain, 1969).

In a study on embryotoxicity in three-day chicken embryos, benzoyl peroxide caused malformations at moderate frequency (Korhonen et al., 1984).

Treatment with 200 mg/kg bisphenol A resulted in DNA-adduct formation in rat liver, demonstrated by ^{32}P-postlabelling (Atkinson & Roy, 1995). Daily oral treatments of pregnant rats and mice with bisphenol A at doses of 160, 320 and 640 mg/kg bw (for rats) and 500, 750, 1000 and 1250 mg/kg bw (for mice) during gestational days 6–15 caused reduced maternal body weight gain in the rats and up to 18% maternal mortality in the mice, at the high dose. The percentage of resorptions per litter was significantly increased in mice treated with the 1250-mg/kg dose. There was no significant effect of bisphenol A treatment on any of the parameters of developmental toxicity in either species, even at doses that caused significant maternal toxicity or mortality (Morrissey et al., 1987). It appears unlikely that bisphenol A produces toxic responses *in vivo* through its weak oestrogenic activity (Olea et al., 1996).

(ix) *Other materials*

In an assessment of hernia repair meshes made of three types of polypropylene implanted in the abdominal wall of rabbits, histological examination after up to 90 days revealed the accumulation of macrophages and the appearance of connective tissue and white adipose tissue. The tissue response depended on the presence of an intact parietal peritoneum (Bellon et al., 1998).

Various forms of artificially degraded poly(L-lactide) or undegraded low-molecular-weight poly-L-lactide displayed minimal differences in their effects on a mouse macrophage cell line (IC21). Parameters studied included cell number, lactate dehydrogenase, prostaglandin E_2 and morphology. Latex beads and Zymosan were used as controls. The authors concluded that degradation of poly-L-lactide had no effect on its toxicity (Dawes & Rushton, 1997).

(b) *Immunological effects*

(i) *Polydimethylsiloxanes (silicones)*

Concern over the possibility of immune disease arising from the use of silicone gel breast implants stimulated experimental studies of the immunotoxicity of silicones. Extensive analysis of the immunotoxic potential of silicones has failed to reveal any factor that would be likely to promote carcinogenesis. Animal studies have shown that silicones are not significantly immunotoxic but that some can act as adjuvants under experimental conditions; however, they have little potential to elicit specific antibody responses or cell-mediated immunity.

The immunotoxicity of subcutaneously administered materials, including silicone fluid (Dow Corning 360), gel and elastomer (from Silastic breast implants) and polyurethane in female B6C3F$_1$ mice was investigated over 10 and 180 days. A number of positive controls were used to confirm that the assays were able to detect the relevant immunotoxicity parameters. None of the following parameters were significantly altered in silicone-treated mice: body weight, organ weight, haematology, blood chemistry (alanine aminotransferase, urea, glucose, albumin, total protein, serum CH 50 and C3 levels), cellularity of bone marrow and cerebrospinal fluid, antibody response to sheep erythrocytes, proliferative response to concanavalin A, phytohaemagglutinin, lipopolysaccharide and allogenic cells, reticuloendothelial function, serum complement, host resistance to *Streptococcus pneumoniae* and B16F10 tumour cells, distribution of splenic B and T cells, and natural killer cell activity after 10 days. A modest protection to challenge with *Listeria monocytogenes* was observed with all silicones and there was some evidence of inflammatory activity with silicone gel. After 180 days, all the materials tested marginally reduced the level of immunoglobulin-positive cells in the spleen but had no consistent effect on the distribution of T-cell surface markers. A modest depression of natural killer cell activity was observed after 180 days in all silicone-treated groups. In further studies to investigate the dose–response relationships of this effect, the reduction of natural killer cell activity was confirmed following exposure to silicone gel, but not with silicone elastomer. These relatively minor changes in natural killer cell activity, in the absence of any changes in the other parameters tested, indicate that there were no significant immunotoxic effects (Luster, 1993; Bradley *et al.*, 1994a,b).

A number of experimental studies in rats have addressed the ability of silicones to act as immunostimulatory agents or adjuvants. In one study, silicone oil was reported to be a weak adjuvant, while silicone gel showed a strong adjuvant effect (Naim *et al.*, 1993). In contrast, in another study, only weak enhancement of a specific immune response was found, and silicones failed to act as non-specific immunostimulants (Chang, 1993).

None of these findings are indicative of immunotoxic effects that might influence carcinogenicity.

(ii) *Other materials*

An inhibitory effect on immunocompetence was noted in poorly reported studies involving the implantation of various materials into mice. Groups of female C57BL/6 mice (total, 380) were given implants of discs (15 × 2 mm) of poly(ether urethane), silicone elastomer, poly(methyl methacrylate) and an amorphous-phase calcium phosphate ceramic (bioglass) into subcutaneous dorsal pockets. At the same time, tumours were induced by injection of suspensions of 3-methylcholanthrene-induced mouse fibrosarcoma cells, which are known to produce tumours within 28 days. The tumour cell suspension was injected over and around the implant. Controls received tumour cells without implants. Splenic lymphocytes were harvested at 28 days to study the effect of the polymers on immunocompetence. In assays with the mitogens lipopolysaccharide and phytohaemagglutinin, inhibition of lymphoproliferation was caused by the polyurethane and poly(methyl methacrylate), while bioglass and silicone had no effect. Sensitization to M_4 tumour antigen was depressed in lymphocytes from mice implanted with polyurethane, silicone or the ceramic (Habal *et al.*, 1980).

5B.3 Genetic and related effects

5B.3.1 *Humans*

Clastogenicity was clearly associated with worn orthopaedic implants in a limited study of 71 revision arthroplasty patients and 30 primary arthroplasty controls (Case *et al.*, 1996). This study is described in Section 5A.4.1.

5B.3.2 *Experimental systems*

As in the case of metallic devices, non-metallic devices have been tested mainly by the use of extracts. Certain materials used in the preparation of cements have been previously evaluated in *IARC Monographs*: acrylic acid (IARC, 1979c), methyl methacrylate (IARC, 1994b), methyl acrylate and ethyl acrylate (IARC, 1986).

(a) In-vitro genotoxicity assays

The majority of the studies have been performed with dental materials.

Twenty-seven dental materials were tested in a battery of three in-vitro assays: the bacterial *umu*-test, the eukaryotic DNA synthesis inhibition test in HeLa cells and the alkaline filter elution technique for detection of strand breaks in the DNA of gills taken from exposed clams. Some dental materials were tested as single substances present in dental devices (monomers, inhibitors, co-initiators or photo-initiators) or as extracts of materials. Frequently the materials consisted of about 10–20 single ingredients (root canal filling material, composites or ionomer cements). The dental materials were extracted in serum, culture medium or dimethyl sulfoxide (DMSO) for 24 h at 37°C. The extracts of two widely used root-filling dental materials (Vitrebond® and AH26®) produced dose-dependent effects in all three test systems (Heil *et al.*, 1996).

The mutagenicity observed in various assays with the epoxy resin sealer AH26 was attributed to formaldehyde released from decomposition of hexamethylene tetramine, a component of this endodontic material (Geurtsen & Leyhausen, 1997). A DMSO extract of AH26 was reported to be mutagenic in *Salmonella typhimurium* strain TA100 and its epoxy-bisphenol A resin component was associated with the mutagenic properties of this sealer (Ørstavik & Hongslo, 1985). Extracts of the dental material N2®, which contains paraformaldehyde, showed genotoxic activity in the bacterial *umu*-test (Heil *et al.*, 1996). Several of the substances present in some dental materials demonstrated a mutagenic effect when tested separately, but extracts of dental materials that contain mutagenic components did not always show mutagenicity.

Two of six orthodontic direct-bonding resin systems tested were shown to be mutagenic in *S. typhimurium* strain TA100 both before and after curing using aqueous and DMSO extracts. No metabolic activation was necessary. The mutagenic agent(s) were not chemically identified, but when the formulation of one of the mutagenic bonding resins was changed by the manufacturer, the product was no longer mutagenic (Cross et al., 1983).

The mutagenic potential of saline and DMSO extracts of another dental adhesive, Syntac®, was demonstrated in *S. typhimurium* strains TA102 and TA104. Glutaraldehyde, an ingredient of this type of adhesive, was mutagenic in these same strains. In the same study and using the same protocol, two other dentin-bonding agents, Pertac® and Prisma® Universal Bound, did not show mutagenic activity (Schweikl et al., 1994). A physiological saline extract of Prisma Universal Bond 3 adhesive, which contains glutaraldehyde, was strongly mutagenic in *S. typhimurium* TA102 (Schweikl et al., 1996).

Compounds of commercially available dental material kits were tested for mutagenicity in *S. typhimurium*. One of these materials, Gluma 3, contains glutaraldehyde and 2-hydroxyethyl methacrylate and was highly mutagenic in strains TA100 and TA104 (Li et al., 1990). DMSO extracts of Gluma 3 and two other glutaraldehyde-containing dentin-bonding agents, Syntac adhesive and Prisma Universal Bond 3 adhesive, were reported to cause mutations in the *hprt* locus of Chinese hamster lung V79 cells (Schweikl & Schmalz, 1997).

Components of three glass ionomer cements were mixed and allowed to polymerize for one hour or one week. Extracts were prepared by incubation of 1 g of the material in 5 mL phosphate-buffered saline for three days at 37°C. The extracts were tested for induction of sister chromatid exchanges in human lymphocytes *in vitro*, in the presence or absence of a metabolic activation system (microsomal S9 fraction). One of the extracts obtained one hour after polymerization caused induction of sister chromatid exchanges, while the other two showed weak or no activity. The extract obtained from the first material after one week showed activity, while those from the two other preparations were inactive in inducing sister chromatid exchanges. In general, the activity of the extracts in this assay was higher in the absence of S9 than in its presence. The composition of the dental cements was not given (Stea et al., 1998).

Non-shrinking dental epoxy-copolymers, containing spiroorthocarbonates and various epoxy derivatives, were tested for mutagenicity in *S. typhimurium*. The weak mutagenic activity found with strain TA97a was attributed to the epoxy formulation rather than to the spiroorthocarbonate component (Yourtee et al., 1994).

Saline (0.9% sodium chloride) extracts of thermoplastic polyurethanes, used as insulating materials for cardiac pacemaker leads, did not show mutagenic activity in *S. typhimurium* (Pande, 1983).

Methanolic extracts of three segmented polyurethanes, one non-segmented polyurethane and silicone containing 25% silica were tested for induction of chromosomal aberrations in Chinese hamster lung cells. No activity was found (Nakamura et al., 1992).

Alumina ceramic and ultra-high molecular weight polyethylene are used in the manufacture of pivot bearings in centrifugal blood pumps for cardiopulmonary bypass. Extracts were prepared by incubation of these materials in saline for 72 h at 50°C, and tested for mutagenicity in *S. typhimurium* strains TA97a, TA98, TA100, TA102 and TA1535, with or without metabolic activation. No mutagenicity was detected (Takami *et al.*, 1997).

A bioresorbable membrane (Soprafilm), made of hyaluronic acid and carboxymethyl cellulose, was tested for mutagenic activity in *S. typhimurium* using extracts in saline, DMSO and saline/ethanol. No mutagenic activity was detected (Burns *et al.*, 1997). [The Working Group noted that the method used to prepare the extract and the conditions of testing were not clearly presented.]

Kevlar®49 (a poly-*para*-phenylene-terephthalimide) was tested for mutagenic activity. Test samples were the raw material (ground powder), and extracts in chloroform or ethanol. None of the samples showed mutagenic activity in the six *S. typhimurium* strains tested. In a mammalian mutagenicity assay, Kevlar®49 extracts obtained by incubation of the materal in cell culture medium or in DMSO for seven days at 37°C, did not show mutagenicity at the *hprt* locus in Chinese hamster lung V79 cells (Wening *et al.*, 1995).

A bone cement containing methyl methacrylate, *N,N*-dimethyl-*para*-toluidine and hydroquinone (Surgical simplex P) was tested in an in-vitro micronucleus assay with human lymphocytes from 15 different donors. Clearly positive results were demonstrated with freshly polymerized cement and with cement that had been preincubated in cell culture medium for five days before the assay (Bigatti *et al.*, 1994). The same material was reported to be inactive in an assay to determine sister chromatid exchanges in cultured human lymphocytes, but in those experiments a significant decrease in the cell proliferation index was observed (Bigatti *et al.*, 1989).

In a DNA synthesis inhibition test with HeLa cells, the effects of bis-GMA were masked by the cytotoxicity of the chemical, although no mutagenic activity was observed in the bacterial *umu*-microtest (Leyhausen *et al.*, 1995). A total of 27 acrylate esters, among which 1,4-butanediol dimethacrylate, diethylene glycol dimethacrylate and 1,6-hexanediol dimethacrylate were reported to be non-mutagenic in *S. typhimurium* when tested with five strains with and without metabolic activation (Waegemaekers & Bensink 1984). Tetraethylene glycol dimethacrylate, identified as an impurity in composite dental materials, was found to be genotoxic in several *in vitro* assays: the micronucleus test, the chromosomal aberration test and the mouse lymphoma mutagenicity test with cultured L5178Y cells (Dearfield *et al.*, 1989).

The genetic effects of benzoyl peroxide, used as a polymerization initiator, have recently been reviewed (IARC, 1999b).

The bone cement polymerization accelerator *N,N*-dimethyl-*para*-toluidine was weakly mutagenic (Miller *et al.*, 1986) or non-mutagenic in *S. typhimurium* strains TA97, TA98 and TA100 with rat and hamster S9 (Taningher *et al.*, 1993; Cameron, 1993). However, this compound was positive in the mouse lymphoma test (Cameron, 1993), induced micronuclei *in vitro* in V79 hamster cells with an increase of non-disjunction (at doses of 0.9 and 1.9 mM), and gave rise to DNA damage *in vivo* in mouse liver (at 1 mmol/kg i.p.) and rat liver (at 4 and 8 mmol/kg i.p. and 8 mmol p.o.) as determined in the alkaline elution assay (Taningher *et al.*, 1993). The photosensitizer camphorquinone was non-mutagenic in *S. typhimurium* TA 100 strain and in a battery of different bacterial strains with or without activating systems (Cameron, 1993). Inhibition of DNA synthesis in HeLa cells by camphorquinone was masked by the cytotoxicity of the compound (Leyhausen *et al.*, 1995). The inhibitor *p*-methoxyphenol was non-mutagenic in different strains of *S. typhimurium* (Haworth *et al.*, 1983). The UV stabilizer 2-hydroxy-4-methoxybenzophenone did not show mutagenic activity in five strains of *S. typhimurium* with or without rat S9 (Bonin *et al.*, 1982). These results were later confirmed by Zeiger *et al.* (1987). The dental composite additive triphenyl antimony inhibited DNA synthesis in HeLa cells but had no mutagenic activity in the bacterial *umu*-microtest (Leyhausen *et al.*, 1995).

N-Acryloyl-*N'*-phenylpiperazine (Acr NPP) is a promoter of redox reactions that has been proposed as a polymerization activator of acrylic resins for biomedical use. It was tested in a battery of genotoxicity tests. No mutagenic activity was detected in three strains of *S. typhimurium* (TA97, TA98 and TA100) with or without metabolic activation. However, because of bacterial toxicity, the highest level tested was only 0.3 μmol/plate. In the DNA damage–alkaline elution test with hamster V79 cells treated in culture for 24 h with 10 mM of this compound and with liver cells isolated from mice 24 h after in-vivo treatment by i.p. injection with 1 mmol/kg bw, a weak but statistically significant increase in DNA fragmentation was observed, but this effect was associated with a high level of cytotoxicity. In the micronucleus test with cultured V79 hamster cells, Acr NPP showed a dose-dependent effect that reached about 25-fold the level of the background controls. Immunofluorescent staining with antibodies against kinetochore proteins revealed that micronuclei were due to an aneugenic mechanism and not to a clastogenic effect, as confirmed by the alkaline DNA elution test. Acr NPP is to be regarded as an aneugen (Taningher *et al.*, 1992).

Liu *et al.* (1997) tested a nonceramic hydroxylapatite, used as a calcium phosphate cement, for gene mutation in *S. typhimurium* TA98 and TA100, for unscheduled DNA synthesis in Chinese hamster ovary cells using a scintillation method and in a mouse bone marrow micronucleus induction assay. Crushed and ground specimens were extracted with physiological saline (1:2, w:v) for 24 h at 37°C. There was no determination of the chemical composition of the extracts or of their physicochemical properties (pH, osmolality). No effects were demonstrated in any of the assays, but there was no evidence that anything had been extracted from the material.

(b) Cell transformation test

Cells growing *in vitro* from explants of subcutaneous connective tissue from adult BALB/c mice were grown for 18 or more days before being implanted while attached to a plastic plate. Tumours formed after 24–79 weeks, the latent period before tumour appearance being correlated inversely with the time period during which the cells were cultured *in vitro*. Tumours appeared to be composed of histologically undifferentiated sarcoma cells that were transplantable without plates. When inoculated in saline suspension, the cells did not form tumours until they had been in tissue culture for 12 weeks. The plastic plates alone did not induce tumour formation within more than 1.5 years of implantation. The authors concluded that a smooth surface was acting as a carcinogen first *in vitro* and then *in vivo* and that factors related to the geometry and mechanics of cell attachment to a flat surface play a role in this process (Boone *et al.*, 1979). A BALB/c 3T3 cell transformation assay gave positive results when the cells were cultured with glass dishes coated with poly(ether urethanes) in the presence of *O*-tetradecanoylphorbol 13-acetate (TPA) (Tsuchiya *et al.*, 1996).

(c) *In-vivo genotoxicity assays*

Diaminotoluenes have been studied because of their industrial use as intermediates in polyurethane synthesis and because of their potential release by degradation from the poly(ester urethane) covering of some breast implants (see Section 5B.1.1(*a*)). The extent of DNA damage induced by these compounds was determined in female Fischer 344 rats fed 10, 40, 80 or 180 ppm 2,4-diaminotoluene, a carcinogenic isomer, for up to six weeks, or in rats receiving subcutaneous implants of poly(ester urethane) foam (67 or 267 mg/kg) in mammary fat pad. DNA adducts and mutations at the *hprt* gene were determined in spleen T-lymphocytes of rats fed 40 or 80 ppm of 2,4-diamino-toluene for six weeks. No increase in either marker was observed at 1, 6, 12, 20, 28 and 42 weeks after the start of feeding. In the liver and mammary glands, a single major DNA adduct was detected in animals fed 10–180 ppm 2,4-diaminotoluene, while two minor DNA adducts were occasionally observed. DNA adduct levels in the liver reached a plateau three to six weeks after the start of feeding. A similar plateau with DNA adduct levels generally 1.5–4-fold lower than those observed in the liver was seen in the mammary gland. The major DNA adduct was present in the mammary gland up to 43 weeks after implantation. Implantation of poly(ester urethane) foam did not increase DNA adducts in liver, mammary gland or spleen or mutations at the *hprt* gene in spleen T-lymphocytes at the same sampling times (Delclos *et al.*, 1996).

In an abstract, results were summarized of three in-vivo tests, the mouse bone marrow micronucleus assay, the mouse sperm morphology test and the Chinese hamster bone marrow sister chromatid exchange assay. Three uncured dental materials were tested in mice by addition at 50 ppm in the drinking-water for 14 weeks. [The basis for this dose selection was not stated.] One preparation ('Right-On Adhesive') induced sister chromatid exchanges (Dunipace *et al.*, 1990).

Saline extracts of two bone waxes were given to Swiss albino mice on two consecutive days via the intraperitoneal route at doses of up to 50 mL/kg bw per day. The mouse bone marrow micronucleus test, performed 24 or 36 h after the second dosing, revealed no genotoxic effect with either extract (Mohanan & Rathinam, 1996). [The Working Group noted that no information about the composition of the waxes or the extracts was provided.]

(d) *Cytogenetic effects in tumour cells*

A cytogenetic analysis was performed of cells from implantation site sarcomas from CBA/H and CBA/H-T6 mice implanted with double films of unplasticized vinyl chloride–vinyl acetate copolymer. The principal findings were numerical chromosomal abnormalities in preneoplastic lesions during the early foreign-body reaction and structural abnormalities of specific chromosomes found as stable cell markers during late preneoplasia (Rachko & Brand, 1983).

5B.4 Mechanistic studies of implantation-site sarcomagenesis in rodents

5B.4.1 *Major factors that affect tumour incidence in solid-state carcinogenesis*

Foreign-body carcinogenesis in rodent species has, for many years, been recognized as a classic model of multistage endogenous tumorigenesis that requires half to two-thirds of the lifespan for tumour development. A number of studies have demonstrated that physical and not chemical characteristics are responsible for this phenomenon and that a dose–response relationship is evident with respect to implant size and tumour frequency (Schoen, 1987). The major physical factors that affect the occurrence of tumours in response to foreign bodies in rodents are discussed extensively in Section 4B.22.1.

5B.4.2 *Biological factors*

(a) *Fibrous tissue capsule formation and continued presence of implant*

There has been a general consensus that the process of foreign-body tumorigenesis requires two sequential preconditions: (a) fibrous tissue capsule formation in linear circumferential fashion; and (b) continued presence of the implant in the capsule during the latent period (Oppenheimer *et al.*, 1961; Brand *et al.*, 1975c; Schoen, 1987; Brand, 1994).

Polystyrene films (15 × 15 × 0.01 mm) were implanted subcutaneously into rats. During each month thereafter, film and surrounding capsule or film only were removed. Three groups of animals were observed: Group 1, rats that retained both film and capsule; Group 2, rats with capsules but no films; and Group 3, rats with neither capsules nor films. Six per cent of the animals in Group 1 developed tumours; no tumours were found in Group 2 when the films were removed before six months, while 11% of the animals developed tumours when the films were removed after six months; no tumour development was found in Group 3 independent of the time of removal of film and capsule (Oppenheimer *et al.*, 1958).

The same experiments were carried out with cellophane films. As with polystyrene, no tumours were induced when the capsule was removed as well as the film. However, when films alone were removed during the early months, there was a marked reduction in the number of tumours, although a difference was observed between cellophane and polystyrene: with polystyrene, removal of the film within six months entirely precluded tumour formation, whereas with cellophane, five tumours (8.6%) arose when the film was removed during the first six months (Oppenheimer *et al.*, 1964).

In another experiment, when a glass cover-slip implanted on the right side in rats was removed from the tissue capsule after four months, no sarcomas developed, whereas six sarcomas occurred on the left side in association with glass cover-slips that were left in place (Oppenheimer et al., 1961).

The effect of film removal was also observed after subcutaneous implantation of non-perforated poly(vinyl chloride) films (22 × 15 × 0.2 mm) in mice. At twelve months after implantation, the number of sarcomas per number of surviving animals was 17/30 (56.6%) when the film was left in place, and 0/20 (0%) and 1/29 (3.6%) when the film was removed after 3.5 months or 6.5 months, respectively (Moizhess & Vasiliev, 1989).

(b)   The role of perforation in the reduction of tumorigenicity

Series of Millipore filter disks with eight different pore sizes were subcutaneously implanted in mice. One, three, five and 10 months after implantation, histological and ultrastructural studies were carried out on specimens composed of the implants and the surrounding tissue. Filters with pore sizes equal to and larger than 0.22 μm were non-tumorigenic and induced tissue reactions characterized by invasion of filters by macrophages and by presence of phagolysosomes within macrophages as evidence of phagocytic activity. In tissue reactions induced by tumorigenic filters, which had pore sizes of less than 0.22 μm, these features were always missing; instead, there were more fibrous capsules (Karp et al., 1973).

Similar marked histological differences in the long-term tissue reactions were observed between flat and foamed polyurethane films (Nakamura et al., 1995).

(c)   Species and strain differences

The results of several studies suggest that species and strains of animals differ in susceptibility to foreign-body sarcoma development. However, the data on species other than mice and rats are limited.

Poly(methyl methacrylate) discs were implanted intramuscularly into rats and guinea-pigs. Tumours were observed in rats in association with large and medium-sized discs, whereas no tumours were found in guinea-pigs. In the latter species, a considerable decrease in the thickness of the capsule surrounding the implant was observed during the course of the 30-month experiment (Stinson, 1964).

Following subcutaneous implantation of poly(2-hydroxyethyl methacrylate) films, five tumours developed in 10 rats that survived for more than 12 months, whereas no tumours were found in hamsters or guinea-pigs. The occurrence of tumours was associated with the presence of a thick capsule surrounding the implant (Imai & Masuhara, 1982). [The Working Group noted the small numbers of animals.]

Striking differences in tumour response to subcutaneous implantation of vinyl chloride–vinyl acetate copolymer films were found among 18 strains of mice: the incidence of tumours was 90–100% in CBA/H and CBA/H-T6 females, AKR/J males, BALB/cJ and BALB/c Wat females, C57BL/10ScSn females and (C57BL/10ScSc

× CBA/H)F₁ males and females, whereas no tumour was induced in males of strain I/LnJ or strain SJL/J. The incidence in other strains was intermediate (Brand et al., 1977).

5B.4.3 Timing and location of preneoplastic events

The process of foreign-body tumorigenesis was extensively studied by Brand and coworkers using the techniques of transplantation of fibrous capsules and/or explanted films from strain CBA/H mice into the co-isogenic strain, CBA/H-T6. The presence or absence of the T6 marker chromosome was used to distinguish CBA/H-T6 from CBA/H cells (Brand et al., 1967a,b, 1971, 1973, 1975a,b,c; Thomassen et al., 1975; Brand, 1976).

Groups of implant-carrying mice were treated every two weeks or monthly as follows: film implants (double pieces of 15 × 22-mm vinyl chloride–vinyl acetate copolymer) and two thirds of the surrounding tissue capsules were removed and cut into 7 × 15-mm pieces. (a) One film pair and the corresponding tissue were separately implanted into fresh recipient animals, either at different sites (left and right flank) of the same animal or into different recipients; (b) another third of the film pair was reimplanted into the capsule pocket that had been left in the original carrier; (c) the last third of the film and tissue capsule was examined by karyological, histological and in-vitro culture methods.

The results of these experiments were summarized as four main findings. (i) If the capsule or implanted film was transferred after a latent period lasting two to nine months, tumours developed from transplanted film pieces only, not from capsule tissue. Capsule transfer was tumorigenic only in the latest phase of premalignancy, i.e. about four weeks before tumour development in the original animals. (ii) Tumours in the original and corresponding recipient animals were identical, especially in chromosome number, but occasionally also with regard to ploidy level. (iii) Tumours appeared in the original and corresponding recipient animals up to nine months after transfer at almost exactly the same time (within two weeks). (iv) Tumours developed in animals always on one side, either right or left. No independent multiple tumours on both sides were ever recorded. Furthermore, tumours developed regularly from one side of the implant only, either the upper or the lower surface. Film transfer experiments showed that tumours in the original and corresponding recipient animals always developed from the same side of the film fragments. Thus, it was evident that the premalignant cell clone was restricted to only one side of the film.

From these results, it was concluded that: (1) premalignant cells can first be demonstrated five to six months after initial implantation of the plastic film; (2) premalignant cells are firmly attached to the plastic implant at least up to nine months before tumour appearance; (3) premalignant cells are on the film surface in multiple foci, since film cuttings carry equal tumorigenicity; (4) there seems to be no cell division among the film-attached premalignant population; (5) the capsule tissue is free of transplantable premalignant cells until about one month before tumour development; (6) since the tumours in the original and corresponding recipient animals appear at the same time and are composed karyologically of the same stemline, a specific cell clone must reside on the film at transfer; (7) individual premalignant clones must also exist, because premalignant cells are found only at one implant site and only on one side of the implant; and (8) the specific and stable individuality of the premalignant cell clone suggests that the parent cell may have been already endowed with the clonal characteristics of karyotype and premalignant determination (Brand *et al.*, 1967a,b).

A different paper reported that some animals of the 8.5- and 9.5-month transfer groups developed late tumours from tissue capsules remaining after the implants were removed. These late tumours were always heterologous to those developing from corresponding film segments transferred to recipient animals (Thomassen *et al.*, 1975).

A more precise transplantation study was carried out to clarify the timing and location of preneoplastic events: the implants and mouse strains used were the same as above, and two main experimental designs were adopted. In the first (Experiment 1), whole unopened film/capsule complexes were exchanged at one, two, three, four or five months after implantation, between animals with and without the T6 marker chromosome; in the second (Experiment 2) only the implanted films were exchanged after 2.5, 3.0, 3.5, 4.0, 4.5, 5.0, 5.5 or 6.0 months, between pairs of animals with and without the T6 marker; capsules remained *in situ* but were opened to remove and replace the films.

The results of Experiment 1 showed that, within one month after implantation, transferable preneoplastic cells appeared at the site of the foreign-body reaction in 33% of the animals, and the rate increased rapidly with time to over 70%. In the two-month transfer groups, as well as in later transfer groups, several instances of karyologically identical 'homologous tumours' (descending from a common parent cell) were recorded in recipient and original animals. This was considered to be unequivocal evidence that, before the time of transfer, not only were preneoplastic cells present in the original implant carrier but the parent cell had already expanded into a clone.

Early opening and cutting of capsule and film disturb the conditions to the extent that preneoplastic cells at that stage have little chance of surviving the transfer operation or establishing themselves in the new host where a fresh foreign-body reaction occurs. However, in a few instances (1/4) in Experiment 2, exchange of films between unexcised capsules of different animals was successful. This suggests that preneoplastic cells may settle on implant surfaces at least within 2.5 months after implantation (Brand *et al.*, 1971).

The following conclusions were drawn from these results. Tumours arose from cells with the same neoplastic specificity, which indicated their clonal nature. Specific tumour properties must have been predetermined and fixed in these clonal cells before the implants were cut and transferred. The demonstration of such clones implied the prior existence of 'parent cells' in which the initial determining event had already taken place (Brand, 1976).

In order to determine how many preneoplastic parent cells are induced by film implants of a given size, the time-to-tumour data following subcutaneous implantation of vinyl chloride–vinyl acetate copolymer films (7 × 15 and 15 × 22 mm) into CBA mice were analysed statistically. Animals were declared 'tumour-negative' when > 30 months without tumour development elapsed before death. It was calculated that the most probable number of 'preneoplastic parent cells' must be 1 in response to a 7 × 15-mm implant and 3 in response to a 15 × 22-mm implant (Brand et al., 1973). These values agreed with those obtained by direct counts (Thomassen et al., 1975).

5B.4.4 Origin of preneoplastic parent cells

To determine the origin (progenitor cell) of foreign-body tumorigenesis, histological and electron microscopic studies were carried out with sarcomas induced in CBA or AKR mice by subcutaneous implantation of unplasticized vinyl chloride–vinyl acetate copolymer films and with cultured cells from preneoplastic capsule tissue (Johnson et al., 1973a; Buoen et al., 1975; Johnson et al., 1977, 1980).

In spite of the heterogeneity of sarcoma types obtained, all sarcomas were characterized by (a) a pericellular, periodic acid–Schiff-positive, argyrophilic and filamentous substance resembling basal lamina; (b) a sparsity of collagen production; and (c) prominent cytoplasmic accumulation of 6-nm microfilaments in 60–100% of the cells from each sarcoma. Sarcomas from six mice with leiomyomatous cells, in which extensive concentrations of microfilaments were observed ultrastructurally, also had many acid fuchsin-positive cells when examined with the light microscope. The consistent presence of these morphological characteristics despite the variability of histological sarcoma type suggested that a pluripotential mesenchymal cell type other than the fibroblast is the common progenitor cell (Johnson et al., 1973a).

Preneoplastic foreign-body segments (film removed from capsule) or reactive capsule tissue were excised at 1, 1.5, 2, 5 or 10 months after implantation of unplasticized vinyl chloride–vinyl acetate copolymer in CBA mice. Reactive capsule tissue was minced and treated for 30 min with 0.3% collagenase at 37°C. The cells were cultured in 35-mm plastic culture dishes (with an 11 × 22 mm glass coverslip on the floor of each dish) in medium with antibiotics and 20% fetal calf serum. Cell-laden film implants were placed directly in 35-mm culture dishes containing the culture medium. The cultures were passaged routinely (after trypsinization) as soon as monolayers reached confluence (i.e., after approximately four to six days for capsule-derived primary cultures and three to five weeks for film-attached primary cultures). Cells isolated in vitro were found to conform to four cell-type categories on the basis of light microscopic morphology, pattern of in-vitro appearance, in-vitro topographical relationships and certain karyotype similarities. Euploid type I (macrophage-like) and type II (fibroblast-like) cells predominated in primary cultures and early passages (passages 1 and 2) of cells derived from reactive capsule tissue. The observation of small numbers of type III cells (unidentified cell type with unknown karyotype characteristics) in passages 1 and 2 of cells derived from reactive capsule tissue coincided with the deterioration of euploid type II cell populations and preceded the appearance of type IV (endothelial-like) cells. Type IV cells had a pronounced growth advantage over cell types I, II and III, resulting in cultures composed only of type IV cells after three passages. Cultures derived from cells attached to the surfaces of implant segments also conformed to the criteria established for type IV cells. Of the four cell types, type IV cells were determined to have special importance regarding the nature of the progenitor cell in foreign-body tumorigenesis, in that they were aneuploid and eventually produced homologous sarcomas when injected as a suspension into compatible hybrid recipient mice that carried the T6 marker chromosome. [The Working Group noted that details of the experiment on type IV cell injection were not reported.] The growth characteristics of type IV cells were significantly different from those of type II cells, in that the former grew to confluence, forming a monolayer with little or no evidence of piling up or cell overlap. These morphological features and the tendency to form monolayers of uniformly spaced cells in pavement-like or mosaic patterns are consistent with the characteristics reported for cultured endothelial cells *in vitro*. The findings were considered to be consistent with the hypothesis that cells of the local microvasculature are the likely progenitor or parent cells from which foreign-body sarcomas are derived (Johnson *et al.*, 1977).

The submicroscopic features of the aneuploid type IV cells included: (1) numerous microfilaments (diameter, 6–9 nm); (2) many plasmalemmal (pinocytotic) vesicles; (3) many surface microvilli, ruffles or blebs; (4) formation of intercellular gap junctions; and (5) relatively extensive smooth-surfaced endoplasmic reticulum and significantly less rough-surfaced endoplasmic reticulum (Johnson *et al.*, 1980).

5B.4.5 *Stages in foreign-body tumorigenesis*

On the basis of the results described above, foreign-body tumorigenesis was considered by Brand *et al.* (1975c) and Brand (1976) to be a multistage process. In Stage 1, the foreign body surface was covered with a macrophage monolayer by the 12th day after implantation. Within four to eight weeks, preneoplastic parent cells could be seen in the loose cellular foreign body reactive tissue, but not on the foreign body surface. In Stage 2, a fibrous capsule around the foreign body was formed during the second month after implantation. Preneoplastic cells were then present as clones in the capsule and in the loose connective tissue around it, but still not on the foreign body surface. In Stage 3, preneoplastic clonal cells began to settle on the foreign body surface. The fibrotic consolidation of the capsule was complete between the fourth and sixth months. The macrophage-type cells that still predominated on the foreign body surface appeared ultrastructurally inactive and dormant. However, foreign-body contact was not at that time a necessary condition for preneoplastic cell maturation. In Stage 4, direct foreign-body contact became a requirement for completion of preneoplastic maturation. Homologous preneoplastic cells in the capsule would not give rise to tumours upon transfer of the capsule unless a new foreign body was inserted. In Stage 5, the preneoplastic cells had acquired autonomy. The proliferating cells detached from the foreign body surface and invaded the capsule tissue. Capsule transfer at this stage could induce tumours in recipient animals. [The Working Group noted that because of the inadequacy of reporting, it is not possible to determine to what extent these conclusions are based on evidence or are conjectural. Their validity cannot always be determined.]

5B.4.6 *Other data on the role of capsule and implant on tumour promotion/ progression*
   (a) *Different roles of an implant during early and late stages of carcinogenesis*

As described in Section 4B.22, the presence of an implant of continuous surface in a tissue capsule is essential for induction of malignant tumours at the site of implantation. However, the data in Table 58 show that the implanted foreign body plays different roles during the early and later stages of carcinogenesis. Non-perforated poly(vinyl chloride) (PVC) film (A) induced local tumours at a significantly higher rate than perforated PVC film having 50–60 holes (0.3 mm wide) per cm^2 (D) or Millipore filter with 0.45-µm pores (E); a significant decrease in local tumour development was seen

Table 58. Replacement of non-perforated poly(vinyl chloride) film by perforated poly(vinyl chloride) film or by Millipore filters

Implant		No. of sarcomas/ no. of mice alive 12 months after implantation	Tumour incidence (%)[a]	Minimal latent period (months after first implantation)
A	Non-perforated film (no replacement)	17/30	56.6	11.5
B	Non-perforated film (removed after 3.5 months)	0/20	0	–
C	Non-perforated film (removed after 6.5 months)	1/29	3.6	10.0
D	Perforated film (no replacement)	3/29	10.3	13.0
E	Millipore filter (no replacement)	1/34	2.9	6.0
F	Non-perforated film → Millipore filter (replaced at 3.5 months)	6/28	21.4	11.0
G	Non-perforated film → perforated film (replaced at 1.5 months)	5/35	14.3	13.5
H	Non-perforated film → perforated film (replaced at 3.5 months)	10/27	37.0	14.0

[a] D and E, significantly less than A ($p \leq 0.0005$); F, significantly greater than E ($p = 0.007$; H, significantly greater than D ($p = 0.011$); B and C, significantly less than A ($p < 0.005$)
Adapted from Moizhess & Vasiliev (1989)

when the non-perforated PVC film (A) was removed after 6.5 months from the capsule formed (B and C). However, when the non-perforated PVC film was replaced with a perforated PVC film (H) or Millipore filter (F) after 3.5 months, the local tumour incidence was significantly higher than that found with perforated PVC film (D) or Millipore filter (E) implanted from the beginning (Moizhess & Vasiliev, 1989).

These data suggest that preneoplastic clones formed in the micro-environment of non-perforated film can continue their neoplastic evolution in the micro-environment of weakly carcinogenic foreign bodies (perforated film, Millipore filter). To test this suggestion, the following experiments were performed. In Experiment 1, non-perforated film implanted into CBA mice (donors) was surgically removed from the capsule and minced into 12–15 fragments. These fragments with attached cells were implanted into F_1(CBA × C57BL) mice (recipients). Five out of 34 recipient mice developed sarcomas at the site of implantation. All these sarcomas were transplantable to CBA and F_1 mice but not to C57BL mice. In the control group, 'intact (fresh)' minced film alone was implanted into F_1 mice and none of 26 mice surviving after 12 months developed sarcomas. In Experiment 2, the capsules that formed around non-perforated film were removed four months after implantation. These capsules were minced into small fragments, mixed with fragments of Millipore filters (fresh) and transplanted subcutaneously into F_1 mice. Five out of 12 recipients developed tumours and all these tumours were of donor origin. Thus, 'preneoplastic' cells present in the capsule around non-perforated film were able to develop into sarcomas when placed into the environment around fragmented Millipore filter. In Experiment 3, the non-perforated film with surrounding capsule was excised after four months in CBA mice and transplanted into F_1 mice. Fourteen days later, the film was surgically removed from the capsule. After another four months, Millipore filters were implanted at the same site. Three tumours developed in 28 mice of this group and they were of CBA origin. No tumours were observed in the control group, in which Millipore filters were not implanted after removal of the film. Thus, film fragments alone were not carcinogenic, but they promoted the development of tumours from the donor cells attached to the film surface before fragmentation (Moizhess & Vasiliev, 1989).

(b) *Promotion by an implant of subcutaneous carcinogenesis initiated by irradiation or a chemical carcinogen*

The results presented in Table 59 show that total-body γ-irradiation alone, as well as implantation of perforated film alone, induced a low frequency of subcutaneous sarcomas. Implantation of perforated film 2.5 months after total irradiation induced sarcomas at a considerably higher incidence. This incidence decreased to that of control groups when the film was implanted 1.5 months after irradiation and removed four months after implantation. Thus, the continued presence of the implanted film in the subcutaneous tissue of irradiated mice was needed for efficient tumour formation. Minimal latent periods of tumour formation were shorter in the group of mice irradiated before implantation than in the control group (Moizhess & Vasiliev, 1989).

Table 59. Induction of sarcomas by subcutaneous implantation of perforated poly(vinyl chloride) film after total-body γ-irradiation

Experiment	Experimental conditions	No. of sarcomas/ no. of mice alive after 12 months (%)	Minimal latent period (months)
1A	Perforated film alone	2/33 (6.0)	22
1B	γ-Irradiation (8.2 Gy + bone marrow) + perforated film implanted 2.5 months later	10/34 (29.5)	12
2A	Perforated film alone	8/34 (23.5)	13
2B	γ-Irradiation (7.5 Gy) alone	1/21 (4.2)	16
2C	γ-Irradiation (7.5 Gy) + perforated film implanted 1.5 months later	15/29 (51.7)	8.5
2D	γ-Irradiation (7.5 Gy) + perforated film implanted 1.5 months later and removed after four months	1/24 (4.7)	14

1A, significantly less than 1B ($p < 0.0001$); 2A, significantly less than 2 C ($p < 0.0005$); 2B, significantly less than 2C ($p < 0.00005$); 2D, significantly less than 2 C ($p < 0.00005$)
Adapted from Moizhess & Vasiliev (1989)

In other experiments, a single intraperitoneal injection of N-ethyl-N-nitrosourea (ENU) was given to CBA mice; 2.5 months later, two foreign bodies were implanted into each mouse: minced PVC film was implanted into the subcutaneous space on the left flank and perforated film on the right flank. Because many CBA mice developed multiple lung adenomas at 9–10 months and died in a preliminary test, in order to increase the observation period, the implanted foreign bodies with surrounding tissues from ENU-treated and from control CBA mice were transplanted into intact two- to three-month-old F_1 mice (CBA × C57BL/6) 9.5 months after the implantation. The incidence of tumours was much higher around the implants from ENU-treated animals than around the implants from non-treated animals, as shown in Table 60. The tumours arising in new hosts were of donor origin (Moizhess & Vasiliev, 1989).

5B.4.7 Effect of different implant materials on inhibition of gap-junctional intercellular communication as an index of tumour promotion

Many tumour-promoting chemicals inhibit cell–cell communication mediated by gap junctions (Swierenga & Yamasaki, 1992; Budunova & Williams, 1994). The inhibition of gap-junctional intercellular communication (GJIC) by tumour promoters is thought to play an important role in carcinogenesis (Holder et al., 1993; Mesnil & Yamasaki, 1993).

Table 60. Induction of sarcomas by 'non-carcinogenic' film after injection of N-ethyl-N-nitrosourea (ENU)

ENU	Film	No. of sarcomas/ no. of implants at 12 months	Tumour incidence (%)	Minimal latent period (months)
+	–	0/28	–	–
–	Perforated	5/30	16.6	23
–	Minced	1/27	3.7	19
+	Perforated	12/30	40	10.5
+	Minced	10/31	32.2	10.5

Adapted from Moizhess & Vasiliev (1989)

A short-term GJIC assay, the V79 metabolic cooperation test (Trosko et al., 1982) was used to assess the putative tumour-promoting activity of various non-metallic materials. In these experiments, culture medium extracts from the materials were tested. The test samples were pure poly(ether urethane) (PEU), pure silicone (I-Silicone) and their 1 : 1 blend films (PEU/I-Silicone), the tumorigenic potential of which had previously been evaluated in vivo (Nakamura et al., 1992; see Section 4B.2.1). One gram of these materials was cut into small pieces and extracted with 10 mL of the culture medium for 24 h at 37°C, and the extracts were diluted serially with the medium. Undiluted extracts from I-Silicone, PEU/I-Silicone or PEU showed a clear inhibitory effect on GJIC, but their activity varied: the lowest effective dilutions of PEU, PEU/I-Silicone and I-Silicone were 12.5, 25 and 50%, respectively (Tsuchiya et al., 1995a). These in-vitro activities correlated well with the in-vivo long-term (two-year) tissue responses including tumour development following implantation of these materials in rats (Nakamura et al., 1992).

The parameters to describe the histological response, including tumour development and cell proliferation with or without preneoplastic change following implantation in rats of three PEUs of the same chemical composition but of different molecular weight (Nakamura et al., 1992) did not correlate with the lowest effective concentrations of methanol extracts of these materials in the metabolic cooperation inhibition test. However, they were highly correlated ($r = 0.99$) with the inhibitory activity of the materials themselves when they were used to coat culture dishes at 2 mg per 22-mm diameter dish. In the same studies, various amounts of S-silicone (an uncured vinylmethylpolysiloxane mixed with 25% silica) were coated on the surface of glass dishes for the metabolic cooperation assay. The results with S-silicone were equivocal, indicating that the inhibitory potential of the S-silicone-coated dish was weaker than those of the PEU-coated dishes (Tsuchiya & Nakamura, 1995).

Components of the PEU were tested to identify which chemical structure(s) inhibited GJIC. A carbamate, 4,4'-di(ethoxycarboamide)diphenylmethane (MDU), which is considered to be a model of the hard segment of PEUs, was not active in this assay while 1,4-butanediol (a chain extender of polyurethane) inhibited metabolic cooperation only at very high concentrations (> 600 µg/mL). Four different kinds of poly-(tetramethylene oxide) (PTMO) (a component monomer of the soft segment) were active at lower concentrations than 1,4-butanediol. At a concentration of 10 µg/mL, the PTMO of the lowest molecular weight tested had the highest activity (Tsuchiya & Nakamura, 1995; Tsuchiya et al., 1995a).

Other types of polyurethane (PUs), such as fluoropolyether glycol (FPEG)-PU, polybutadiene (PBD)-PU, and hydrogenated PBD (HPBD)-PU, were tested by the coated dish method. Surprisingly, these materials were either inactive or were very weak inhibitors of GJIC. The lowest effective amount of FPEG-PU was 8 mg per 22-mm diameter dish, which was 10-fold greater than that of the most active of the PEUs tested above. FPEG-PU possesses a side-chain substituted with fluoride, and this side-chain might hinder oxidation and reduce biodegradability (Takahara et al., 1991). PBD-PU and HPBD-PU, which contain no polyether moiety, showed no inhibitory activity in the assay. From these results, it was speculated that the polyether moiety such as PTMO is a key structural feature in the inhibition of GJIC by PEUs (Tsuchiya et al., 1995b). No in-vivo tumorigenicity data for these materials are available.

The GJIC of V79 cells was inhibited on the surface of polyethylene film, but this inhibitory activity was markedly decreased when the surface of the polyethylene film was immobilized with collagen. This decrease was dependent on the amount of immobilized collagen on the polyethylene film (Nakaoka et al., 1997). On the other hand, collagen immobilization greatly reduced the tumour incidence induced by polyethylene sponges in a one-year subcutaneous implantation study (Kinoshita et al., 1993). Again, a good in-vivo/in-vitro correlation was obtained.

In contrast, the GJIC inhibitory activity of polyethylene film in the metabolic cooperation assay was only slightly reduced when the polyethylene was immobilized either with bovine serum albumin or with Arg-Gly-Asp-Ser (RGDS) peptide, a known sequence of the cell attachment domain in extracellular matrix proteins. This indicates that cell attachment to the polymer via the RGDS peptide was not a dominant factor for GJIC. The reduction of the inhibitory activity of GJIC by collagen immobilization seems to be due not only to improvement of the cell adherence onto polyethylene film via an RGDS sequence but also to some other interaction between collagen and cells which is essential for normal assembly and function of connexins. Generally, the surface modification of polyethylene by means of collagen immobilization may provide an environment suitable for maintaining normal cell function (Nakaoka et al., 1997).

It has been reported that collagen immobilization on silicone elastomer before subcutaneous implantation into rats led to strong adhesion with the surrounding tissue and prevented down-growth of epidermal tissue and bacterial infection (Okada & Ikada, 1995).

On the basis of these results, a hypothesis concerning the tumorigenic potential of polymeric materials has been presented. The genotoxic activities of these materials are probably weak but their tumour-promoting activities may be significant and may differ between materials. Greater promoting activity will affect tumorigenic potential by shortening the latency period and increasing tumour incidence, and may be mediated by differences in the GJIC-inhibiting potential of the surfaces of the materials (Tsuchiya & Nakamura, 1995; Tsuchiya, 1998; Tsuchiya et al., 1998).

5B.4.8 What initiates the formation of preneoplastic parent cells?

It has been hypothesized that, in mice, a primary 'transforming' event takes place before the fourth to eighth week of the foreign-body reaction, and that such transformation may occur at sites distant from the foreign body, in a single or a few mesenchymal pluripotential stem cells of the microvasculature (Brand, 1976) [The Working Group noted that the existence of such cells is no longer believed]. Several possibilities for the nature of this initiating event were proposed: (a) a genome change caused either by mutation or activation of indigenous viral genes, (b) chromosome defects or imbalance and (c) aberrant epigenic differentiation (Brand, 1976).

Viruses or viral genomes have been sought in cells of foreign body-induced tumours, but no convincing evidence of a causal relationship has been found.

The possibility that mutagenic chemicals leach out of the materials and initiate parent cells by a process of chemical carcinogenesis seems unlikely in most cases, because the conventional mutagenicity assays (bacterial gene mutation and mammalian cell chromosomal aberration assays) gave negative results with PEUs, PVC, poly(2-hydroxyethyl methacrylate) and silicone, when the leachables obtained by extraction with organic solvents followed by evaporation were tested (Nakamura et al., 1992). This conclusion is supported by the finding that subcutaneous implantation of powdered polymers did not induce tumours, although leaching of chemicals from pulverized polymers is accelerated.

Possible tumour-initiating activities of polyurethane materials were tested using the two-stage BALB/c 3T3 cell transformation assay. Firstly, methanol extracts of PEU were tested in the presence or absence of TPA, a potent tumour promoter. The extract alone did not increase the number of transformed foci, but did in the presence of TPA. These results indicate that leachable substances from PEU can act as a weak tumour initiator, while transforming activity was found only in the presence of TPA. In the same series of experiments, chemical models of component units of PEUs were tested to identify a chemical moiety that might induce the initiation of cell transformation. 1,4-Butanediol induced no significant increase in transformed cell foci up to a concentration of 20 mg/mL. PTMO of average molecular weight 1000 also showed no transforming activity, whereas MDU induced transformation at a concentration of 0.2 µg/mL. Therefore, it is possible that substances containing a phenyl-carbamate structure act as tumour initiators. In order to clarify the effects of direct interaction of cells with the coated materials on cell transformation, one half of the surface of a set of test dishes was coated with PEUs. The number of foci on the area coated with PEU increased significantly in the presence of TPA, whereas no increase was found on the non-coated area. These results imply that initiation may be caused not only by the leachable substances but also by biodegradable substances present on the surface of PEUs. Comparison of the potencies of tumour-initiating and -promoting activity of the PEUs in the various assays indicated that the promoting activities of the PEUs are stronger than the initiating activities.

From the results described, it was speculated that the mechanism of tumorigenesis induced by PEUs involves (1) initiation caused by the hard segment, with a chemical structure like that of MDU (this chemical moiety is present in the leachable and biodegradable oligomers) and (2) promotion mainly through the action of a polyether soft segment moiety such as PTMO in inhibiting GJIC. This soft segment moiety is derived from the leachable oligomers and degradation through a direct cell/material interaction (Tsuchiya et al., 1996).

Various tumour promoters have been shown to inhibit GJIC by phosphorylation of connexin proteins. The effects of PEUs were investigated on connexin 43 (Cx43), a major gap-junction protein of both V79 and BALB/c 3T3 clone A31-1-1 cells. Cx43 in the A31-1-1 cells after transformation by PEUs was phosphorylated at tyrosine, serine and threonine residues and GJIC was inhibited, according to the dye-transfer assay. Both hard and soft segment models induced phosphorylation of Cx43 and also inhibited GJIC, which is considered to play an important role in tumour promotion (Tsuchiya et al., 1998). Thus, a post-translational modification or a defect in gene expression, but not a mutation in the coding sequence of the *Cx43* gene is probably involved in the PEU-induced inhibition of GJIC during tumorigenesis *in vitro* (Tsuchiya et al., 1999). However, since it is not clear how GJIC regulates cell growth, further studies on the molecular mechanism of the inhibitory action on GJIC by interaction of cells with biomaterials are needed.

5B.4.9 *Possible genotoxic mechanisms underlying solid-state carcinogenesis*

To investigate the relationship between inflammatory processes and foreign-body carcinogenesis, groups of 20 male Fischer 344 rats, four months old, were given implants of discs (15 mm diameter × 0.2 mm) of silicone elastomer prepared with dichlorobenzoyl peroxide catalyst, as used in breast implants (Dow Corning), or cellulose acetate filters (Millipore) with pore sizes of < 0.02 μm ('impermeable', positive control) or > 0.65 μm ('porous', negative control) into a dorsal interscapular subcutaneous pocket (James et al., 1997). Groups of 10 rats were killed one week or two months after implantation. Each implant and tissue capsule was divided for histopathological examination, for immunohistochemical determination of leukocyte antigen expression and cell proliferation and for in-situ 3'-OH-end-labelling to measure DNA strand breaks in DNA-damaged viable cells and in apoptotic cells. Inflammatory response and capsular thickness were assessed blind, using qualitative scales. Similar acute inflammatory responses, seen in both the silicone and positive-control groups, comprised a discontinuous layer of macrophages adjacent to the implants and a loosely organized capsule of collagen fibres interspersed with numerous spindle cells and neovascularization after one week. The response in the negative-control group comprised a continuous layer of macrophages, mainly multinucleated syncytial giant cells, closely adherent to the implants, with fibrillar processes penetrating the pores and only a weak fibrotic response. By two months, dense capsules of linearly aligned collagen fibres with minimal vascularization, numerous spindle cells and minimal lymphocytes or macrophages were evident in the silicone and positive-control groups. In the negative-control group, the macrophage layer and degree of fibrosis were similar to those observed before. A significant ($p < 0.001$) difference in capsular thickness was observed between the negative-control group (0.08 mm) and the other groups (0.27 and 0.21 mm for the silicone and positive-control groups, respectively).

There were no clear differences in the expression of leukocyte antigen epitopes at one week; CD11b/c (a marker for phagocytic cells exposed to cytokines) was strongly expressed in the macrophage layer in all groups. CD4 and CD8 epitopes (expressed by T helper/inducer and T cytotoxic/suppressor cells, respectively) were scattered throughout the capsule. After two months, expression of CD11b/c, CD4 and CD8 was reduced in the silicone and positive-control groups but remained broadly similar to that seen in week 1 in the porous-filter group, indicating that the high level of these inflammatory markers was maintained with the non-carcinogenic material only.

Serial sections of formalin-fixed tissue were labelled and stained for 3′-OH of DNA strands by in-situ end-labelling (see Table 61). The percentage incidence of stained spindle cells was determined in fields adjacent to the implant and in the multinuclear giant-cell layer. At one week, DNA fragmentation was common in viable cells in capsules surrounding the silicone and positive-control materials (52 and 53.3%, respectively) but rare in the negative-control group (0.2%; $p < 0.01$ relative to other groups). Labelled cells were interspersed throughout the capsule but did not

Table 61. Percentage of viable and apoptotic cells detected by in-situ end-labelling of DNA in connective tissue adjacent to implants

		Silicone	Positive control	Negative control
1 week	% viable cells with DNA strand breaks	52.0 ± 8.4	53.3 ± 3.3	0.2 ± 0.1[a]
	% apoptotic bodies	4.7 ± 1.0	12.1 ± 1.4	2.1 ± 0.6[a]
2 months	% viable cells with DNA strand breaks	50.8 ± 5.9	49.8 ± 6.9	0.1 ± 0.02[a]
	% apoptotic bodies	11.0 ± 1.2	4.9 ± 0.2	0.9 ± 0.2[a]

[a] $p < 0.01$ relative to silicone and positive control
Adapted from James et al. (1997)

coincide with markers for leukocyte antigen epitopes, such as CD11b/c. A similar pattern was evident at two months. These DNA-damaged cells were assumed to originate from connective tissue.

A similar method was used to quantify cell proliferation through immunohistochemical analysis of proliferating cell nuclear antigen (PCNA). After one week, cell proliferation was higher in spindle cells and macrophages in capsules surrounding the silicone and positive-control materials (36.1 and 33.7%, respectively, for spindle cells) in comparison with the negative-control group (13.9%). By two months, the proportion of proliferating cells had decreased to about 6% (1.6% in negative controls), and these were predominantly spindle cells within the well-defined capsule.

The authors concluded that cell proliferation, apoptosis and DNA strand breaks were significantly increased in tissue adjacent to carcinogenic implants. Conversely, in the presence of non-carcinogenic implants, DNA strand breaks were negligible and associated with reduced levels of proliferation and apoptosis. [The Working Group noted that the presence of DNA strand breaks was not confirmed by a separate assay. The immunohistochemical detection system used (Apotag) is usually interpreted as indicating DNA fragmentation related to apoptosis, not to genotoxicity, as suggested by the authors].

The authors of these studies emphasized the similarity of the pathology observed in the silicone and positive-control group, in which the acute inflammatory response was attenuated and replaced by fibrosis, and the different cellular response produced by the porous material, in which the inflammatory response was chronically maintained and associated with minimal fibrosis. The frustrated phagocytic response, typified by syncytial giant-cell aggregation around the porous material, was in contrast to the fibrotic response towards impenetrable materials, directed at isolation of the foreign body. The authors hypothesized that this could be the result of specific cytokine release. It was further postulated that the loss of vasculature associated with capsule formation would lead to an environment known to promote carcinogenicity. The authors concluded that the results suggest that the micron-scale surface morphology of the implant determines the nature of the subsequent cellular response, which may predispose to tumour development (James *et al.*, 1997).

Further work on tumour development, reported in an abstract, investigated the incidence of mutations in the *p53* gene in human tissue. Experimental groups were apparently similar to those reported above, with implants of silicone elastomer and non-porous cellulose acetate, although no further information on this was given. Within 12 months of implantation, hyperplastic inflammatory foci were observed within the fibrous tissue adjacent to the carcinogenic implants. These foci stained positive for both mutant p53 protein and DNA strand breaks, as tested by *in situ* end-labelling. Fibrosarcomas developed in all rats in these groups within two years of implantation. No tumours developed in negative controls. Polymerase chain reaction (PCR) amplification and single-strand conformation polymorphism (SSCP) analysis of DNA from tumour tissue samples indicated that 40% of tumours (6/15) exhibited abnormal band migration patterns consistent with *p53* gene mutation. Reamplification and direct sequencing of an abnormal SSCP band revealed a double mutation in exon 6 of the gene (C→T, G→T). Further analysis revealed a hot-spot mutation in 50% of the tumours with *p53* mutations, comprising GCT→CCC (Ala→Pro), at codon 201 of exon 6. The authors concluded that these results suggest, for the first time, that indirect genotoxic mechanisms resulting in *p53* mutations are involved in foreign-body carcinogenesis (Pogribna *et al.*, 1997). [The Working Group noted that *p53* mutations may arise during the later stages of tumour development.]

5C. OTHER FOREIGN BODIES

5C.1 Degradation in biological systems
No data were available to the Working Group.

5C.2 Distribution and excretion
The potential for components of implanted bullets and shell fragments to be mobilized (solubilized or degraded by phagocytosis) and distributed to distant parts of the body is relevant to the systemic carcinogenicity of such foreign bodies. Of the possible metals in these objects, lead and depleted uranium are those of greatest concern.

5C.2.1 *Lead*

   (a) *Humans*

That lead is distributed from the site of retained bullets to other areas of the body has been clearly demonstrated from the number of case reports of lead toxicity in individuals with retained bullets.

Machle (1940) reported in detail on two cases in which clinical diagnoses of lead poisoning were correlated with retained bullets. He further reviewed 40 other cases that had been described in the literature from 1867 to 1938 and was impressed with the paucity of cases compared with the frequency of gunshot wounds and of bullets that had been permitted to remain in the body. Bird and buck shot accounted for a fairly high proportion of the cases, even though it is likely that many more persons had implanted artillery shrapnel and rifle bullets from the First World War. The interval between lodgment of the bullets (including buckshot) and initial lead poisoning symptoms varied considerably (from 12 days to 48 years), although among the 13 cases in which the symptoms developed in less than one year, only two would be considered cases of lead poisoning at the present time. The location of lodgment seemed important, as more than half of the bullet-related lead poisoning cases consisted of bullets retained within bones or joints.

Since Machle's review, a number of individual case reports of bullet-related lead poisoning have been published. In 1982, Linden *et al.* (1982) presented three additional bullet-lead poisoning cases plus a review of 13 other cases. Additional sporadic reports of bullet retention and resultant lead poisoning have been reported since that time.

In a more recent review and critical analysis of lead poisoning associated with retained bullets, Magos (1994) analysed the data presented by Machle (1940), Linden *et al.* (1982) and other published reports. On the basis of this extensive review, the author concluded that while it is likely that only a fraction of persons with implanted lead projectiles actually develop lead poisoning, it is even more likely that only a fraction of those with bullet-related lead poisoning were actually diagnosed with the condition. The number of mild lead poisoning cases is probably quite high but many were missed by the examining clinicians due to (1) non-specificity of signs and symptoms of lead poisoning, (2) general lack of awareness and familiarity as to the toxicity of lead and (3) inappropriate use of laboratory tests of lead indicators (blood, serum, urine analysis). Mobilization of lead from retained bullets and shot may be influenced by several factors, depending on mobilization from either the projectile itself or from the surrounding tissues and other secondary storage sites. The factors that can be considered most important are indicated in Table 62. On the basis of the cases reviewed, the risk of lead poisoning and the latent period could not be predicted, but it was noted that the number of known clinical cases was small in relation to the actual number of persons carrying lead-containing bullets (Magos, 1994).

(b) *Experimental systems*

Discs of lead (enriched with two natural isotopes) were implanted into the knee joints or leg (thigh) muscle of two mongrel dogs. The animals were monitored by mass spectrometry for release of lead in blood over a three-year period. ^{206}Pb served as a marker for the discs implanted into the synovium, while ^{208}Pb served as the marker for lead implanted in the muscle. The knee implant underwent vigorous attack by the synovial fluid and blood lead levels reached a maximum in four to six months, declining thereafter as the remaining fragments became encapsulated. In contrast, there was only minor mobilization of lead from the discs placed in the muscle during the first month and even less thereafter as the discs became encapsulated. Very little physical change was noted in the muscle implants, whereas the joint implants had disintegrated after six months into a number of particles with corroded outlines. The smaller particles subsequently became encapsulated within the joint (Manton & Thal, 1986).

5C.2.2 *Depleted uranium*

(a) *Humans*

The distribution of uranium was determined radiochemically in tissues obtained at autopsy of a man who had been employed in the uranium processing industry for 26 years. The deposition of uranium in human tissues followed the order: skeleton > liver > kidney, with concentration ratios of 63:2.8:1. This study indicates that the long-term storage compartment for uranium in the skeleton may be greater than previously estimated (Kathren *et al.*, 1989).

Table 62. Factors that may affect the mobilization of lead from retained bullets

Mobilization from the projectile (lead bullet)	
Surface area	Dissolution is faster from multiple pellets than from an equal mass of a single bullet and is faster from fragmented bullets than from non-fragmented ones.
Location	Bullets retained in soft tissues tend to become encapsulated by fibrous tissue which impedes release of lead.
Mechanical effects	Impact of bullet with bone creates abrasive effect on bullet lodged in a joint, which promotes disintegration of the bullet.
Acidity	Low pH of synovial and bursal fluids promotes dissolution, with high lead concentrations in the fluids and surrounding tissues.
Mobilization from surrounding tissues and other secondary storage sites	
Inflammation	Lead taken up by the surrounding tissues may cause synovitis and arthritis, which will promote dispersal of lead to other areas. Cell migration and increased blood flow may also play a role.
Impaired use of limbs	Inactivity due to painful arthritis can promote mobilization of lead from bones.
Hypermetabolic conditions	Alcoholic acidosis, hyperthyroidism and fever may promote lead mobilization and increase sensitivity to lead.

Modified from Magos (1994)

(b)   Experimental systems

The distribution of implanted depleted uranium was studied with Sprague-Dawley rats using three dose levels (low, medium, high: 4, 10, 20 pellets). The implants consisted of 99.25% depleted uranium and 0.75% titanium with the uranium isotopes amounting to 99.75% ^{238}U and 0.2% ^{235}U and trace levels of ^{234}U. [The Working Group noted that the authors did not consider the radioactivity of the residual ^{235}U and ^{234}U isotope as a major concern.] The pellets were implanted into the gastrocnemius muscle of male Sprague-Dawley rats and tissue samples were analysed at day 1 and at 1, 6, 12 and 18 months. Within one day, uranium had appeared in the kidney and bone. By six months, the uranium level had reached a plateau in the kidney but continued to rise in bone throughout the 18-month period in the high-dose group. The urine concentration of uranium reached a maximum at 12 months and had declined by 18 months. A dose- and time-related increase in uranium levels was found in many tissues. The greatest concentrations were found in the kidney and bone, the primary reservoirs for uranium redistributed from intramuscularly embedded depleted uranium fragments. Many tissues other than muscle had significant concentrations of uranium, including the brain, liver, spleen, lung, lymph nodes and testes (Pellmar et al., 1999).

The effects of implantation of depleted uranium pellets were studied in Sprague-Dawley rats. Groups of animals received 20 depleted uranium pellets (high dose), 10 depleted uranium pellets and 10 tantalum (inert control) pellets (medium dose), or four depleted uranium and 16 tantalum pellets (low dose). The control group received 20 tantalum pellets. At 6, 12 and 18 months after implantation, the concentrations of uranium in urine were significantly increased in all dose groups, peak concentrations being observed at 12 months (Miller et al., 1998a). In the same study, mutagenicity in urine was investigated (see Section 5C.4.2).

5C.3 Tissue responses and other expressions of toxicity

5C.3.1 Lead

The toxicity of systemically distributed lead is well known and has been reviewed by IARC (1980) and elsewhere. The toxic effects in humans involve several different organ systems with subtle clinical symptoms in most cases. In adults, the main organs affected are the neurological system, the haem-synthesizing system and the kidneys. With excess occupational exposure or accidental exposures to lead, the most evident effects have been peripheral neuropathy and chronic nephropathy. The most sensitive effects in adults may be hypertension and anaemia. Less commonly, lead-induced toxicity may affect the gastrointestinal and reproductive systems (sterility and neonatal deaths).

5C.3.2 Depleted uranium

In humans, the kidney and bone are the primary target organs of internal exposure to uranium, regardless of the route of exposure. Most of the absorbed uranium is cleared from the blood stream and excreted in the urine within 24 h. The uranium that is not excreted is reabsorbed by the proximal tubules of the kidney, where it causes its primary toxic effects (Kathren et al., 1989; Pellmar et al., 1999). Chronically exposed uranium mill workers showed mild dysfunction of the kidney and increased urinary excretion of beta-2-microglobulin (Thun et al., 1985). In one case study, neurological effects were seen (Goasguen et al., 1982). These data indicate that embedded fragments of depleted uranium may lead to neural damage, which may affect both cognitive and motor functions.

Preliminary results have been published of toxicity studies in rats with implanted depleted uranium. Depleted uranium pellets (1 × 2 mm) consisting of 99.25% depleted uranium and 0.75% titanium by weight were implanted at three dose levels (4, 10 and 20 pellets) into the gastrocnemius muscle of male Sprague-Dawley rats. Clinical and laboratory analyses are being performed to detect kidney, behavioural and neural toxicity. Six months after implantation, decreased weight gain, a dose-related increase in levels of depleted uranium in the kidneys, bone and urine, and a decrease in neuronal excitation in the hippocampus were reported. However, while uranium was found in the brain, no behavioural toxicity was observed at six months after implantation. The authors indicated that the kidney toxicity was less than would be expected on the basis of the uranium levels in the kidneys (Pellmar et al., 1998).

A preliminary report was given of an ongoing study to assess the potential carcinogenicity of long-term exposure of rats to implants of depleted uranium (DU), such as shrapnel in wounds. Groups of 50 male Wistar rats were given implants into the thigh muscle of $5.0 \times 5.0 \times 1.5$-mm or $2.5 \times 2.5 \times 1.5$-mm DU squares composed of 99.25% uranium and 0.75% titanium. Other groups were given implants of 2.0×1.0-mm diameter DU pellets, tantalum squares (negative controls) and thorotrast (thorium dioxide) injections (positive controls). After 15 months of the planned 24-month exposure period, a marked local tissue reaction (including fibrous capsule formation) had developed around the DU and tantalum implants, the capsules being much thicker around the uranium implants. There was also a decrease in weight of the group that received the largest mass of DU, although survival was not affected in any of the groups. Carcinogenic response is not yet known (Hahn et al., 1999).

5C.4 Genetic and related effects

5C.4.1 *Lead*

The genetic and related effects of lead have been reviewed (IARC, 1987c).

5C.4.2 *Depleted uranium*

(a) *Humans*

No data were available to the Working Group.

(b) *Experimental systems*

Mutagenicity induced by depleted uranium implants has been demonstrated in experiments with male Sprague-Dawley rats. Urine and serum of these animals were evaluated for mutagenic potential using the Ames *Salmonella* mutation assay. The implants consisted of pellets implanted into the gastrocnemius muscle at three dose levels. Tantalum was used as a negative control. Urine and blood were collected at 0, 6, 12 and 18 months for the mutagenicity assay. While no mutagenicity was observed with the sera, a substantial dose- and time-dependent increase in mutagenicity was seen with urine samples. Positive results were obtained with *S. typhimurium* strain TA98 and the Ames II™ mixed strains (TA7001-7006). A significant elevation in mutagenic potential was observed in TA98 strain and Ames II™ tests with the Amberlite XAD-4 and XAD-8 column fractions of urine, which was dependent on both the length of time since implantation and the number of uranium pellets implanted. Urine from animals that had tantalum implants showed no increase in mutagenicity. A strongly positive correlation was observed between urinary mutagenicity and urinary uranium levels at 6, 12 or 18 months after pellet implantation (Miller et al., 1998a).

A doubling of sister chromatid exchanges was found in human osteoblast-like cells treated with 10 µM of depleted uranium-uranyl chloride for 24 h. This was a greater response than that found with the positive control, nickel sulfate (Miller et al., 1998b).

In the same series of experiments, in-vivo transformation of human osteoblast-like cells with depleted uranium was demonstrated. Human osteosarcoma cells (HOS TE85, clone F-5) were treated with depleted uranium-uranyl chloride (10 µM) for 24 h, at which time the cells were rinsed, trypsinized and seeded onto tissue culture dishes. The dishes were incubated for five weeks and examined for the appearance of transformed foci. Morphologically, the uranium-exposed cells developed into diffused type II foci. A 10-fold increase in transformation frequency was observed in the treated compared to the non-treated cells. The transformation response was stronger with depleted uranium than with the positive controls (nickel sulfate or lead acetate). The transformed cells showed increased expression of the K-*ras* oncogene, and suppression of the phosphorylation of the Rb protein. Transformation was confirmed by injection of 1×10^6 or 5×10^6 of uranyl chloride-treated cells subcutaneously into four- to five-week-old female athymic mice. Tumours developed within four weeks. The histological appearance resembled a carcinoma characterized by an undifferentiated, sheet-like growth (Miller et al., 1998b).

6. SUMMARY OF DATA REPORTED AND EVALUATION

6.1 Exposure data

A wide range of metals and their alloys, polymers, ceramics and composites are used in surgically implanted medical devices and prostheses and dental materials. Most implanted devices are constructed of more than one kind of material (implants of complex composition). Since the early 1900s, metal alloys have been developed for these applications to provide improved physical and chemical properties, such as strength, durability and corrosion resistance. Major classes of metals used in medical devices and dental materials include stainless steels, cobalt–chromium alloys and titanium (as alloys and unalloyed). In addition, dental casting alloys are based on precious metals (gold, platinum, palladium or silver), nickel and copper and may in some cases contain smaller amounts of many other elements, added to improve the alloys' properties.

Orthopaedic applications of metal alloys include arthroplasty, osteosynthesis and in spinal and maxillofacial devices. Metallic alloys are also used for components of prosthetic heart valve replacements, and pacemaker casings and leads. Small metallic parts may be used in a wide range of other implants, including skin and wound staples, vascular endoprostheses, filters and occluders. Dental applications of metals and alloys include fillings, prosthetic devices (crowns, bridges, removable prostheses), dental implants and orthodontic appliances.

Polymers of many types are used in implanted medical devices and dental materials. Illustrative examples are silicones (breast prostheses, pacemaker leads), polyurethanes (pacemaker components), polymethacrylates (dental prostheses, bone cements), poly(ethylene terephthalate) (vascular grafts, heart valve sewing rings, sutures), polypropylene (sutures), polyethylene (prosthetic joint components), polytetrafluoroethylene (vascular prostheses), polyamides (sutures) and polylactides and poly(glycolic acids) (bioresorbables).

Ceramic materials based on metal oxides (alumina, zirconia) find use in joint replacements and dental prostheses. Other materials based on calcium phosphate are used as bone fillers and implant coatings. Pyrolytic carbon applications include heart valves and coatings for implants. Composites are used mainly in dental fillings.

Although precise numbers are not available, many millions of people worldwide have implanted devices, which may remain in place for years.

Foreign bodies, such as bullets and pellets from firearms and metallic fragments from explosions, may penetrate and remain in human tissues for long periods of time. Internal exposure to constituents, including lead (from bullets and pellets) and depleted uranium (from shell and missile fragments), may result.

6.2 Human carcinogenicity data

Sixteen case reports have described neoplasms originating from bone or soft connective tissue in the region of metal implants. An analytical study did not report an increased risk for soft-tissue sarcoma after metal implants. No association with dental amalgam was found in a case–control study in Australia.

The 30 case reports of breast cancer following silicone implants for cosmetic breast augmentation appear unlikely to correspond to an excess of breast cancer. All five cohort studies involving a total of more than 18 000 women treated with surgical prostheses made of silicone (or polyurethane-coated silicone) for cosmetic breast augmentation conducted in Canada, Denmark, Sweden and the United States consistently found no evidence of increased risk of breast cancer. The combined results of the four largest cohort studies show a 25% reduction in risk. Similar results were reported by a large case–control study including more than 2000 cases and 2000 controls in the United States. All cohort studies were based on subjects exposed to implanted silicone at an early age, usually between the ages of 30 and 40 years, so that the number of breast cancer cases observed in each study was relatively small. Except for the case–control study in the United States, only limited allowance was made for potential confounding factors, although no clear evidence has emerged as to the relevance of any such factor to a possible association between implanted silicone and breast cancer risk.

Three of the studies considered the issue of latency, with observation periods of up to 10 years or more, but even in the group of women with follow-up of 10 years or more, there was no suggestion of increased risk. The risk of cancer following surgical implantation of silicone prostheses for breast reconstruction after breast cancer was considered in a study in France. The results of this study suggest no excess risk of second primary breast or other cancer, distant metastases, local recurrence or death from breast cancer. The reduced risks for breast cancer found in the cohort and case–control studies are unlikely to be due to chance, and no bias that would explain these findings has been identified. Four cohort studies of women with surgical breast implants in Denmark, Sweden and the United States reported on cancers at sites other than the breast. None of these studies found an increased risk for all cancers combined. Two studies reported increased risk for lung cancer, but these results were based on a total of only nine observed cases. For no other cancer site was there consistent evidence of an increased risk, although the statistical power to detect an increased risk of rare neoplasms, including soft-tissue sarcomas, was small.

Out of the large number of patients with orthopaedic implants of complex composition (metal with bone cement with or without polyethylene), a total of 35 cases have been reported of malignant neoplasms arising from the bone or the soft tissue in the region of an implant. Fourteen cohort studies of patients following total knee or total hip replacement from six countries were performed to investigate cancer incidence in these populations. Two of the studies from Finland and two studies from Sweden were partially overlapping. One study included only patients with metal-on-metal implants, five studies included only patients with polyethylene-on-metal implants, while the remaining studies included patients with mixed or unspecified types of implant. One study showed a small increase in overall cancer incidence, while the remaining studies showed overall decreases. Four of these studies suggested an excess risk for specific cancers, including Hodgkin's disease, non-Hodgkin lymphoma, leukaemia and kidney cancer. However, results of the other studies were not consistent with this observation. In one small cohort study from Denmark of patients with a finger or hand implant, an increased risk of lymphohaematopoietic cancer was observed. Additionally, two case–control studies, one including cases with soft-tissue sarcoma and the other including lymphoma and leukaemia, were carried out in the United States. The latter overlaps with one of the cohort studies. Neither of these studies showed an association with the presence of implants of complex composition. Most of the studies did not have information on possible confounding variables such as immunosuppressive therapy or rheumatoid arthritis for the lymphomas and analgesic drugs for kidney cancer. The follow-up in most of the studies may have been too short to evaluate cancer occurring many years after exposure; in some studies with longer follow-up, the numbers of long-term survivors were low.

Thirteen cases of breast cancer and one case of plasmacytoma have been reported in patients with cardiac pacemakers. Ten cases of different neoplasms have been reported at the site of non-metallic foreign bodies. Eight cases of sarcoma have been reported at the site of vascular grafts. No conclusions can be drawn from these case reports.

Twenty-three cases of sarcomas, twenty-three cases of carcinomas and seven cases of brain tumours have been reported at the site of metallic foreign bodies, mainly bullets and shrapnel fragments.

6.3 Veterinary studies

Despite the large number and variety of both metallic and non-metallic internal fixation devices used in dogs in recent decades, only about 60 cases of sarcomas, primarily of bone, have been reported. In addition, four cases of sarcomas at the site of other foreign bodies have been reported in dogs. One case–control study found no association between metallic implants used to stabilize fractures in dogs and the development of bone or soft-tissue tumours.

In contrast, at least 563 cases of vaccine-associated sarcomas in cats have been reported in just six years, with an estimated annual incidence of 1–13 per 10 000 vaccinated cats. Vaccine-associated sarcomas have been mostly associated with administration of recently introduced feline vaccines containing adjuvant. Tumours that develop at vaccination sites are morphologically different from those that develop at non-vaccination sites. A cohort study found that cats developed sarcomas in a shorter time at sites used for vaccination than at non-vaccination sites and that there was an increased risk for sarcoma development with increased numbers of vaccines at a given site.

6.4 Animal carcinogenicity data

Chromium metal powder was tested in rats by intramuscular and intrarenal administration, in mice and rats by intrapleural and intraperitoneal administration, in rats and rabbits by intraosseous implantation and in mice, rats and rabbits by intravenous injection. No increase in tumour incidence was observed in these studies, although most studies had limitations in design, duration or reporting.

Cobalt metal powder was tested in rats by intramuscular or intrathoracic injection, producing sarcomas at the injection site. Studies in rats by intrarenal injection and in rabbits by intraosseous injection had limitations in design, duration or reporting.

Nickel metal powder was tested by inhalation exposure in mice, rats and guinea-pigs, by intratracheal instillation in rats and Syrian hamsters, by intramuscular injection in rats and hamsters and by intrapleural, intraperitoneal, intraosseous and intrarenal injection in rats. It was also tested by intravenous injection in mice and rats. Nickel metal pellets were tested by subcutaneous administration in rats. The studies by inhalation exposure were inadequate for an evaluation of carcinogenicity. After intratracheal instillation of nickel, significant numbers of squamous-cell carcinomas and adenocarcinomas of the lung were observed in rats; one adenocarcinoma of the lung was observed in hamsters. Intrapleural injections induced sarcomas in rats. Subcutaneous administration of nickel metal pellets induced sarcomas in rats; intramuscular injection of nickel powder induced sarcomas in rats and hamsters; and intraperitoneal injections induced local carcinomas, mesotheliomas and sarcomas in rats. No significant increase in the incidence of local kidney tumours in rats was seen following intrarenal injection. Studies by the intraosseous and intravenous routes were inadequate for evaluation.

Titanium metal was tested in rats by intramuscular implantation of rods and by intraosseous administration of powder, rods or wire. No local tumours occurred.

Most *nickel-based alloys* that have been tested for carcinogenicity in animals are not actually used in clinical devices, and carcinogenicity data are not available for a number of alloys which are commonly used, including nickel–titanium.

Metal alloys containing a preponderance of *nickel* in combination with varying amounts of chromium, iron, gallium, copper, aluminium and manganese have been tested as powder or pellets by subcutaneous or intraperitoneal administration to rats and by intratracheal administration to hamsters. In these studies, local sarcomas were consistently found at the injection site in the treated animals and were absent in vehicle controls. One of the nickel-based alloys (which contained approximately 66–67% nickel, 13–16% chromium and 7% iron) was tested independently by two laboratories, using different species (hamsters and rats) and different routes of administration (intratracheal and intraperitoneal). In both studies, local tumours were seen in proportion to the dose of alloy. Local tumours were also observed in two bioassays in which rats received identification ear tags made of an alloy that contained 67% nickel, 30% copper, 2% iron and 1% manganese.

Most other nickel-containing alloys tested as powder and rods in rats by intramuscular, intraperitoneal, intrarenal and intraosseous administration gave negative or equivocal results for induction of tumours at the injection site. One study in hamsters by intratracheal administration of an alloy powder containing approximately 27% nickel, 39% iron and 16% chromium also gave negative results.

One clinically relevant alloy, Ni35Co35Cr20Mo10 (MP35N alloy), gave negative results for carcinogenicity when tested in two studies by intramuscular implantation in rats as rods, but produced local sarcomas in one study following intramuscular administration to rats as a powder.

Titanium-based alloys were tested in rats by intramuscular administration of rods and by intraosseous administration of rods and intra-articular administration of wear-debris. No local tumours were observed at the injection site in these experiments, except in one study by intraosseous administration in which a titanium/aluminium/vanadium alloy implanted into the femur as hemi-cylinders produced a high incidence of local tumours, especially where there was loosening of the implant.

Cobalt-based alloys were tested in rats by intramuscular administration. Local tumours were induced by a powder (particle size, 0.1–1 μm) in horse serum but not by dry powders (particle size, 0.5–50 and 100–250 μm) or by polished rods. No local tumours were observed in guinea-pigs following intramuscular injection of cobalt as a dry powder (particle size, 0.5–50 μm). A low incidence of local tumours was observed in rats following intraosseous administration of two cobalt-based alloys given as powder or wire. Local tumours did not occur following intraosseous implantation of rods of two other cobalt-containing alloys. No local tumours occurred in rats following intra-articular administration of a cobalt alloy powder.

Stainless steels containing 13–17% chromium were tested by intratracheal administration of powder to hamsters, intrabronchial administration of wire to rats and by intramuscular administration of rods and discs to rats and intraosseous administration of rods and powder to rats. No local tumours were observed, except in rats receiving stainless steel discs.

Thin foils of silver, gold, platinum, tin, steel, Vitallium (CoCrMo alloy) and tantalum were tested by subcutaneous implantation in rats. All of these foils produced local sarcomas.

In one study in rats, subcutaneous implantation of discs of aluminium oxide ceramic produced local sarcomas. In a few studies in mice and rats, local sarcomas were observed following subcutaneous implantation of glass sheets.

Numerous polymeric materials have been tested for carcinogenicity in mice and rats, most frequently by subcutaneous, intramuscular or intraperitoneal injection. Many materials—cellophane, ε-caprolactone-L-lactide copolymer, polyamide (Nylon), poly-(ethylene terephthalate), polyethylene, poly-L-lactide, poly(2-hydroxyethylmethacrylate), poly(methyl methacrylate), polypropylene, polystyrene, polytetrafluoroethylene, polyurethane, poly(vinyl alcohol), poly(vinyl chloride), polymethylsiloxane (silicone) film or polysilicone gum and vinyl chloride–vinyl acetate copolymers—produced sarcomas at the site of implantation with varying incidence. When several polymers were tested in rats according to the same experimental protocol, sarcoma incidences ranged from 70% (polypropylene) to 7% (silicone). A low incidence of local tumours was seen with silicone in five separate experiments using rats.

A few experiments with various polymeric materials have been reported using small number of other animal species, such as rabbits, guinea-pigs and hamsters, with generally negative findings.

Polymeric materials with a large surface area and a flat and smooth surface morphology generally induced a significantly increased incidence of sarcomas at the site of implantation. In most studies, perforated or foam materials or textiles induced lower incidences of sarcomas in comparison with flat films. Some studies suggest that surface roughening decreases local sarcoma incidence. The diameter and number of transmembrane channels (pores) per unit surface area are critical for this trend of decrease in sarcoma incidence. Segmenting or pulverizing polymeric materials significantly decreases local sarcoma incidences, often to nil.

For biodegradable polymers, the degradation rate is critical for local tumour induction in rodents. No local tumours were observed with poly(glycolic acid), which is quickly degraded within two months, whereas local sarcomas were induced by poly-L-lactide and ε-caprolactone-L-lactide copolymer which degraded more slowly (the polylactide degraded but was dimensionally unchanged at 24 months; ε-caprolactone-L-lactide copolymer fragmented after six months).

6.5 Other relevant data

The mutagenicity and carcinogenicity of a biomaterial are influenced by the exact composition of the biomaterial or extract(s); the composition and rates of release of leachable materials into the biological environment; degradation, which may lead to the formation of compounds with different mutagenic properties or leachability; the physical environment; and the surface properties. Much of the information available for assessment is inadequate in these respects, and methods are often not validated.

Wear and corrosion of metal implants result in the generation and release of a wide range of degradation products. The composition of the material surface or particles can vary as individual components are selectively removed or chemically modified. In the case of alloys, the release of one type of metal ion can be strongly influenced by the identity of other metals in the alloy. Most studies provide inadequate characterization data, but there is potential for the release of chemical species of known mutagenicity or carcinogenicity.

Experimental studies have shown that the potential for lead toxicity as a complication of lead projectile or bullet injury appears to be related to the surface area of the bullet (the greater the surface area, the greater the absorption), the location of the bullet (muscle or joint tissues), the presence of synovial fluid and length of time that the bullet resided in the body.

Available studies are inadequate to permit reliable and accurate estimates of long-term effects of depleted uranium in humans. Because of the low specific radioactivity of depleted uranium, the long-term toxicity is thought to be due to chemical rather than radiation effects.

Inflammatory (fibrotic) reactions have been observed with several non-metallic implant materials, including silicones and polyurethanes. Depending on the physical properties of the biomaterial, its presence can be associated with implantation-site sarcomas in rodents. There are insufficient data to conclude that a genotoxic mechanism operates in solid-state carcinogenesis. There are in-vitro data demonstrating the inhibitory effects of polyurethane, polyethylene and poly(ethylene terephthalate) on gap junctional intercellular communication.

Mutagenic properties of some biomaterial extracts have been demonstrated in some studies. The compounds shown or suspected to be responsible for this are components of the biomaterial, unreacted monomers or products of secondary reactions.

Data on the local and systemic availability of chemical species have been reported for only a limited number of biomaterials. In the case of poly(ester urethane) foam, biodegradation results in the generation of 2,4-diaminotoluene. This compound induces hepatocellular carcinomas when fed to mice and rats. There is no evidence that chemical carcinogenesis due to this compound plays a direct role in the mechanism of implant-site sarcoma development. There is no convincing evidence for the biodegradation of polydimethylsiloxanes (silicones).

Cytotoxicity of freshly cured dental composite materials and bonding agents has been demonstrated. Also, the components of resin composites all cause significant toxicity in direct contact with fibroblasts. However, the hazard for the dental pulp depends on the quantities which permeate the dentin and accumulate in the pulp.

A limited number of animal studies have shown pulpal responses to acid etching and bonding agents, which indicates a possible risk of pulpal reactions in patients. Composite materials may give rise to biological effects, but microleakage and bacterial infection complicate the evaluation of pulpal effects of composites.

Clinical reports on the adverse effects of composite filling materials indicate that pulpal and mucosal reactions rarely occur.

With few exceptions, the amounts of individual chemicals to which professionals and patients are exposed from adhesive agents and composite dental filling materials seem to be insufficient to cause clear, systemic toxic effects. Some constituents of adhesive agents and composite materials may have genotoxic potential. For most compounds of dental composites, there is little information on toxicity. With the exception of methyl methacrylate, no relevant data are available to compare local concentrations of released compounds with levels that produce toxic effects.

Formaldehyde has been shown to be released from some dental polymers *in vitro*, but the levels appear to be low.

6.6 Evaluation

There is *evidence suggesting lack of carcinogenicity* in humans of breast implants, made of silicone, for female breast carcinoma.

There is *inadequate evidence* in humans for the carcinogenicity of implanted prostheses made of silicone for neoplasms other than female breast carcinoma.

There is *inadequate evidence* in humans for the carcinogenicity of non-metallic implants other than those made of silicone.

There is *inadequate evidence* in humans for the carcinogenicity of metallic implants and metallic foreign bodies.

There is *inadequate evidence* in humans for the carcinogenicity of orthopaedic implants of complex composition and of cardiac pacemakers.

No epidemiological data relevant to the carcinogenicity of ceramic implants or dental alloys of precious metals were available.

There is *sufficient evidence* in experimental animals for the carcinogenicity of implants of metallic cobalt, metallic nickel and for nickel alloy powder containing approximately 66–67% nickel, 13–16% chromium and 7% iron.

There is *limited evidence* in experimental animals for the carcinogenicity of implants of alloys containing cobalt and alloys containing nickel, other than the specific aforementioned alloy.

There is *inadequate evidence* in experimental animals for the carcinogenicity of implants of chromium metal, stainless steel, titanium metal, titanium-based alloys and depleted uranium.

There is *sufficient evidence* in experimental animals for the carcinogenicity of polymeric and metallic materials in the form of thin films, foils or sheets when implanted into connective tissues of rodents.

There is *inadequate evidence* in experimental animals for the carcinogenicity of poly(glycolic acid) implants.

There is *inadequate evidence* in experimental animals for the carcinogenicity of polymeric materials in the form of powders when inserted into connective tissues of rodents.

There is *inadequate evidence* in dogs for the carcinogenicity of metallic implants and metallic and non-metallic foreign bodies.

There is *limited evidence* in cats for the carcinogenicity of certain feline vaccines containing adjuvants.

Overall evaluation

Organic polymeric materials as a group are *not classifiable as to their carcinogenicity to humans (Group 3)*.

Polymeric implants prepared as thin smooth films (with the exception of poly(glycolic acid)) are *possibly carcinogenic to humans (Group 2B)*.

Orthopaedic implants of complex composition and cardiac pacemakers are *not classifiable as to their carcinogenicity to humans (Group 3)*.

Silicone breast implants are *not classifiable as to their carcinogenicity to humans (Group 3)*.

Metallic implants prepared as thin smooth films are *possibly carcinogenic to humans (Group 2B)*.

Implanted foreign bodies of metallic cobalt, metallic nickel and an alloy powder containing 66–67% nickel, 13–16% chromium and 7% iron are *possibly carcinogenic to humans (Group 2B)*.

Implanted foreign bodies of metallic chromium or titanium and of cobalt-based, chromium-based and titanium-based alloys, stainless steel and depleted uranium are *not classifiable as to their carcinogenicity to humans (Group 3)*.

Dental materials are *not classifiable as to their carcinogenicity to humans (Group 3)*.

Ceramic implants are *not classifiable as to their carcinogenicity to humans (Group 3)*.

APPENDIX

Cancer has been induced in rodents by the inhalation, instillation or implantation of solid materials, including mineral fibres, crystalline silica and other poorly-soluble particulates. In this section, hypotheses that seek to explain the mechanisms of cancer induction by these substances are reviewed with the objective of identifying whether they provide any insight to mechanisms that might be involved in the induction of cancer by other types of solid, implanted materials.

Asbestos fibres

Naturally occurring asbestos fibres, talc containing asbestiform fibres and non-asbestiform fibres (erionite) have been classified as carcinogenic to humans (IARC, 1977, 1987a,d). Inhalation of these fibrous minerals causes scarring and cancer of the lungs and pleura (reviewed in Kane, 1996a). The histopathology and pathogenesis of these fibrotic and carcinogenic processes in the lungs and mesothelium are somewhat different. Inhalation of asbestos and erionite fibres at high doses causes diffuse interstitial fibrosis or asbestosis that is usually more prominent in the lower lobes of the lungs. This fibrotic reaction develops slowly but progressively, beginning 10 years after the initial exposure. It is hypothesized that oxidants and proteases released from alveolar macrophages activated by phagocytosis of fibres damage the alveolar epithelial lining. In addition, fibres may become translocated across the damaged epithelium into the interstitium of the alveolar walls. This injury is repaired by a combination of epithelial regeneration by Type II alveolar cells plus proliferation of fibroblasts with collagen deposition in the interstitium. Up-regulation of growth factor expression has been observed at sites of asbestos fibre deposition in rat lungs: platelet-derived growth factor (PDGF) and transforming growth factor (TGF)-β are hypothesized to trigger fibroblast proliferation and collagen synthesis, respectively, while TGF-α is mitogenic for alveolar epithelial cells (reviewed in Brody *et al.*, 1997b). Fibres also translocate to the pleural space following inhalation and accumulate near lymphatic openings on the parietal pleura and dome of the diaphragm (Boutin *et al.*, 1996); these are the anatomical sites where fibrotic or calcified pleural plaques develop. Pleural plaques are considered as a marker of prior asbestos exposure; they can occur even in the absence of asbestosis. Diffuse fibrosis of the visceral pleura can also occur, usually following repeated episodes of pleural effusion that is also called benign asbestos pleurisy. It is hypothesized that asbestos-induced pleural effusions are caused by release of chemokines such as interleukin (IL)-8 from mesothelial cells (Boylan *et al.*, 1992). Pleural fibrosis and pleural plaques are hypothesized to develop after injury to mesothelial cells and destruction of the basement membrane. This injury is then repaired by mesothelial and submesothelial cell proliferation and deposition of collagen (Davila & Crouch, 1993).

Inhalation of asbestos fibres contributes to the development of lung cancer arising from the bronchial and alveolar epithelium. Asbestos and cigarette smoke most likely act as co-factors in the induction of lung cancer (Table 63). The anatomical location, histological type of tumour and molecular alterations in oncogenes and tumour-suppressor genes in smokers who have also been exposed to asbestos are similar to those of lung cancers that arise in smokers with no history of exposure to asbestos (Lee et al., 1998). No reports are available that describe the pathology and molecular lesions in asbestos-related lung cancers that are not associated with cigarette smoking. The point mutations in the K-ras oncogene (Husgafvel-Pursiainen et al., 1993) and p53 tumour-suppressor gene (Wang et al., 1995), as well as deletions at the chromosome 3p14 locus are consistent with the known mutagenic spectrum of carcinogens in cigarette smoke (Nelson et al., 1998). The molecular mechanisms leading to the development of lung cancer and diffuse malignant mesothelioma after asbestos exposure are probably different. Human malignant mesotheliomas do not have point mutations in the ras oncogene or p53 tumour-suppressor gene; 40% of cases have mutations at the NF2 tumour-suppressor gene locus and 70–100% show co-deletions of the p15 and p16 tumour-suppressor genes (reviewed in Lechner et al., 1997). The molecular alterations

Table 63. Direct mechanisms of asbestos fibre carcinogenesis

Mechanism	Experimental end-points	References
Genotoxic	Oxidized bases	Chao et al. (1996); Fung et al. (1997a)
	DNA breaks	Reviewed in Jaurand (1996)
	Aneuploidy	Reviewed in Jaurand (1996); Jensen et al. (1996)
	Mutations	Park & Aust (1998)
Non-genotoxic		
Mitogenic	Target cell proliferation	BéruBé et al. (1996); Goldberg et al. (1997); Mishra et al. (1997)
	Binding to or activation of surface receptors	Boylan et al. (1995); Pache et al. (1998)
	Growth factor expression	Liu et al. (1996); Brody et al. (1997b); Kane et al. (1997)
	Intracellular signalling pathways	Zanella et al. (1996); Fung et al. (1997b); Mossman et al. (1997)
Cytotoxic	Apoptosis	Broaddus et al. (1996); Goldberg et al. (1997); Levresse et al. (1997)
	Necrosis	Reviewed in Kane (1996a)

characteristic of lung tumours and malignant mesotheliomas induced by asbestos may develop during later stages of tumour progression and may not reflect the direct genotoxic effect of fibres on the target cell population.

The mechanisms leading to the induction of lung cancers and malignant mesothelioma by exposure to asbestos fibres are unknown. Both physical and chemical parameters of fibres are related to their biological activity: fibre geometry and dimensions, biopersistence in the lungs, chemical composition and surface reactivity (reviewed in Everitt, 1994; Kane, 1996a, 1998). Asbestos fibres may act as direct or indirect carcinogens (see Tables 63 and 64). Direct genotoxic and mitogenic effects of asbestos, as well as of some man-made fibres, have been detected in in-vitro assays. These assays have been widely used because they are relatively inexpensive, simple and rapid. However, they have limitations and often produce conflicting results depending on the cell type, species and conditions of exposure. The most serious shortcoming is that direct exposure of target cells to high doses of fibres *in vitro* may not accurately reflect responses of the same target cells in the lung under conditions of chronic, low-dose exposure. Surface modification of fibres and mechanical dissolution or breakage that have been observed *in vivo* are not easily reproduced in in-vitro models (reviewed in Kane *et al.*, 1996). However, some recent studies using animal models have confirmed the results of some of the in-vitro assays (Table 64). For example, hydroxyl (Schapira *et al.*, 1994) and lipid radicals have been measured in rat lungs after intratracheal instillation of asbestos fibres (Ghio *et al.*, 1998). Up-regulation of the nuclear factor (NF)-κB transcription factor has been detected in rat lung epithelial and mesothelial cells after short-term inhalation of asbestos (Janssen *et al.*, 1997), as has increased expression of c-*fos* and c-*jun* proto-oncogenes in rat pleural mesothelial cells and c-*jun* in Syrian hamster tracheal epithelial cells (Heintz *et al.*, 1993). Target cell proliferation and up-regulation of growth factor expression in proliferating cells have been confirmed in the lungs and mesothelium after in-vivo exposure (Table 64). Persistent proliferation of mesothelial cells observed after direct intraperitoneal injection of asbestos fibres in mice has been correlated temporally and spatially with persistence

Table 64. Indirect mechanisms of asbestos fibre carcinogenesis

Mechanism	References
Co-factor with cigarette smoke	Reviewed in Kane (1996a); Lee *et al.* (1998)
Co-factor with SV40 virus	Carbone *et al.* (1997); Testa *et al.* (1998)
Persistent inflammation with secondary genotoxicity	Donaldson (1996); Reviewed in Driscoll *et al.* (1997); Vallyathan & Shi (1997)
Persistent inflammation with release of cytokines and growth factors	Rosenthal *et al.* (1994); Brody *et al.* (1997b); reviewed in Driscoll *et al.* (1997); Kane *et al.* (1997); Simeonova *et al.* (1997)

of fibres and persistent inflammation (Macdonald & Kane, 1997). In chronic inhalation studies in rats, fibre persistence is also correlated with induction of lung tumours (Hesterberg et al., 1996). These recent chronic inhalation studies include man-made fibres such as ceramic fibres that were previously classified as possibly carcinogenic to humans (Group 2B) (IARC, 1988).

These recent in-vitro and in-vivo studies provide consistent evidence that persistent, nondegradable fibres can trigger proliferation of target cells in the lungs and pleura of rodents. Three mechanisms have been proposed for the mitogenic effects of fibres: direct activation of growth factors or their receptors followed by triggering of intracellular signalling pathways and induction of proto-oncogene expression; compensatory cell proliferation in response to apoptosis or necrosis; and indirect stimulation of cell proliferation by cytokines and growth factors released from inflammatory cells. It is likely that several mechanisms contribute to the proliferative effects of fibres, although it is uncertain to what extent each of these mechanisms may become activated under conditions of low-dose, chronic exposure in humans (reviewed in Kane et al., 1996).

Mineral fibres have been shown to catalyse the formation of reactive oxygen species (ROS) and reactive nitrogen species (RNS) in cell-free models and in-vitro cell cultures (reviewed in Fubini, 1996). Ex-vivo studies have confirmed generation of RNS by rat alveolar macrophages after inhalation of asbestos fibres (Quinlan et al., 1998). Fibres may catalyse the generation of oxidants directly from molecular oxygen, or indirectly from ROS and RNS generated by inflammatory cells in the lungs or mesothelial lining. Some of the genotoxic, mitogenic and cytotoxic activities of asbestos fibres have been shown to be mediated by oxidants generated by target cells directly in the absence of inflammatory cells (Table 64). Surface reactivity and availability of iron to catalyse formation of hydroxyl radicals are important determinants of the biological activity of fibres as assessed in in-vitro systems (Fubini, 1996; Park & Aust, 1998). In addition to asbestos and erionite fibres, man-made fibres including ceramic and silicon carbide can generate free radicals in cell-free assays. No data are available for graphite fibres (Fubini, 1996). Ceramic and silicon carbide fibres are carcinogenic when injected intraperitoneally or intrapleurally in rats (Pott et al., 1987; Johnson & Hahn, 1996); no data are available for graphite or carbon fibres. The surface reactivity can be modified by coating asbestos or man-made fibres with IgG, surfactant or lung lining fluid. Adsorption of these macromolecules to the surface of fibres can either enhance (Chao et al., 1996) or diminish their ability to stimulate oxidant generation (Brown et al., 1998). It is uncertain whether sufficient oxidant generation occurs *in vivo* to induce genotoxicity in target cells. Inhalation of asbestos fibres by rats induces antioxidant defences (Holley et al., 1992; Janssen et al., 1992); in mesothelial cells *in vitro*, exposure to asbestos also induces expression and activity of a DNA repair enzyme and redox factor, apurinic/apyrimidinic (AP)-endonuclease or redox factor 1 (Fung et al., 1998). Changes in glutathione content of lung epithelial cells, alveolar macrophages and bronchoalveolar lavage fluid were variable after inhalation of asbestos or anhydrous gypsum by rats (Clouter et al., 1997). *In vitro*, asbestos exposure caused efflux of glutathione from human lung epithelial cells (Golladay et al., 1997). These conflicting data raise questions about the roles of oxidant stress and induction of antioxidant defences in the pathogenesis of lung tumours and malignant mesotheliomas induced by exposure to asbestos in humans. Polymorphisms of glutathione-*S*-transferases (GSTs) are frequent in human populations and the null phenotype has been reported to be associated with an increased risk of lung cancer and malignant mesothelioma following exposure to asbestos (Anttila et al., 1995).

The *p53* tumour-suppressor gene is an important regulator of apoptosis and induction of cell-cycle arrest and repair in response to DNA damage (reviewed in Kane, 1996a). Short-term inhalation of asbestos fibres in rats induced expression of p53 protein at sites of fibre deposition in the lungs (Mishra et al., 1997). This is the first evidence that exposure to asbestos may induce DNA damage in target cells of the lung after in-vivo exposure. Although point mutations or deletions of the *p53* gene are rare in human malignant mesotheliomas (reviewed in Lechner et al., 1997) or in rat mesotheliomas induced by direct intraperitoneal injection of asbestos fibres (Unfried et al., 1997), the p53 protein is frequently over-expressed in human malignant mesotheliomas (Mayall et al., 1992; Ramael et al., 1992). In some cases, SV40 T-antigen has been detected by immunohistochemistry (Testa et al., 1998). This viral oncoprotein has been reported to bind to p53 protein, prolong its half-life, and inhibit p53 functional activity (reviewed in Carbone et al., 1997). Whether SV40 virus can act as a co-factor with asbestos in the induction of malignant mesothelioma in humans is highly controversial (Galateau-Salle et al., 1998). SV40 virus has also been found in spontaneous human osteosarcomas, as well as in brain and pituitary tumours.

Crystalline silica

Workplace exposures to silicates and crystalline quartz are common (IARC, 1997a). Inhalation of silicate minerals (for example, pure talc, mica, kaolinite, wollastonite) that usually occur in sheets or platy forms causes a minimal fibrotic reaction in the lungs. Silicosis is characterized by irregular stellate lung scars composed of macrophages and multinucleated giant cells surrounding dust particles with mild chronic inflammation and deposition of collagen. In contrast, inhalation of crystalline silica can cause severe acute or chronic lung injury. Inhalation of freshly-fractured quartz is especially hazardous, resulting in extensive lung epithelial injury and accumulation of protein and lipid debris in the alveolar spaces. Acute silicosis or alveolar proteinosis is hypothesized to be mediated by free radicals generated at the surfaces of freshly-fractured quartz (Vallyathan et al., 1995). Chronic exposure to crystalline silica causes a characteristic fibrotic lesion, predominantly in the upper lobes of the lungs. Silicotic nodules are firm, round lesions with a central core of dense collagen surrounded by inflammatory cells and fibroblasts. This lesion is diagnostic of chronic or nodular silicosis. These nodules may enlarge and coalesce with formation of cavities; this is characteristic of progressive massive fibrosis. In contrast to workers exposed to asbestos fibres or silicates, occupational exposure to crystalline silica greatly increases the risk of superimposed infection with *Mycobacterium tuberculosis* or fungi. The mechanisms responsible for formation of these nodular lesions are unknown; chronic release of cytokines such as tumour necrosis factor (TNF)-α is postulated to play a role (Piguet & Vesin, 1994). An imbalance between pro-inflammatory and anti-inflammatory cytokines has also been proposed to perpetuate the pulmonary fibrotic reaction and compromise lung defences against mycobacteria and fungi (reviewed in Kane, 1996b; Huaux et al., 1998).

Most silicates have been categorized by IARC as unclassifiable as to carcinogenicity to humans (Group 3). In contrast, inhaled crystalline silica (in the form of quartz or cristobalite from occupational sources) has been classified in Group 1 (carcinogenic to humans) (IARC, 1997a). The mechanisms responsible for induction of lung cancer under some conditions of occupational exposure to crystalline silica are unknown. It has been hypothesized that these are scar cancers associated with fibrosis, although the anatomical location and histopathological characteristics of nodular silicosis are quite distinct from diffuse interstitial pulmonary fibrosis or asbestosis. As with asbestos fibres, a role for ROS generated at the surfaces of crystalline silica has been proposed (reviewed in Vallyathan & Shi, 1997). Finally, an indirect mechanism for induction of lung cancer by crystalline silica has been proposed (Figure 2). This indirect mechanism is supported by chronic inhalation studies in rats that show a correlation between high lung burdens of particles, persistent inflammation, epithelial proliferation, fibrosis and late development of lung cancer. Oxidative stress has been proposed to increase expression of proinflammatory cytokines in the lungs of rats exposed to particulates. As with asbestos fibres, particulate-induced oxidant stress activates the NF-κB transcription factor that increases expression of cytokines such as TNF-α and chemokines, including macrophage inflammatory protein (MIP)-2 and IL-8. Persistent activation and recruitment of inflammatory cells into the lungs after chronic exposure to particulates trigger the chronic release of growth factors for epithelial cells and ROS and RNS that are genotoxic. The genotoxic effects of ROS released from neutrophils collected after in-vivo exposure to α-quartz has been documented (Driscoll et al., 1997). Chronic exposure of rats to crystalline silica elicits an influx of neutrophils into the lungs (30–50% of cells collected by bronchoalveolar lavage) compared with approximately 5% of neutrophils in bronchoalveolar lavage fluids obtained from human silicotics (IARC, 1997a). Therefore, it is uncertain whether this indirect inflammatory mechanism contributes to the increased incidence of lung cancer observed in some cohorts of workers exposed to crystalline silica.

Recent molecular studies of *p53* tumour-suppressor gene mutations and p53 protein expression in the lungs of patients with lung cancer and occupational exposure to crystalline silica and other dusts have been conducted. Mutations in the *p53* gene were detected at a frequency similar to those in smoking-related lung cancers (Husgafvel-Pursiainen et al., 1997). Expression of p53 protein can be detected by immunohistochemistry in preneoplastic epithelial lesions in the lungs of smokers. In patients with

Figure 2. Proposed mechanism for induction of lung cancer by nongenotoxic particulates[a]

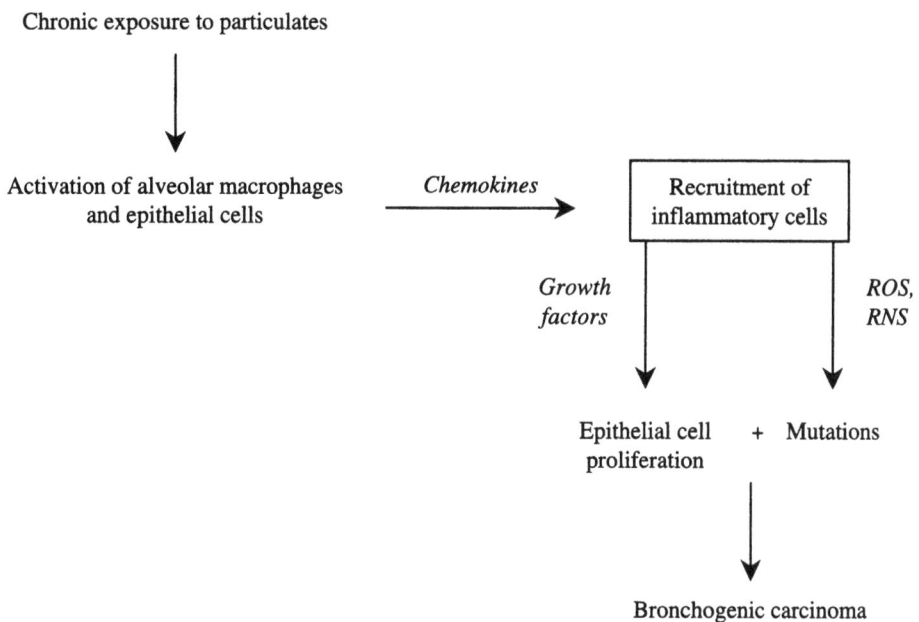

[a] Modified from Oberdörster (1997)
ROS, reactive oxygen species
RNS, reactive nitrogen species

radiographic evidence of pneumoconiosis including silicosis, p53 protein expression was more widespread in bronchiolar dysplasias than in patients without pneumoconiosis (Katabami et al., 1998). Most of the patients in both of these studies were current or former smokers. Similarly to the molecular studies in asbestos workers with lung cancer, no genetic lesion specifically associated with exposure to crystalline silica has been identified in human lung cancers.

Poorly-soluble particulates (PSPs) or low-toxicity dusts

Low-toxicity dusts such as carbon black, coal dust and titanium dioxide have been shown to induce lung tumours when administered at high doses in rats, but not in mice or hamsters. An indirect inflammatory mechanism has been proposed for induction of lung tumours by PSPs in rats (Figure 2). In contrast to crystalline silica, very high exposures to these particulates are required to induce lung tumours in rats. It is hypothesized that these high doses overwhelm lung clearance mechanisms and antioxidant defences, resulting in persistent inflammation and oxidant stress (Morrow et al., 1996; Driscoll et al., 1997; Warheit et al., 1997). The reasons for the species differences in induction of lung tumours by PSPs are unknown. Several mechanisms have been proposed: diminished antioxidant defences, decreased adaptive responses, increased expression of pro-inflammatory cytokines and chemokines, decreased expression of anti-inflammatory cytokines, altered DNA repair mechanisms (reviewed in Oberdörster, 1997) and differences in generation of nitric oxide by alveolar macrophages (Jesch et al., 1997). The relevance of the rat inhalation model to assessment of the risk of PSPs in humans is controversial and was recently reviewed (ILSI Risk Science Institute Workshop Consensus Report, 2000). Coal dust and amorphous silica are not classifiable as to their carcinogenicity to humans (IARC, 1997a,d). Coal miners with prolonged exposure to bituminous coal develop stellate aggregates of dust macules in the centriacinar regions of the lungs with little inflammation or fibrosis. Under heavy exposures, these macules may coalesce into larger lesions called complicated coal workers' pneumoconiosis. Even these workers do not show an increased incidence of lung cancer (ILSI Risk Science Institute Workshop Consensus Report, 2000).

The tumours that develop in rats exposed to carbon black rarely show mutations in the K-*ras* oncogene or *p53* tumour-suppressor gene (Swafford et al., 1995). In contrast, human lung cancers show frequent mutations in K-*ras* and *p53* that are consistent with the genetic spectrum of chemical carcinogens present in cigarette smoke (reviewed in Perera, 1996).

Relevance of these mechanisms for evaluation of the carcinogenicity of surgical implants and prosthetic devices

Many of the materials that have been associated with solid-state carcinogenesis have been fabricated into surgical implants and prosthetic devices. In the experimental model of foreign-body carcinogenesis in rats and mice (Brand, 1982), non-metallic implants with smooth, continuous surfaces induce subcutaneous or intraperitoneal sarcomas. The mechanisms responsible for the induction of foreign-body tumours in this model are speculative and the biochemical and molecular events leading to the development of these tumours have not been identified. When similar materials are implanted subcutaneously or intraperitoneally in particulate form, they stimulate variable degrees of acute inflammation and fibrosis depending on the anatomical site and species. No tumours have been induced by these particulate non-metallic materials (Rigdon, 1975). Any analogy between foreign-body carcinogenesis in rats and mice and carcinogenicity of surgical implants and prosthetic devices in humans is limited by the following considerations. First, smooth films implanted subcutaneously or intraperitoneally in rodents induce sarcomas by an unknown mechanism. Isolated cases of sarcomas induced by surgical implants and prosthetic devices in humans have been reported; however, these have not provided any mechanistic information. Second, inflammatory and fibrotic reactions to foreign materials are common in experimental animals and humans. Despite the well-documented associations between chronic inflammatory conditions and carcinomas in humans (Table 65), it is uncertain whether this mechanism can be extrapolated to sarcomas induced by surgical implants and prosthetic devices. Human cancers associated with chronic inflammation are usually carcinomas (rather than sarcomas) that

Table 65. Some chronic inflammatory conditions that have been associated with cancer in humans[a]

Predisposing condition	Cancer
Chronic hepatitis[b]	Hepatocellular carcinoma
Chronic cystitis[c]	Bladder carcinoma
Ulcerative colitis	Colon carcinoma
Helicobacter pylori gastritis[d]	Gastric carcinoma and lymphoma
Chronic osteomyelitis	Cutaneous squamous-cell carcinoma
Chronic pancreatitis	Pancreatic cancer

[a] Reviewed in Brand (1982, 1987)
[b] Hagen *et al*. (1994), IARC (1994c)
[c] Kawai *et al*. (1993)
[d] IARC (1994d); Mannick *et al*. (1996)

develop at sites of repeated episodes of cell necrosis or apoptosis, followed by epithelial regeneration (for example, hepatocellular carcinoma associated with persistent viral infection, as discussed by Nakamoto *et al*., 1998). In these predisposing conditions, inflammation accompanied by local release of cytokines and oxidants is postulated to contribute to genotoxicity in proliferating epithelial cell populations (Kawai *et al*., 1993; Hagen *et al*., 1994; Mannick *et al*., 1996). In the examples of chronic inflammation associated with persistent viral infection (Nakamoto *et al*., 1998), bacterial infection (Mannick *et al*., 1996) or parasitic infestation (Brand, 1982), host immune defence mechanisms amplify tissue injury by inducing apoptosis of epithelial cells and exacerbating cytokine release. Nitric oxide has been proposed as an important mediator of chronic inflammation and DNA damage under these conditions; however, it may also be tumoricidal (Wink *et al*., 1998).

Asbestos fibres are established human carcinogens that cause lung cancer and malignant mesothelioma in humans and rodents (IARC, 1977, 1987a). Despite numerous experimental studies *in vitro* and *in vivo*, the mechanisms responsible for the development of these cancers are unknown. Fibrous minerals such as asbestos appear to be especially effective in inducing malignant mesotheliomas after inhalation or direct intrapleural or intraperitoneal injection. High doses of non-metallic particulates do not cause mesotheliomas even when injected intraperitoneally in rats (Pott *et al*., 1987). Asbestos fibres show genotoxic and mitogenic activities in several in-vitro systems; some of these activities have been confirmed in in-vivo models. However, a major limitation of all of these models is the use of high-dose exposures to produce tumours. It is uncertain whether the same mechanisms operate under conditions of chronic, low-dose inhalation exposure in humans. Lung carcinomas and malignant mesotheliomas are produced after inhalation of fibres; therefore, it is unwarranted to predict whether similar materials in fibrous form or incorporated into composites would be carcinogenic when implanted at other anatomical sites (Rigdon, 1975).

Correlations between persistence of fibres or particulates in the lungs, inflammation and fibrosis have been made in several model systems, especially in the rat. While these studies show consistent temporal associations, there has been no rigorous proof of a causal relationship between these parameters and the development of lung cancer (Kane *et al.*, 1996). Rats appear to be extremely susceptible to induction of lung cancer by PSPs; extrapolation of this response to humans exposed to similar materials by inhalation must be done cautiously (ILSI Risk Science Institute Workshop Consensus Report, 2000). It would be premature to apply the proposed mechanism for the induction of rat lung tumours by PSPs to the evaluation of carcinogenicity of similar materials implanted at other anatomical sites in humans.

REFERENCES

Aboulafia, A.J., Littelton, K., Shmookler, B. & Malawer, M.M. (1994) Malignant fibrous histiocytoma at the site of hip replacement in association with chronic infection. *Orthop. Rev.*, **23**, 427–432

AEPI (1995) *Health and Environmental Consequences of Depleted Uranium Use in the US Army: Technical Report*, Atlanta, GA, United States Army Environmental Policy Institute

Agency for Toxic Substances and Disease Registry (1988) *Toxicological Profile for Lead*, Atlanta, GA, United States Department of Health and Human Services

Agency for Toxic Substances and Disease Registry (1998) *Toxicological Profile for Uranium*, Atlanta, GA, United States Department of Health and Human Services

Agins, H.J., Alcock, N.W., Bansal, M., Salvati, E.A., Wilson, P.D., Pellicci, P.M. & Bullough, P.G. (1988) Metallic wear in failed titanium-alloy total hip replacements. *J. Bone Joint Surg.*, **70A**, 347–356

Alban, L.E. (1981) Metal surface treatments (case hardening). In: Mark, H.F., Othmer, D.F., Overberger, C.G. & Seaborg, G.T., eds, *Kirk-Othmer Encyclopedia of Chemical Technology*, Vol. 15, 3rd Ed., New York, John Wiley, pp. 313–324

Al-Dawood, A. & Wennberg, A. (1993) Biocompatibility of dentin bonding agents. *Endod. dent. Traumatol.*, **9**, 1–7

Amin, P., Wille, J., Shah, K. & Kydonieus, A. (1993) Analysis of the extractive and hydrolytic behaviour of microthane poly(ester-urethane) foam by high pressure liquid chromatography. *J. biomed. Mater. Res.*, **27**, 655–666

Andreopoulos, A.G. & Evangelatou, M. (1994) Evaluation of various reinforcements for maxillofacial silicone elastomers. *J. Biomater. Appl.*, **8**, 344–360

Angervall, L., Kindblom, L.-G. & Merck, C. (1977) Myxofibrosarcoma. A study of 30 cases. *Acta pathol. microbiol. scand., Sect. A*, **85**, 127–140

Anon. (1992) Summary of the report on silicone-gel-filled breast implants. *Can. med. Assoc. J.*, **147**, 1127

Anttila, S., Luostarinen, L., Hirvonen, A., Elovaara, E., Karjalainen, A., Nurminen, T., Hayes, J.D., Vainio, H. & Ketterer, B. (1995) Pulmonary expression of glutathione S-transferase M3 in lung cancer patients: association with GSTM1 polymorphism, smoking, and asbestos exposure. *Cancer Res.*, **55**, 3305–3309

Anusavice, K.J. (1996) *Phillips' Science of Dental Materials*, 10th Ed., Philadelphia, W.B. Saunders

Arden, G.P. & Bywaters, E.G.L. (1978) Tissue reaction. In: Arden, G.P. & Ansell, B.M., eds, *Surgical Management of Juvenile Chronic Polyarthritis*, London, Academic Press, pp. 257–275

Argani, P., Ghossein, R. & Rosai, J. (1998) Anthracotic and anthracosilicotic spindle cell pseudotumors of mediastinal lymph nodes: report of five cases of a reactive lesion that simulates malignancy. *Hum. Pathol.*, **29**, 851–855

Aronoff, M.S. (1995) Market study: biomaterials supply for permanent medical implants. *J. biomater. Appl.*, **9**, 205–261

Ashammakhi, N. & Rokkanen, P. (1997) Absorbable polyglycolide devices in trauma and bone surgery. *Biomaterials*, **18**, 3–9

Assad, M., Yahia, L.H., Rivard, C.H. & Lemieux, N. (1998) *In vitro* biocompatibility assessment of a nickel–titanium alloy using electron microscopy in situ end-labeling (EM-ISEL). *J. biomed. Mater. Res.*, **41**, 154–161

ASTM (1998) F 748 Standard practice for selecting generic biological test methods for materials and devices. In: *ASTM Annual Book of Standards*, Vol. 13.01, Medical devices and services, Philadelphia, American Society for Testing and Materials, pp. 193–197

Athanasiou, K.A., Niederauer, G.G., Agrawal, C.M. & Landsman, A.S. (1995) Applications of biodegradable lactides and glycolides in podiatry. *Clin. podiat. Med. Surg.*, **12**, 475–495

Atkinson, A. & Roy, D. (1995) In vivo DNA adduct formation by bisphenol A. *Environ. mol. Mutagen.*, **26**, 60–66

Autian, J., Singh, A.R., Turner, J.E., Hung, G.W., Nunez, L.J. & Lawrence, W.H. (1975) Carcinogenesis from polyurethanes. *Cancer Res.*, **35**, 1591–1596

Autian, J., Singh, A.R., Turner, J.E., Hung, G.W., Nunez, L.J. & Lawrence, W.H. (1976) Carcinogenic activity of a chlorinated polyether polyurethan. *Cancer Res.*, **36**, 3973–3977

Bagó-Granell, J., Aguirre-Canyadell, M., Nardi, J. & Tallada, N. (1984) Malignant fibrous histiocytoma of bone at the site of a total hip arthroplasty. A case report. *J. Bone Joint Surg.*, **66B**, 38–40

Baker, S., Brooks, S.C. & Walker, D.M. (1988) The release of residual monomeric methyl methacrylate from acrylic appliances in the human mouth: an assay for monomer in saliva. *J. dent. Res.*, **67**, 1295–1299

Banks, W.C., Morris, E., Herron, M.R. & Green, R.W. (1975) Osteogenic sarcoma associated with internal fracture fixation in two dogs. *J. Am. vet. med. Assoc.*, **167**, 166–167

Bardos, D.I. (1979) High strength Co-Cr-Mo alloy by hot isostatic pressing of powder. *Biomater. Med. Devices artif. Organs*, **7**, 73–80

Barnett F (1992) Pulpal response to restorative procedures and materials. *Curr. Opin. Dent.*, **2**, 93–98

Barry, M., Thomas, S.M., Rees, A., Shafighian, B & Mowbray, M.A. (1995) Histological changes associated with an artificial anterior cruciate ligament. *J. clin. Pathol.*, **48**, 556–559

Bartels, M.J., Timchalk, C. & Smith, F.A. (1993) Gas chromatographic/tandem mass spectrometric identification and quantification of metabolic 4-acetyltoluene-2,4-diamine from the F344 rat. *Biol. mass Spectrom.*, **22**, 194–200

Bates, B.R. & Klein, M. (1966) Importance of a smooth surface in carcinogenesis by plastic film. *J. natl Cancer Inst.*, **37**, 145–151

Bauer, K. & Frey, R. (1955) *Geschwulst und Trauma. Handbuch der gesamten Unfallheilkunde*, Stuttgart, S. Hirzel Verlag

Bayne, S.C. (1992) Dental composites/glass ionomers: clinical reports. *Adv. dent. Res.*, **6**, 65–77

Bechtol, C.O., Ferguson, A.B., Jr & Laing, P.G. (1959) *Metals and Engineering in Bone and Joint Surgery*, Baltimore, Williams & Wilkins

Beck, G., Beyer, H.-H., Gerhartz, W., Hanßelt, J. & Zimmer, U. (1995) *Edelmetall-Taschenbuch*, Heidelberg, Hüthing-Verlag, pp. 58–59

Beekman, W.H., Feitz, R., van Diest, P.J. & Hage, J.J. (1997) Migration of silicone through the fibrous capsules of mammary prostheses. *Ann. plast. Surg.*, **38**, 441–445

Behling, C.A. & Spector, M. (1986) Quantitative characterization of cells at the interface of long-term implants of selected polymers. *J. biomed. Mater. Res.*, **20**, 653–666

Bell, R.S., Hopyan, S., Davis, A.M., Kandel, R. & Gross, A.E. (1997) Sarcoma of bone–cement membrane: a case report and review of the literature. *Can. J. Surg.*, **40**, 51–55

Bellón, J.M., Contreras, L.A., Buján, J., Palomares, D. & Carrera-San Martín, A. (1998) Tissue response to polypropylene meshes used in the repair of abdominal wall defects. *Biomaterials*, **19**, 669–675

Ben-Izhak, O., Kerner, H., Brenner, B. & Lichtig, C. (1992) Angiosarcoma of the colon developing in a capsule of a foreign body. Report of a case with associated hemorrhagic diathesis. *Am. J. clin. Pathol.*, **97**, 416–420

Bennett, D., Campbell, J.R. & Brown, P. (1979) Osteosarcoma associated with healed fractures. *J. small Anim. Pract.*, **20**, 13–18

Benoit, F.M. (1993) Degradation of polyurethane foams used in the Même breast implant. *J. biomed. Mater. Res.*, **27**, 1341–1348

Bering, E.A., Jr & Handler, A.H. (1957) The production of tumors in hamsters by implantation of polyethylene film. *Cancer*, **10**, 414–415

Bering, E.A. Jr, McLaurin, R.L., Lloyd, J.B. & Ingraham, F.D. (1955) The production of tumors in rats by the implantation of pure polyethylene. *Cancer Res.*, **15**, 300–301

Berkel, H., Birdsell, D.C. & Jenkins, H. (1992) Breast augmentation: a risk factor for breast cancer? *New Engl. J. Med.*, **326**, 1649–1653

Bernstein, K.E. & Lattes, R. (1982) Nodular (pseudosarcomatous) fasciitis, a nonrecurrent lesion: clinicopathologic study of 134 cases. *Cancer*, **49**, 1668–1678

Berry, J.P., Galle, P., Poupon, M.F., Pot-Deprun, J., Chouroulinkov, I., Judde, J.G. & Dewally, D. (1984) Electron microprobe in vitro study of interaction of carcinogenic nickel compounds with tumour cells. In: Sunderman, F.W., Jr, ed., *Nickel in the Human Environment* (IARC Scientific Publications No. 53), Lyon, IARC, pp. 153–164

BéruBé, K.A., Quinlan, T.R., Moulton, G., Hemenway, D., O'Shaughnessy, P., Vacek, P. & Mossman, B.T. (1996) Comparative proliferative and histopathologic changes in rat lungs after inhalation of chrysotile and crocidolite asbestos. *Toxicol. appl. Pharmacol.*, **137**, 67–74

Bhandarkar, D.S., Bewu, A.D.M. & Taylor, T.V. (1993) Carcinoma of the breast at the site of migrated pacemaker generators. *Postgrad. med. J.*, **69**, 883–885

Bigatti, M.P., Lamberti, L., Cannas, M. & Rossi, E. (1989) Lack of sister-chromatid exchange induction by polymethyl methacrylate bone cement in human lymphocytes cultured in vitro. *Mutat. Res.*, **227**, 21–24

Bigatti, M.P., Lamberti, L., Rizzi, F.P., Cannas, M. & Allasia, G. (1994) In vitro micronucleus induction by polymethyl methacrylate bone cement in cultured human lymphocytes. *Mutat. Res.*, **321**, 133–137

Billmeyer, F.W. (1989) Polymers. In: Grayson, M., Mark, H.F., Othmer, D.F. & Othmer, D.F. eds, *Kirk-Othmer Concise Encyclopedia of Chemical Technology*, Vol. 18, 3rd Ed., New York, John Wiley, p. 934

Bingham, H.G., Copeland, E.M., Hackett, R.R. & Caffee, H.H. (1988) Breast cancer in a patient with silicone breast implants after 13 years. *Ann. plast. Surg.*, **20**, 236–237

Biran, S., Keren, A., Farkas, T. & Stern, S. (1979) Development of carcinoma of the breast at the site of an implanted pacemaker in two patients. *J. surg. Oncol.*, **11**, 7–11

Birdsell, D.C., Jenkins, H. & Berkel, H. (1993) Breast cancer diagnosis and survival in women with and without breast implants. *Plast. reconstr. Surg.*, **92**, 795–800

Birnmeyer, G. (1963) The fate of metallic foreign bodies in the frontal sinus. *Laryng.-Rhinol.-Otol.*, **42**, 778–785 (in German)

Bischoff, F. & Bryson, G. (1964) Carcinogenesis through solid state surfaces. *Progr. Exp. Tumor Res.*, **5**, 85–133

Bischoff, F. & Bryson, G. (1977) Intraperitoneal foreign body reaction in rodents. *Res. Commun. chem. Pathol. Pharmacol.*, **18**, 201–214

Björk, V.O. (1985) The development of artificial heart valves: introduction and historical perspective. In: Morse, D., Steiner, R.M. & Fernandez, J., eds, *Guide to Prosthetic Cardiac Valves*, New York, Springer-Verlag, pp. 1–4

Black, J. (1992) Implant materials: properties. In: Black, J., ed., *Biological Performance of Materials, Fundamentals of Biocompatibility*, New York, Marcel Dekker, pp.110–122

Black, J. (1994) Biological performance of tantalum. *Clin. Mater.*, **16**, 167–173

Blackwell, G. & Käse, R. (1996) Technical characteristics of light curing glass-ionomers and compomers. *Dent. Mat.*, **12**, 77–88

Blake, J.M. (1943) Primary carcinoma of the bronchus associated with foreign body. *Am. Rev. Tuberc.*, **47**, 109–111

Blakely, H.W. (1952) Shrapnel, semantics and such. *Combat Forces. J.*, **March**

Bleiweiss, I.J. & Copeland, M. (1995) Capsular synovial metaplasia and breast implants. *Arch. Pathol. Lab. Med.*, **119**, 115–116

Blümlein, H. (1957) Malignant tumours after gunshot injury. *Arch. Ohren.-Nasen.-Kehlk. Heilk.*, **171**, 239–244 (in German)

Bolewska, J., Hansen, H.J., Holmstrup, P., Pindborg, J.J. & Stangerup, M. (1990a) Oral mucosal lesions related to silver amalgam restorations. *Oral Surg. Oral Med. Oral Pathol.*, **70**, 55–58

Bolewska, J., Holmstrup, P., Møller-Madsen, B., Kenrad, B., & Danscher, G. (1990b) Amalgam associated mercury accumulations in normal oral mucosa, oral mucosal lesions of lichen planus and contact lesions associated with amalgam. *J. Oral Pathol. Med.*, **19**, 39–42

Bonin, A.M., Arlauskas, A.P., Angus, D.S., Baker, R.S.U., Gallagher, C.H., Greenoak, G., Lane Brown, M.M., Meher-Homji, K.M. & Reeve, V. (1982) UV-absorbing and other sun-protecting substances: genotoxicity of 2-ethylhexyl *p*-methoxycinnamate. *Mutat. Res.*, **105**, 303–308

Boone, C.W., Takeichi, N., Eaton, S.D.A. & Paranjpe, M. (1979) 'Spontaneous' neoplastic transformation *in vitro*: a form of foreign body (smooth surface) tumorigenesis. *Science*, **204**, 177–179

Borg, E.L. (1979) Ethylene-propylene. In: Mark, H.F., Othmer, D.F., Overberger, C.G. & Seaborg, G.T., eds, *Kirk-Othmer Encyclopedia of Chemical Technology*, Vol. 8, 3rd Ed., New York, John Wiley, pp. 492–500

Borgmeijer, P.J., Kreulen, C.M., van Amerongen, W.E., Akerboom, H.B.M. & Gruythuysen, R.J.M. (1991) The prevalence of postoperative sensitivity in teeth restored with Class II composite resin restorations. *J. Dent. Child.*, **58**, 378–383

Bouchard, P.R., Black, J., Albrecht, B.A., Kaderly, R.E., Galante, J.O. & Pauli, B.U. (1996) Carcinogenicity of CoCrMo (F-75) implants in the rat. *J. biomed. Mater. Res.*, **32**, 37–44

Bouillaguet, S., Virgillito, M., Wataha, J., Ciucchi, B. & Holz, J. (1998) The influence of dentine permeability on cytotoxicity of four dentine bonding systems, *in vitro*. *J. oral Rehabilitation*, **25**, 45–51

Boutin, C., Dumortier, P., Rey, F., Viallat, J.R. & De Vuyst, P. (1996) Black spots concentrate oncogenic asbestos fibers in the parietal pleura. *Am. J. resp. crit. Care Med.*, **153**, 444–449

Bowers, D.G., Jr & Radlauer, C.B. (1969) Breast cancer after prophylactic subcutaneous mastectomies and reconstruction with silastic prostheses. *Plast. reconstr. Surg.*, **44**, 541–544

Boylan, A.M., Ruegg, C., Kim, K.J., Hebert, C.A., Hoeffel, J.M., Pytela, R., Sheppard, P., Goldstein, I.M. & Broaddus, V.C. (1992) Evidence of a role for mesothelial cell-derived interleukin-8 in the pathogenesis of asbestos-induced pleurisy in rabbits. *J. clin. Invest.*, **89**, 1257–1267

Boylan, A.M., Sanan, D.A., Sheppard, D. & Broaddus, V.C. (1995) Vitronectin enhances internalization of crocidolite asbestos by rabbit pleural mesothelial cells via the integrin $\alpha v \beta 5$. *J. clin. Invest.*, **96**, 1987–2001

Bradley, S.G., Munson, A.E., McCay, J.A., Brown, R.D., Musgrove, D.L., Wilson, S., Stern, M., Luster, M.I. & White, K.L., Jr (1994a) Subchronic 10 day immunotoxicity of polydimethylsiloxane (silicone) fluid, gel and elastomer and polyurethane disks in female B6C3F1 mice. *Drug chem. Toxicol.*, **17**, 175–220

Bradley, S.G., White, K.L., Jr, McCay, J.A., Brown, R.D., Musgrove, D.L., Wilson, S., Stern, M., Luster, M.I. & Munson, A.E. (1994b) Immunotoxicity of 180 day exposure to polydimethylsiloxane (silicone) fluid, gel and elastomer and polyurethane disks in female B6C3F1 mice. *Drug chem. Toxicol.*, **17**, 221–269

Branchaud, R.M., Garant, L.J. & Kane, A.B. (1993) Pathogenesis of mesothelial reactions to asbestos fibers. Monocyte recruitment and macrophage activation. *Pathobiology*, **61**, 154–163

Brand, K.G. (1976) Diversity and complexity of carcinogenic processes: conceptual inferences from foreign-body tumorigenesis. *J. natl Cancer. Inst.*, **57**, 973–976

Brand, K.G. (1982) Cancer associated with asbestosis, schistosomiasis, foreign bodies, and scars. In: Becker, F.F., ed., *Cancer: A Comprehensive Treatise*, 2nd Ed., New York, Plenum Press, pp. 661–692

Brand, K.G. (1987) Solid state carcinogenesis. In: Butterworth, B.E. & Slaga, T.J., eds, *Nongenotoxic Mechanisms in Carcinogenesis* (Banbury Report 25), Cold Spring Harbor, CSH Press, pp. 205–213

Brand, K.G. (1994) Do implanted medical devices cause cancer? *J. biomater. Appl.*, **8**, 325–343

Brand, K.G., Buoen, L.C. & Brand, I. (1967a) Carcinogenesis from polymer implants: new aspects from chromosomal and transplantation studies during premalignancy. *J. natl Cancer Inst.*, **39**, 663–679

Brand, K.G., Buoen, L.C. & Brand, I. (1967b) Premalignant cells in tumorigenesis induced by plastic film. *Nature*, **213**, 810

Brand, K.G., Buoen, L.C. & Brand, I. (1971) Foreign body tumorigenesis: timing and location of preneoplastic events. *J. natl Cancer Inst.*, **47**, 829–836

Brand, K.G., Buoen, L.C. & Brand, I. (1973) Foreign-body tumorigenesis in mice: most probable number of originator cells, *J. natl Cancer Inst.*, **51**, 1071–1074

Brand, K.G., Buoen, L.C., Johnson, K.H. & Brand, I. (1975a) Etiological factors, stages, and the role of the foreign body in foreign body tumorigenesis: a review. *Cancer Res.*, **35**, 279–286

Brand, K.G., Buoen, L.C. & Brand, I. (1975b) Foreign-body tumorigenesis induced by glass and smooth and rough plastic; comparative study of preneoplastic events. *J. natl Cancer Inst.*, **55**, 319–322

Brand, K.G., Buoen, L.C. & Brand, I. (1975c) Foreign-body tumorigenesis by vinyl chloride vinyl acetate copolymer: no evidence for chemical cocarcinogenesis. *J. natl Cancer Inst.*, **54**, 1259–1262

Brand, I., Buoen, L.C. & Brand, K.G. (1977) Foreign-body tumors of mice: strain and sex differences in latency and incidence. *J. natl Cancer Inst.*, **58**, 1443–1447

Brånemark, P.I. (1983) Osseointegration and first experimental background. *J. prosth. Dent.*, **3**, 399–410

Bratel, J., Hakeberg, M. & Jontell, M. (1996) Effect of replacement of dental amalgam on oral lichenoid reactions. *J. Dent.*, **24**, 41–45

Brick, R.M., Pense, A.W. & Gordon, R.B. (1977) *Structure and Properties of Engineering Materials*, New York, McGraw-Hill, pp. 234–241, 337–343, 386–391

Brien, W.W., Salvati, E.A., Healey, J.H., Bansal, M., Ghelman, B. & Betts, F. (1990) Osteogenic sarcoma arising in the area of a total hip replacement. A case report. *J. Bone Joint Surg.*, **72A**, 1097–1099

Brinton, L.A. & Brown, S.L. (1997) Breast implants and cancer. *J. natl Cancer Inst.*, **89**, 1341–1349

Brinton, L.A., Malone, K.E., Coates, R.J., Schoenberg, J.B., Swanson, C.A., Daling, J.R. & Stanford, J.L. (1996) Breast enlargement and reduction: results from a breast cancer case-control study. *Plast. reconstr. Surg.*, **97**, 269–275

Briscoe, C.M., Lipscomb, T.P. & McKinney, L. (1998) Pulmonary metastasis of a feline vaccination site fibrosarcoma. *J. vet. Diagn. Invest.*, **10**, 79–82

Broaddus, V.C., Yang, L., Scavo, L.M., Ernst, J.D. & Boylan, A.M. (1996) Asbestos induces apoptosis of human and rabbit pleural mesothelial cells via reactive oxygen species. *J. clin. Invest.*, **98**, 2050–2059

Brody, R.I., Ueda, T., Hamelin, A., Jhanwar, S.C., Bridge, J.A., Healey, J.H., Huvos, A.G., Gerald, W.L. & Ladanyi, M. (1997a) Molecular analysis of the fusion of *EWS* to an orphan nuclear receptor gene in extraskeletal myxoid chondrosarcoma. *Am. J. Pathol.*, **150**, 1049–1058

Brody, A.R., Liu, J.-Y. Brass, D. & Corti, M. (1997b) Analyzing the genes and peptide growth factors expressed in lung cells *in vivo* consequent to asbestos exposure and *in vitro*. *Environ. Health Perspect.*, **105** (Suppl. 5), 1165–1171

Brorson, T., Skarping, G. & Sango, C. (1991) Biological monitoring of isocyanates and related amines. IV. 2,4- and 2,6-Toluenediamine in hydrolysed plasma and urine after test-chamber exposure of humans to 2,4- and 2,6-toluene diisocyanate. *Int. Arch. occup. environ. Health*, **63**, 253–259

Brown, S.A. & Lemons, J.E. (1996) Overview. In: Brown, S.A. & Lemons, J.E., eds, *Medical Applications of Titanium and its Alloys: The Material and Biological Issues*, STP 1272, West Conshohocken, PA, Association of Standard Testing Materials, pp. ix–xii

Brown, S.A., Farnsworth, L.J., Merritt, K. & Crowe, T.D. (1988) In vitro and in vivo metal ion release. *J. biomed. Mater. Res.*, **22**, 321–338

Brown, S.A., Zhang, K., Merritt, K. & Payer, J.H. (1993) In vivo transport and excretion of corrosion products from accelerated anodic corrosion of porous coated F75 alloy. *J. biomed. Mater. Res.*, **27**, 1007–1017

Brown, D.M., Roberts, N.K. & Donaldson, K. (1998) Effect of coating with lung lining fluid on the ability of fibres to produce a respiratory burst in rat alveolar macrophages. *Toxicol. In Vitro*, **12**, 15–24

Brunnberg, V.L., Gunsser, I. & Hänichen, T. (1980) Bone tumours in dogs after trauma and osteosynthesis. *Kleintier Prax.*, **25**, 143–152 (in German)

Brunner, H. (1959) Experimental formation of tumours by implantation of polymethyl methacrylate in rats. *Arzneim. Forsch.*, **9**, 396–399 (in German)

Bryant, H. & Brasher, P. (1995) Breast implants and breast cancer—reanalysis of a linkage study. *New Engl. J. Med.*, **332**, 1535–1539

Bryant, H., Brasher, P., van de Sande, J.H. & Turc, J.M. (1994) Review of methods in 'breast augmentation: a risk factor for breast cancer?' (Letter to the Editor) *New Engl. J. Med.*, **330**, 293

Brydson, J.A. (1979) *Plastics Materials*, 3rd Ed., London, Butterworths

Bryson, G. & Bischoff, F. (1969) The limitations of safety testing. *Prog. exp. Tumor Res.*, **11**, 100–133

Budunova, I.V. & Williams, G.M. (1994) Cell culture assays for chemicals with tumor-promoting or tumor-inhibiting activity based on the modulation of intercellular communication. *Cell Biol. Toxicol.*, **10**, 71–116

Buoen, L.C., Brand, I. & Brand, K.G. (1975) Foreign-body tumorigenesis: In vitro isolation and expansion of preneoplastic clonal cell populations. *J. natl Cancer Inst.*, **55**, 721–723

Bürkle de la Camp, H. (1958) Failure and hazards of alloplastics in bones and joint surgery. *Langenbecks Arch. Klin.*, **289**, 463–475 (in German)

Burns, W.A., Kanhouwa, S., Tillman, L., Saini, N. & Herrmann, J.B. (1972) Fibrosarcoma occurring at the site of a plastic vascular graft. *Cancer*, **29**, 66–72

Burns, J.W., Colt, M.J., Burgess, L.S. & Skinner, K.C. (1997) Preclinical evaluation of Seprafilm™ bioresorbable membrane. *Eur. J. Surg.*, **577**, 40–48

Burns-Naas, L.A., Mast, R.W., Meeks, R.G., Mann, P.C. & Thevenaz, P. (1998) Inhalation toxicology of decamethylcyclopentasiloxane (D5) following a 3-month nose-only exposure in Fischer 344 rats. *Toxicol. Sci.*, **43**, 230–240

Butterworth, B.E., Popp, J.A., Conolly, R.B. & Goldsworthy, T.L. (1992) Chemically induced cell proliferation in carcinogenesis. In: Vainio, H., Magee, P., McGregor, D. & McMichael, A.J., eds, *Mechanism of Carcinogenesis in Risk Identification* (IARC Scientific Publications No.116), Lyon, IARC, pp. 279–305

Button, M. (1979) Epitheloid sarcoma: A case report. *J. Hand Surg.*, **4**, 368–371

Cameron, T. (1993) *Short-Term Test Program Sponsored by the Division of Cancer Etiology, National Cancer Institute*, Bethesda, MD, National Cancer Institute

Camps, J., Tardieu, C., Déjou, J., Franquin, J.C., Ladaique, P. & Rieu, R. (1997) In vitro cytotoxicity of dental adhesive systems under simulated pulpal pressure. *Dent. Mater.*, **13**, 34–42

Can, Z., Yilmaz, S., Riza, A., Apaydin, E.I. & Kuzu, I. (1998) Sarcoma developing in a burn scar: case report and review of the literature. *Burns*, **24**, 68–71

Carbone, M., Rizzo, P. & Pass, H.I. (1997) Simian virus 40, polio vaccines and human tumors: a review of recent developments. *Oncogene*, **15**, 1889–1894

Carrillo, T., Cuevas, M., Munoz, T., Hinjosa, M. & Moneo, L. (1986) Contact urticaria and rhinitis from latex surgical gloves. *Contact Derm.*, **15**, 69–72

Carter, R.L. & Roe, F.J. (1969) Induction of sarcomas in rats by solid and fragmented polyethylene: experimental observations and clinical implications. *Br. J. Cancer*, **23**, 401–407

Carter, R.L., Roe, F.J. & Peto, R. (1971) Tumor induction by plastic films: attempt to correlate carcinogenic activity with certain physicochemical properties of the implant. *J. natl Cancer Inst.*, **46**, 1277–1289

Case, C.P., Langkamer, V.G., Howell, R.T., Webb, J., Standen, G., Palmer, M., Kemp, A. & Learmonth, I.D. (1996) Preliminary observations on possible premalignant changes in bone marrow adjacent to worn total hip arthroplasty implants. *Clin. Orthop. rel. Res.*, **329** (Suppl.), S269–S279

Castleman, B. & McNeely, B.U. (1965) Case records of the Massachusetts General Hospital. Weekly clinicopathological exercises. Case 38-1965. Presentation of case. *New Engl. J. Med.*, **273**, 494–504

Caughman, W.F., Caughman, G.B., Shiflett, R.A., Rueggeberg, F. & Schuster, G.S. (1991) Correlation of cytotoxicity, filler loading and curing time of dental composites. *Biomaterials*, **12**, 737–740

Cesarman, E. & Knowles, D.M. (1997) Kaposi's sarcoma-associated herpesvirus: a lymphotropic human herpesvirus associated with Kaposi's sarcoma, primary effusion lymphoma, and multicentric Castleman's disease. *Semin. diagn. Pathol.*, **14**, 54–66

Chan, J.C.K. (1996) Inflammatory pseudotumor: a family of lesions of diverse nature and etiologies. *Adv. anat. Pathol.*, **3**, 156–171

Chan, J.C.K. (1997) Proliferative lesions of follicular dentric cells an overview including a detailed account of follicular dentritic cell sarcoma a neoplasms with many faces and uncommon etiologic associations. *Adv. anat. Pathol.*, **4**, 387–411

Chan, S.C., Birdsell, D.C. & Gradeen, C.Y. (1991a) Detection of toluenediamines in the urine of a patient with polyurethane-covered breast implants. *Clin. Chem.*, **37**, 756–758

Chan, S.C., Birdsell, D.C. & Gradeen C.Y. (1991b) Urinary excretion of free toluenediamines in a patient with polyurethane-covered breast implants *Clin. Chem.*, **37**, 2143–2145

Chang, Y.-H. (1993) Adjuvanticity and arthritogenicity of silicone. *Plast. reconstr. Surg.*, **92**, 469–473

Chao, C.-C., Park, S.-H. & Aust, A.E. (1996) Participation of nitric oxide and iron in the oxidation of DNA in asbestos-treated human lung cells. *Arch. Biochem. Biophys.*, **326**, 152–157

Charnley, J. (1970) The reaction of bone to self-curing acrylic cement. A long-term histological study in man. *J. Bone Joint Surg.*, **52B**, 340–353

Charnley, J. & Cupic, Z. (1973) The nine and ten year results of the low-friction arthroplasty of the hip. *Clin. Orthop.*, **95**, 9–25

Charosky, C.B., Bullough, P.G. & Wilson, P.D., Jr (1973) Total hip replacement failures. A histological evaluation. *J. Bone Joint Surg.*, **55A**, 49–58

Chivers, C.P. (1972) Two cases of occupational leucoderma following contact with hydroquinone monomethyl ether. *Br. J. ind. Med.*, **29**, 105–107

Chung, E.B. & Enzinger, F.M. (1975) Proliferative fasciitis. *Cancer*, **36**, 1450–1458

Chung, E.B. & Enzinger, F.M. (1983) Malignant melanoma of soft parts. A reassessment of clear cell sarcoma. *Am. J. surg. Pathol.*, **7**, 405–413

Clayton, G.D. & Clayton. F.E., eds (1993) *Patty's Industrial Hygiene and Toxicology*, II Part A, Toxicology, New York, John Wiley, pp. 485–486

Clouter, A., Houghton, C.E., Bowskill, C.A., Hibbs, L.R., Brown, R.C. & Hoskins, J.A. (1997) Effect of inhaled fibers on the glutathione concentration and γ-glutamyl transpeptidase activity in lung type II epithelial cells, macrophages, and bronchoalveolar lavage fluid. *Inhal. Toxicol.*, **9**, 351–367

Cocke, W.M., Jr & Tomlinson, J.A. (1993) Malignant fibrous histiocytoma developing in burn scar of the ear. *Burns*, **19**, 241–243

Coffin, C.M., Watterson, J., Priest, J.R. & Dehner, L.P. (1995) Extrapulmonary inflammatory myofibroblastic tumor (inflammatory pseudotumor). A clinicopathologic and immunohistochemical study of 84 cases. *Am. J. surg. Pathol.*, **19**, 859–872

Coindre, J.M. (1993) Pathology and grading of soft tissue sarcomas. *Cancer Treat. Res.*, **67**, 1–22

Cole, B.J., Schultz, E., Smilari, T.F., Hajdu, S.I. & Krauss, E.S. (1997) Malignant fibrous histiocytoma at the site of a total hip replacement: review of the literature and case report. *Skel. Radiol.*, **26**, 559–563

Coleman, M.P. (1996) Cancer risk from orthopedic prostheses. *Ann. clin. Lab. Sci.*, **26**, 139–146

Collard, S.M., McDaniel, R.K. & Johnston, D.A. (1989) Particle size and composition of composite dusts. *Am. J. Dent.*, **2**, 247–253

Collard, S.M., Vogel, J.J. & Ladd, G.D. (1991) Respirability, microstructure and filler content of composite dusts. *Am. J. Dent.*, **4**, 143–151

Committee on Toxicity of Chemicals in Food Consumer Products and the Environment (1997) *Statement on the Toxicity of Dental Amalgam*, London, Department of Health

Cook, P.D., Osborne, B.M., Connor, R.L. & Strauss J.F. (1995) Follicular lymphoma adjacent to foreign body granulomatous inflammation and fibrosis surrounding silicone breast prosthesis. *Am. J. surg. Pathol.*, **19**, 712–717

Cook, L.S., Daling, J.R., Voigt, L.F., deHart, M.P., Malone, K.E., Stanford, J.L., Weiss, N.S., Brinton, L.A., Gammon, M.D. & Brogan, D. (1997) Characteristics of women with and without breast augmentation. *J. Am. med. Assoc.*, **277**, 1612–1617

Coombes, A.G.A. & Meikle, M.C. (1994) Resorbable polymers as replacements for bone grafts. *Clin. Mater.*, **17**, 35–67

Cooper, C.S. (1996) Translocations in solid tumours. *Curr. Opin. Genet. Dev.*, **6**, 71–75

Costa, M. (1997) Nonmutagenic mechanisms of nickel carcinogenesis: inactivation of critical genes by nickel-induced DNA methylation and chromatin condensation. In: Dungworth, D.L., Adler, K.B., Harris, C.C. & Plopper, C.G., eds, *Correlations Between In Vitro and In Vivo Investigations in Inhalation Toxicology*, Washington DC, ILSI Press, pp. 359–366

Costantino, P.D. (1994) Synthetic biomaterials for soft-tissue augmentation and replacement in the head and neck. *Otolaryngol. Clin. North Am.*, **27**, 223–262

Cox, C.F., Suzuki, S. & Suzuki, S.H. (1995) Biocompatibility of dental adhesives. *J. Calif. Dent. Assoc.*, **23**, 35–41

Coyne, M.J., Postorini-Reeves, N.C. & Rosen, D.K. (1997) Estimated prevalence of injection-site sarcomas in cats during 1992. *J. Am. vet. Med. Assoc.*, **210**, 249–251

Crespi, G. & Luciani, L. (1981) Polypropylene. In: Mark, H.F., Othmer, D.F., Overberger, C.G. & Seaborg, G.T., eds, *Kirk-Othmer Encyclopedia of Chemical Technology*, Vol. 16, 3rd Ed., New York, John Wiley, pp. 453–469

Cross, N.G., Taylor, R.F. & Nunez, L.J. (1983) 'Single-step' orthodontic bonding systems: Possible mutagenic potential. *Am. J. Orthod.*, **84**, 344–350

Crowninshield, R. (1988) An overview of prosthetic materials for fixation. *Clin. Orthop.*, **235**, 166–172

Dahlmann, J. (1951) Traumatic lung carcinoma. *Fortschr. Röntgenstr.*, **75**, 628–635 (in German)

Dalal, J.J., Winterbottam, T., West, R.R. & Henderson, A.H. (1980) Implanted pacemakers and breast cancer (Letter to the Editor). *Lancet*, **ii**, 311

Dalinka, M.K., Rockett, J.F. & Kurth, R.J. (1969) Carcinoma of the breast following simple mastectomy and mammoplasty. *Radiology*, **93**, 914

Dasler, W. & Milliser, R.V. (1963) Induction of tumors in rats by subcutaneous implants of surgical sponges. *Experimentia*, **19**, 424–426

Davila, R.M. & Crouch, E.C. (1993) Role of mesothelial and submesothelial stromal cells in matrix remodeling following pleural injury. *Am. J. Pathol.*, **142**, 547–555

Davis, R.F. (1979) Ceramics (scope). In: Mark, H.F., Othmer, D.F., Overberger, C.G. & Seaborg, G.T., eds, *Kirk-Othmer Encyclopedia of Chemical Technology*, Vol. 5, 3rd Ed., New York, John Wiley, pp. 234–237

Davis, G.W. (1982) Polyester fibers. In: Mark, H.F., Othmer, D.F., Overberger, C.G. & Seaborg, G.T., eds, *Kirk-Othmer Encyclopedia of Chemical Technology,* Vol. 18, 3rd Ed., New York, John Wiley, pp. 531–594

Dawes, E. & Rushton, N. (1997) Response of macrophages to poly(L-lactide) particulates which have undergone various degrees of artificial degradation. *Biomaterials,* **18**, 1615–1623

Deapen, D.M. & Brody, G.S. (1995) Augmentation mammoplasty and breast cancer: a five-year update of the Los Angeles study. *J. clin. Epidemiol.,* **48**, 551-556

Deapen, D.M., Pike, M.C., Casagrande, J.T. & Brody, G.S. (1986) The relationship between breast cancer and augmentation mammoplasty: an epidemiologic study. *Plast. reconstr. Surg.,* **77**, 361–367

Deapen, D.M., Bernstein, L. & Brody, G.S. (1997) Are breast implants anticarcinogenic? A 14-year follow-up of the Los Angeles study. *Plast. reconstr. Surg.,* **99**, 1346–1353

Dearfield, K.L., Millis, C.S., Harrington-Brock, K., Doerr, C.L. & Moore, M.M. (1989) Analysis of the genotoxicity of nine acrylate/methacrylate compounds in L5178Y mouse lymphoma cells. *Mutagenesis,* **4**, 381–393

De Giovanni, J.V. (1995) Medical devices: new regulations, new responsibilities. *Br. Heart J.,* **73**, 401–402

Dei Tos, A.P. & Dal Cin, P. (1997) The role of cytogenetics in the classification of soft tissue tumours. *Virchows Arch.,* **431**, 83–94

Delclos, K.B., Blaydes, B., Heflich, R.H. & Smith, B.A. (1996) Assessment of DNA adducts and the frequency of 6-thioguanine resistant T-lymphocytes in F344 rats fed 2,4-toluenediamine or implanted with a toluenediisocyanate-containing polyester polyurethane foam. *Mutat. Res.,* **367**, 209–218

Delgado, E.R. (1958) Sarcoma following a surgically treated fractured tibia. A case report. *Clin. Orthop.,* **12**, 315–318

del Rosario, A.D., Bui, H.X., Petrocine, S., Sheehan, C., Pastore, J., Singh, J. & Ross, J.S. (1995) True synovial metaplasia of breast implant capsules: a light and electron microscopic study. *Ultrastruct. Pathol.,* **19**, 83–93

Desjacques, R. (1939) Cancer and war injuries (knee sarcoma, 21 years after war injury). *Rev. chir. (Paris),* **58**, 373–375 (in French)

Deva, A.K., Merten, S. & Chang, L. (1998) Silicone in nasal augmentation rhinoplasty: A decade of clinical experience. *Plast. reconstr. Surg.,* **102**, 1230–1237

Devor, D.E., Waalkes, M.P., Goering, P. & Rehm, S. (1993) Development of an animal model for testing human breast implantation materials. *Toxicol. Pathol.,* **21**, 261–273

Dewan, P.A., Owen, A.J. & Byard, R.W. (1995) Long-term histological response to subcutaneously injected Polytef and Bioplastique in a rat model. *Br. J. Urol.,* **76**, 161–164

Dickinson, G.L., Leinfelder, K.F., Mazer, R.B. & Russell, C.M. (1990) Effect of surface penetrating sealant on wear rate of posterior composite resins. *J. Am. dent. Assoc.,* **121**, 251–255

Dietrich, A. (1950) *Krebs im Gefolge des Krieges,* Stuttgart, S. Hirzel Verlag

Dietrich, W. (1958) Trauma and malignant tumour: an expert opinion. *Zentralbl. Chir.,* **83**, 1878–1883 (in German)

Digby, J.M. (1982) Malignant lymphoma with intranodal silicone rubber particles following metacarpophalangeal joint replacements. *Hand*, **14**, 326–328

Di Maio, V.J.M. (1985) *Gunshot Wounds. Practical Aspects of Firearms, Ballistics, and Forensic Techniques*, New York, Elsevier, pp. 19–22, 99–125, 143–146, 175–179

Dodion, P., Putz, P., Amiri-Lamraski, M.H., Efira, A., de Martelaere, E. & Heimann, R. (1983) Immunoblastic lymphoma at the site of an infected vitallium bone plate. *Histopathology*, **6**, 807–813

Donaghy, M., Rushworth, G. & Jacobs, J.M. (1991) Generalized peripheral neuropathy in a dental technician exposed to methyl methacrylate monomer. *Neurology*, **41**, 1112–1116

Donaldson, K. (1996) Short-term animal studies for detecting inflammation, fibrosis and pre-neoplastic changes induced by fibres. In: Kane, A.B., Boffetta, P., Saracci, R. & Wilbourn, J.D., eds, *Mechanisms of Fibre Carcinogenesis* (IARC Scientific Publications No. 140), Lyon, IARC, pp. 97–106

Dontenwill, W. & Graf, R. (1953) Malignant neurinoma after gunshot injury. *Z. Krebsforsch.*, **59**, 381–388 (in German)

Doorn, P.F., Campbell, P.A., Worrall, J., Benya, P.D., McKellop, H.A. & Amstutz, H.C. (1998) Metal wear particle characterization from metal on metal total hip replacements: transmission electron microscopy study of periprosthetic tissues and isolated particles. *J. biomed. Mater. Res.*, **42**, 103–111

Dorado, L., Ruis-Montoya, M.R. & Rodriguez-Mellado, J.M. (1992) A contribution to the study of the structure-mutagenicity relationship for alpha-dicarbonyl compounds using the Ames test. *Mutat. Res.* **269**, 301–306

Doran, A., Law, F.C., Allen, M.J. & Rushton, N. (1998) Neoplastic transformation of cells by soluble but not particulate forms of metals used in orthopaedic implants. *Biomaterials*, **19**, 751–759

Dorland (1998) *Medical and Health Care Market Place*, Philadelphia, Dorland's Directories

Dorne, L., Alikacem, N., Guidoin, R. & Auger, M. (1995) High resolution solid state ^{29}Si NMR spectroscopy of silicone gels used to fill breast protheses. *Magn. Reson. Med.*, **34**, 548–554

Dorr, L.D., Bloebaum, R., Emmanual, J. & Meldrum, R. (1990) Histologic, biochemical, and ion analysis of tissue and fluids retrieved during total hip arthroplasty. *Clin. Orthop. & Related Res.*, **261**, 82–95

Downey, D. (1989) Contact mucositis due to palladium (Short communication). *Contact Derm.*, **21**, 54

Driscoll, K.E., Deyo, L.C., Carter, J.M., Howard, B.W., Hassenbein, D.G. & Bertram, T.A. (1997) Effects of particle exposure and particle-elicited inflammatory cells on mutation in rat alveolar epithelial cells. *Carcinogenesis*, **18**, 423–430

Druckrey, H. & Schmähl, D. (1952) Carcinogenic action of plastic films. *Z. Naturforsch.*, **7**, 353–356 (in German)

Druckrey, H. & Schmähl, D. (1954) Carcinogenicity of polyethylene films in rats. *Z. Krebsforch.*, **96**, 529–530 (in German)

Drut, R. & Barletta, L. (1975) Osteogenic sarcoma arising in an old burn scar. *J. cutan. Pathol.*, **2**, 302–306

Dube, V.E. & Fisher, D.E. (1972) Hemangioendothelioma of the leg following metallic fixation of the tibia. *Cancer*, **30**, 1260–1266

Dubeau, L. & Fraser, R.S. (1984) Long-term effects of pulmonary shrapnel injury. Report of a case with carcinoma and residual shrapnel tract. *Arch. Pathol. Lab. Med.*, **108**, 407–409

Dubielzig, R.R., Hawkins, K.L. & Miller, P.E. (1993) Myofibroblastic sarcoma originating at the site of rabies vaccination in a cat. *J. vet. Diagn. Invest.*, **5**, 637–638

Duffy, D.M. (1990) Silicone: a critical review. *Adv. Dermatol.*, **5**, 93–100

Dukes, C.E. & Mitchley, B.C.V. (1962) Polyvinyl sponge implants: experimental and clinical observations. *Br. J. plast. Surg.*, **15**, 225–235

Dunaif, C.B., Stubenbord, W.T. & Conway, H. (1963) Observations on subcutaneously implanted polyetherurethane sponge in mice. *Surg. Gynecol. Obstet.*, **10**, 454–458

Dunipace, A.J., Noblitt, T.W., Li, Y. & Stookey, G.K. (1990) *In vivo* genotoxic assays for evaluation of dental materials (Abstract). *J. dent. Res.*, **69**, 229

Dupree, W.B. & Enzinger, F.M. (1986) Fibro-osseous pseudotumor of the digits. *Cancer*, **58**, 2103–2109

Duvic, M., Moore, D., Menter, A. & Vonderheid, E.C. (1995) Cutaneous T-cell lymphoma in association with silicone breast implants. *J. Am. Acad. Dermatol.*, **32**, 939–942

Ebert, G. (1954) Sarcoma formation after injury. *Langenbecks Arch. dtch. Z. Chir.*, **278**, 218–228 (in German)

Eckstein, F.S., Vogel, U. & Mohr, W. (1992) Fibrosarcoma in association with a total knee joint prosthesis. *Virchows Arch. A Pathol. Anat.*, **421**, 175–178

Edwards, C.K. III, Ghiasuddin, S.M., Schepper, J.M., Yunger, L.M. & Kelley, K.W. (1988) A newly defined property of somatotropin: priming of macrophages for production of superoxide anion. *Science*, **239**, 769–771

Eistert, B., Glanz, H. & Kleinsasser, O. (1989) Two cases of laryngeal cancer following gunshot injury. *HNO*, **37**, 220–223 (in German)

Ekfors, T.O., Aro, H., Mäki, J. & Aho, A.J. (1984) Cystic osteolysis induced by silicone rubber prosthesis. *Arch. Pathol. Lab. Med.*, **108**, 225–227

Elbaum, R., Pignoly, C. & Brouillet, J.L. (1991) A histologic study of the biocompatibility of a dentinal bonding system. *Quintessence Int.*, **22**, 901–910

Emory, T.S., Scheithauer, B.W., Hirose, T., Wood, M., Onofrio, B.M. & Jenkins, R.B. (1995) Intraneural perineurioma. A clonal neoplasm associated with abnormalities of chromosome 22. *Am. J. clin. Pathol.*, **103**, 696–704

Engel, A., Lamm, S.H. & Lai, S.H. (1995) Human breast sarcoma and human breast implantation: a time trend analysis based on SEER data (1973–1990). *J. clin. Epidemiol.*, **48**, 539–544

Engelhardt, J.P. & Grün, L. (1972) Microbial breakdown of methyl methacrylate, plasticizers and netting agent. *Dtsch. Zahnärztl. Z.*, **27**, 466–473 (in German)

Enzinger, F.M. & Dulcey, F. (1967) Proliferative myositis. Report of thirty-three cases. *Cancer*, **20**, 2213–2223

Enzinger, F.M. & Weiss, S.W., eds (1995) *Soft Tissue Tumors*, 3rd Ed., St Louis, C.V. Mosby

Erlandson, R.A., ed. (1994) *Diagnostic Transmission Electron Microscopy of Tumors with Clinico–Pathological, Immunohistochemical and Cytogenic Correlations*, New York, Raven Press

Esplin, D.G. & Campbell, R. (1995) Widespread metastasis of a fibrosarcoma associated with a vaccination site in a cat. *Feline Pract.*, **23**, 13–16

Esplin, D.G., Jaffe, M.H. & McGill, L.D. (1996) Metastasizing liposarcoma associated with a vaccination site in a cat. *Feline Pract.*, **24**, 20–23

Evans, H.L. (1993) Low–grade fibromyxoid sarcoma. A report of 12 cases. *Am. J. surg. Pathol.*, **17**, 595–600

Evans, D.M.D., Williams, W.J. & Kung, I.T.M. (1983) Angiosarcoma and hepatocellular carcinoma in vinyl chloride workers. *Histopathology*, **7**, 377–388

Everitt, J.I. (1994) Mechanisms of fiber-induced diseases: implications for the safety evaluation of synthetic vitreous fibers. *Regul. Toxicol. Pharmacol.*, **20**, S67–S75

Fehrenbacher, J.W., Bowers, W., Strate, R. & Pittman, J. (1981) Angiosarcoma of the aorta associated with a Dacron graft. *Ann. thorac. Surg.*, **32**, 297–301

Fischer-Wasels, J. (1951) 'Scar-carcinoma' after shrapnel injury with 30 years latency. *Z. Krebsforsch.*, **57**, 379–386 (in German)

Fisher, A.A. (1982) Contact dermatitis in medical and surgical personnel. In: Maibach, H.I. & Gellin, G.A., eds, *Occupational and Industrial Dermatology*, Chicago, Year Book Medical Publishers, pp. 219–228

Fisher, C. (1986) Synovial sarcoma: ultrastructural and immunohistochemical features of epithelial differentiation in monophasic and biphasic tumors. *Hum. Pathol.*, **17**, 996–1008

Fisher, C. (1988) Epithelioid sarcoma: the spectrum of ultrastructural differentiation in seven immunohistochemically defined cases. *Hum. Pathol.*, **19**, 265–275

Fisher, C. (1996) Fibrohistiocytic tumors. *Monogr. Pathol.*, **38**, 162–180

Fisher, C. (1999) Current aspects of the pathology of soft tissue sarcomas. *Semin. Rad. Oncol.* (in press)

Fisher, C., Flood, L.M. & Ramsey, A.D. (1992) The role of electron microscopy in the diagnosis of tumours of the head and neck. *J. Laryngol. Otol.*, **106**, 403–408

Fletcher, C.D.M. (1992) Pleomorphic malignant fibrous histiocytoma: fact or fiction? A critical reappraisal based on 159 tumors diagnosed as pleomorphic sarcoma. *Am. J. surg. Pathol.*, **16**, 213–228

Foley, R.T. & Brown, B.F. (1979) Corrosion and corrosion inhibitors. In: Mark, H.F., Othmer, D.F., Overberger, C.G. & Seaborg, G.T., eds, *Kirk-Othmer Encyclopedia of Chemical Technology*, Vol. 7, 3rd Ed., New York, John Wiley, pp. 113–142

Fontana, M.G. & Greene, N.D. (1978) *Corrosion Engineering*, 2nd Ed., New York, McGraw-Hill, pp. 38–45, 60–63

Fraedrich, G., Kracht, J., Scheld, H.H., Jundt, G. & Mulch, J. (1984) Sarcoma of the lung in a pacemaker pocket—Simple coincidence or oncotaxis? *Thorac. cardiovasc. Surgeon*, **32**, 67–69

Frantz, P. & Herbst, C.A., Jr (1975) Augmentation mammoplasty, irradiation, and breast cancer. A case report. *Cancer*, **36**, 1147–1150

Freilich, M.A., Goldberg, A.J., Gilpatrick, R.O. & Simonsen, R.J. (1992) Three-year occlusal wear of posterior composite restorations. *Dent. Mater.*, **8**, 224–228

Frey, R. & Knauer, W. (1949) Sarcoma and trauma. *Langenbecks Arch. dtsch. Z. Chir.*, **263**, 59–70 (in German)

Friis, S., McLaughlin, J.K., Mellemkjær, L., Kjøller, K.H., Blot, W.J., Boice, J.D., Jr, Fraumeni, J.F., Jr & Olsen, J.H. (1997) Breast implants and cancer risk in Denmark. *Int. J. Cancer*, **7**, 956–958

Fryzek, J.P., Mellemkjaer, L., McLaughlin, J.K., Blot, W.J. & Olsen, J.H. (1999) Cancer risk among patients with finger and hand joint and temporo-mandibular joint prostheses in Denmark. *Int. J. Cancer*, **81**, 723–725

Fubini, B. (1996) Use of physico-chemical and cell-free assays to evaluate the potential carcinogenicity of fibres. In: Kane, A.B., Boffetta, P., Saracci, R. & Wilbourn, J.D., eds, *Mechanisms of Fibre Carcinogenesis* (IARC Scientific Publications No. 140), Lyon, IARC, pp. 35–54

Fubini, B., Aust, A.E., Bolton, R.E., Borm, P.J.A., Bruch, J., Ciapetti, G., Donaldson, K., Elias, Z., Gold, J., Jaurand, M. C., Kane, A. B., Lison, D. & Muhle, H. (1998) Non-animal tests for evaluating the toxicity of solid xenobiotics. *ATLA*, **26**, 579–617

Fujisawa, S., Kadoma, Y. & Masuhara, E. (1986) Effects of photoinitiators for the visible-light resin system on hemolysis of dog erythrocytes and lipid peroxidation of their components. *J. dent. Res.*, **65**, 1186–1190

Fung, H., Kow, Y.W., Van Houten, B. & Mossman, B.T. (1997a) Patterns of 8-hydroxy-deoxyguanosine formation in DNA and indications of oxidative stress in rat and human pleural mesothelial cells after exposure to crocidolite asbestos. *Carcinogenesis*, **18**, 825–832

Fung, H., Quinlan, T.R., Janssen, Y.M.W., Timblin, C.R., Marsh, J.P., Heintz, N.H., Taatjes, D.J., Vacek, P., Jaken, S., & Mossman, B.T. (1997b) Inhibition of protein kinase C prevents asbestos-induced c-*fos* and c-*jun* proto-oncogene expression in mesothelial cells. *Cancer Res.*, **57**, 3101–3105

Fung, H., Kow, Y.W., Van Houten, B., Taatjes, D.J., Hatahet, Z., Janssen, Y.M.W., Vacek, P., Faux, S.P. & Mossman, B.T. (1998) Asbestos increases mammalian AP-endonuclease gene expression, protein levels, and enzyme activity in mesothelial cells. *Cancer Res.*, **58**, 189–194

Furst, A. (1971) Trace elements related to specific chronic diseases: cancer. In: Cannon, H.L. & Hopps, H.C., eds, *Environmental Geochemistry in Health and Disease*, Boulder, CO, Geological Society of America, pp. 109–130

Furst, A. & Cassetta, D. (1973) Carcinogenicity of nickel by different routes (Abstract No. 121). *Proc. Am. Assoc. Cancer Res.*, **14**, 31

Furst, A. & Schlauder, M.C. (1971) The hamster as a model for metal carcinogenesis. *Proc. west. Pharmacol. Soc.*, **14**, 68–71

Furst, A., Cassetta, D.M. & Sasmore, D.P. (1973) Rapid induction of pleural mesothelioma in the rat. *Proc. west. Pharmacol. Soc.*, **16**, 150–153

Fyfe, B.S., Quintana, C.S., Kaneko, M. & Griepp, R.B. (1994) Aortic sarcoma four years after Dacron graft insertion. *Ann. thorac. Surg.*, **58**, 1752–1754

Gabriel, S.E., O'Fallon, W.M., Kurland, L.T., Beard, C.M., Woods, J.E. & Melton, L.J., III (1994) Risk of connective-tissue diseases and other disorders after breast implantation. *New Engl. J. Med.*, **330**, 1697–1702

Gaechter, A., Alroy, J., Andersson, G.B.J., Galante, J., Rostoker, W. & Schajowicz, F. (1977) Metal carcinogenesis: a study of the carcinogenic activity of solid metal alloys in rats. *J. Bone Joint Surg.*, **59A**, 622–624

Galateau-Salle, F., Bidet, P.H., Iwatsubo, Y., Gennetay, E., Renier, A., Letourneux, M., Pairon, J.C., Moritz, S., Brochard, P., Jaurand, M.C. & Freymuth, F. (1998) SV40-like DNA sequences in pleural mesothelioma, bronchopulmonary carcinoma, and non-malignant pulmonary diseases. *J. Pathol.*, **184**, 252–257

Gangal, S.V. (1980) Polytetrafluoroethylene. In: Mark, H.F., Othmer, D.F., Overberger, C.G. & Seaborg, G.T., eds, *Kirk-Othmer Encyclopedia of Chemical Technology*, Vol. 11, 3rd Ed., New York, John Wiley, pp. 1–24

Gargan, T.J., Mitchell, L. & Plaus, W. (1988) Burn scar sarcoma. *Ann. plast. Surg.*, **20**, 477–480

Garrido, L. & Ackerman, J.L. (1996) ^{29}Si NMR and blood silicon levels in silicone gel breast implant recipients. *Magn. Reson. Med.*, **36**, 499–501

Garrido, L., Pfleiderer, B., Papisov, M. & Ackerman, J.L. (1993) In vivo degradation of silicones. *Magn. Reson. Med.*, **29**, 839–843

Geis-Gerstorfer, J. & Pässler, K. (1993) Studies on the influence of Be content on the corrosion behavior and mechanical properties of Ni-25Cr-10Mo alloys. *Dent. Mater.*, **9**, 177–181

Geurtsen, W. & Leyhausen, G. (1997) Biological aspects of root canal filling materials—histocompatibility, cytotoxicity, and mutagenicity. *Clin. oral Invest.*, **1**, 5–11

Ghio, A.J., Kadiiska, M.B., Xiang, Q.-H. & Mason, R.P. (1998) In vivo evidence of free radical formation after asbestos instillation: an ESR spin trapping investigation. *Free Rad. Biol. Med.*, **24**, 11–17

Gill, R.J. (1993) AAS or ICP-OES: Are they competing techniques? *Am. Lab.*, **November**, 24F–24K

Gillespie, W.J., Frampton, C.M.A., Henderson, R.J. & Ryan, P.M. (1988) The incidence of cancer following total hip replacement. *J. Bone Joint Surg.*, **70B**, 539–542

Gillespie, W.J., Henry, D.A., O'Connell, D.L., Kendrick, S., Juszczak, E., McInneny, K. & Derby, L. (1996) Development of hematopoietic cancers after implantation of total joint replacement. *Clin. Orthopaed. rel. Res.*, **329** (Suppl.), S290–S296

Glantz, P.-O. (1998) Biomaterial consideration for the optimized therapy for the edentulous predicament. *J. prost. Dent.*, **79**, 90–92

Glod, D. & Frykberg, R.G. (1990) Foreign body reaction in a Dacron-meshed hemi-implant. *J. Foot Surg.*, **29**, 250–252

Goasguen, J., Lapresle, J., Ribot, C. & Rocquet, G. (1982) Chronic neurological syndrome resulting from intoxication with metallic uranium. *Nouv. Press. Med.*, **11**, 119–121 (in French)

Goldberg, J.L., Zanella, C.L., Janssen, Y.M.W., Timblin, C.R., Jimenez, L.A., Vacek, P., Taatjes, D.J. & Mossman, B.T. (1997) Novel cell imaging techniques show induction of apoptosis and proliferation in mesothelial cells by asbestos. *Am. J. respir. Cell mol. Biol.*, **17**, 265–271

Goldhaber, P. (1962) Further observations concerning the carcinogenicity of Millipore filters (Abstract 96). *Proc. Am. Assoc. Cancer Res.*, **3**, 323

Golladay, S.A., Park, S.-H. & Aust, A.E. (1997) Efflux of reduced glutathione after exposure of human lung epithelial cells to crocidolite asbestos. *Environ. Health Perspect.*, **105** (Suppl. 5), 1273–1277

Golubyeva, V.A. & Mitin, V.N. (1984) Osteogenic sarcoma in a dog at site of a metallic bone-fixing pin. *Arch. Pathol. (Moscow)*, **46**, 34–37

Gott, D.M. & Tinkler, J.J.B. (1994) *Evaluation of Evidence for Association Between the Implantation of Silicones and Connective Tissue Disease*, London, Medical Devices Agency, pp. 1–62

Gottlieb, V., Muench, A.G., Rich, J.D. & Pagadala, S. (1984) Carcinoma in augmented breasts. *Ann. plast. Surg.*, **12**, 67–69

Gould, V.E. (1986) Histogenesis and differentiation: a re-evaluation of these concepts as criteria for the classification of tumors. *Hum. Pathol.*, **17**, 212–215

Granchi, D., Cenni, E., Ciapetti, G., Savarino, L., Stea, S., Gamberini, S., Gori, A. & Pizzoferrato, A. (1998) Cell death induced by metal ions: necrosis or apoptosis? *J. Materials Sci.: Materials in Medicine*, **9**, 31–37

Grantham, P.H., Mohan, L., Benjamin, T., Roller, P.P., Miller, J.R. & Weisburger, E.K. (1979) Comparison of the metabolism of 2,4-toluenediamine in rats and mice. *J. Environ. Pathol. Toxicol.*, **3**, 149–166

Gray, S.J. & Stirling, K. (1950) Tagging of red cells and plasma proteins with radioactive chromium. *J. clin. Invest.*, **29**, 1604–1613

Greim, H., Ahlers, J., Bias, R., Broecker, B., Hollander, H., Gelbke, H.-P., Jacobi, S., Klimisch, H.-J., Mangelsdorf, I., Mayr, W., Schön, N., Stropp, G., Stahnecker, P., Vogel, R., Weber, C., Ziegler-Skylakakis, K. & Bayer, E. (1995) Assessment of structurally related chemicals: toxicity and ecotoxicity of acrylic acid and acrylic acid alkyl esters (acrylates), methacrylic acid and methacrylic acid alkyl esters (methacrylates). *Chemosphere*, **31**, 2637–2659

Gridley, G., McLaughlin, J.K., Ekbom, A., Klareskoo, L., Adami, H.-O., Hacker, D.G., Hoover, R. & Fraumeni, J.F., Jr (1993) Incidence of cancer among patients with rheumatoid arthritis. *J. natl Cancer Inst.*, **85**, 307–311

Grieve, A.R., Alani, A. & Saunders, W.P. (1991) The effects of the dental pulp of a composite resin and two dentine bonding agents and associated bacterial microleakage. *Int. Endod. J.*, **24**, 108–118

Grimsdottir, M.R., Gjerdet, N.R. & Hensten-Pettersen, A. (1992) Composition and in vitro corrosion of orthodontic appliances. *Am. J. Orthod. Dentofac. Orthop.*, **101**, 525–532

Griss, P., Werner, E., Buchinger, R., Büsing, C.-M. & Heimke, G. (1977) Experimental investigation on non-specific foreign body sarcoma induction of Al_2O_3-ceramic implants. *Arch. orthop. Unfall-Chir.*, **90**, 29–40 (in German)

Grote, J.J., van Blitterswijk, C.A. & Kuijpers, W. (1986) Hydroxyapatite ceramic as middle ear implant material: animal experimental results. *Ann. Otol. Rhinol. Laryngol.*, **123** (Suppl.), 1–5

Guyuron, B. & Lasa, C.I., Jr (1992) Reaction to stainless steel wire following orthognathic surgery. *Plast. reconstr. Surg.*, **89**, 540–542

Haag, M. & Adler, C.P. (1989) Malignant fibrous histiocytoma in association with hip replacement. *J. Bone Joint Surg.*, **71B**, 701

Habal, M.B., Powell, M.L. & Schimpff, R.D. (1980) Immunological evaluation of the tumorigenic response to implanted polymers. *J. biomed. Mater. Res.*, **14**, 455–466

Hagen, T.M., Huang, S., Curnutte, J., Fowler, P., Martinez, V., Wehr, C.M., Ames, B.N. & Chisari, F.V. (1994) Extensive oxidative DNA damage in hepatocytes of transgenic mice with chronic active hepatitis destined to develop hepatocellular carcinoma. *Proc. natl Acad. Sci. USA*, **91**, 12808–12812

Hahn, F.F., Guilmette, R.A. & Hoover, M.D. (1999) Toxicity of uranium fragments in Wistar rats (Abstract). *The Toxicologist*, **48 (1-S)**, 333–334

Hallervorden, J. (1948) Oligodendroglioma following brain trauma. *Nervenartz*, **19**, 163–167 (in German)

Hallström, U. (1993) Adverse reaction to a fissure sealant: Report of a case. *J. Dent. Child.*, **60**, 143–146

Hamaker, W.R., Lindell, M.E. & Gomez, A.C. (1976) Plasmacytoma arising in a pacemaker pocket. *Ann. thor. Surg.*, **21**, 354–356

Hanks, C.T., Strawn, S.E., Wataha, J.C. & Craig, R.G. (1991) Cytotoxic effects of resin components on cultured mammalian fibroblasts. *J. dent. Res.*, **70**, 1450–1455

Hardman, B.B. & Torkelson, A. (1989) Silicones. In: Grayson, M., Mark, H.F., Othmer, D.F. & Othmer, D.F., eds, *Kirk-Othmer Concise Encyclopedia of Chemical Technology*, New York, John Wiley, pp. 1062–1065

Hare, T.M. (1979a) Ceramics (thermal treatment). In: Mark, H.F., Othmer, D.F., Overberger, C.G. & Seaborg, G.T., eds, *Kirk-Othmer Encyclopedia of Chemical Technology*, Vol. 5, 3rd Ed., New York, John Wiley, pp. 260–266

Hare, T.M. (1979b) Ceramics (properties and applications). In: Mark, H.F., Othmer, D.F., Overberger, C.G. & Seaborg, G.T., eds, *Kirk-Othmer Encyclopedia of Chemical Technology*, Vol. 5, 3rd Ed., New York, John Wiley, pp. 267–290

Harland, R.W., Sharma, M. & Rosenzweig, D.Y. (1993) Lung carcinoma in a patient with lucite sphere plombage thoracoplasty. *Chest*, **103**, 1295–1297

Harmand, M.-F., Naji, A. & Gonfrier, P. (1994) *In vitro* study of biomaterial biodegradation using human cell cultures. *Clin. Mater.*, **15**, 281–285

Harnirattisai, C. & Hosoda, H. (1991) Pulpal responses to various dentin bonding systems in dentin cavities. *Dent. Mater. J.*, **10**, 149–164

Harris, W.R. (1990) Chondrosarcoma complicating total hip arthroplasty in Maffucci's syndrome. *Clin. Orthop. rel. Res.*, **260**, 212–214

Harris, H.E., Jr & Hawk, W.A. (1969) Laryngeal injection of teflon paste. Report of a case with postmortem study of the larynx. *Arch. Otolaryngol.*, **90**, 194–197

Harrison, J.W., McLain, D.L., Hohn, R.B., Wilson, G.P., Chalman, J.A. & MacGowan, K.N. (1976) Osteosarcoma associated with metallic implants. Report of two cases in dogs. *Clin. Orthop. rel. Res.*, **116**, 253–257

Hartley, J.A., Gibson, N.W., Kilkenny, A. & Yuspa, S.H. (1987) Mouse keratinocytes derived from initiated skin or papillomas are resistant to DNA strand breakage by benzoyl peroxide: a possible mechanism for tumor promotion mediated by benzoyl peroxide. *Carcinogenesis*, **8**, 1827–1830

Hartwig, A., Schlepegrell, R., Dally, H. & Hartmann, M. (1996) Interaction of carcinogenic metal compounds with deoxyribonucleic acid repair processes. *Ann. clin. Lab. Sci.*, **26**, 31–38

Haslhofer, L. (1950) Two cases of late death after war injury. *Wien. klin. Wochenschr.*, **62**, 569–572 (in German)

Haworth, S., Lawlor, T., Mortelmans, K., Speck, W. & Zeiger, E. (1983) Salmonella mutagenicity test results for 250 chemicals. *Environ. Mutagen.*, **5**, *Suppl. 1*, 3–142

Hayman, J. & Huygens, H. (1983) Angiosarcoma developing around a foreign body. *J. clin. Pathol.*, **36**, 515–518

Heath, J.C. (1954) Cobalt as a carcinogen. *Nature*, **173**, 822–823

Heath, J.C. (1956) The production of malignant tumours by cobalt in the rat. *Br. J. Cancer*, **10**, 668–673

Heath, J.C. & Daniel, M.R. (1962) The production of malignant tumours by cobalt in the rat: intrathoracic tumours. *Br. J. Cancer*, **16**, 473–478

Heath, J.C., Freeman, M.A. & Swanson, S.A. (1971) Carcinogenic properties of wear particles from prostheses made of cobalt-chromium alloy. *Lancet*, **i**, 564–566

Heil, J., Reifferscheid, G., Waldmann, P., Leyhausen, G. & Geurtsen, W. (1996) Genotoxicity of dental materials. *Mutat. Res.*, **368**, 181–194

Heintz, N.H., Janssen, Y.M. & Mossman, B.T. (1993) Persistent induction of *c-fos* and *c-jun* expression by asbestos. *Proc. natl Acad. Sci. USA*, **90**, 3299–3303

Heitmann, T. & Unterbrink, G. (1995) Direct pulp capping with a dentinal adhesive resin system: a pilot study. *Quint. Int.*, **26**, 765–770

Hendrick, M.J., Goldschmidt, M.H., Shofer, F.S., Wang, Y.-Y. & Somloy, A.P. (1992) Postvaccinal sarcomas in the cat: epidemiology and electron probe microanalytical identification of aluminum. *Cancer Res.*, **52**, 5391–5394

Hendrick, M., Shofer, F., Goldschmidt, M., Haviland, J.C., Schelling, S.H., Engler, S.J. & Gliatto, J.M. (1994) Comparison of fibrosarcomas that developed at vaccination sites and at nonvaccination sites in cats: 239 cases (1991–1992). *J. Am. vet. Med. Assoc.*, **205**, 1425–1429

Hensten-Pettersen, A. (1992) Casting alloys: side-effects. *Adv. dent. Res.*, **6**, 38–43

Hensten-Pettersen, A. & Jacobsen, N. (1991) Perceived side effects of biomaterials in prosthetic dentistry. *J. prosthet. Dent.*, **65**, 138–144

Hester, T.R., Jr, Ford, N.F., Gale, P.J., Hammett, J.L., Raymond, R., Turnbull, D., Frankos, V.H. & Cohen, M.B. (1997) Measurement of 2,4-toluenediamine in urine and serum samples from women with Même or Replicon breast implants. *Plast. reconstr. Surg.*, **100**, 1291–1298

Hesterberg, T.W., Miller, W.C., Musselman, R.P., Kamstrup, O., Hamilton, R.D. & Thevenaz, P. (1996) Biopersistence of man-made vitreous fibers and crocidolite asbestos in the rat lung following inhalation. *Fundam. appl. Toxicol.*, **29**, 267–279

Hierholzer, S. & Hierholzer, G. (1984) Metal allergy as a pathogenetic factor in bone infection following osteosynthesis. *Unfallheilkunde*, **87**, 1–6 (in German)

Himmer, O., Lootvoet, L., Deprez, P., Monfort, L. & Ghosez, J.-P. (1991) Case report of angiosarcoma following total knee prosthesis. *Rev. Chir. orthop.*, **77**, 125–128 (in French)

Hinsull, S.M., Bellamy, D., Franklin, A. & Watson B.W. (1979) The inhibitory influence of metal–plastic implant on cellular proliferation patterns in an experimental tumour compared with normal tissue. *Eur. J. Cancer*, **16**, 159–166

Hizawa, K., Inaba, H., Nakanishi, S., Otsuka, H. & Izumi, K. (1984) Subcutaneous pseudosarcomatous polyvinylpyrrolidone granuloma. *Am. J. surg. Pathol.*, **8**, 393–398

Holder, J.W., Elmore, E. & Barrett, J.C. (1993) Gap junction and cancer. *Cancer Res.*, **53**, 3475–3485

Holley, J.A., Janssen, Y.M.W., Mossman, B.T. & Taatjes, D.J. (1992) Increased manganese superoxide dismutase protein in type II epithelial cells of rat lungs after inhalation of crocidolite asbestos or cristobalite silica. *Am. J. Pathol.*, **141**, 475–485

Holmberg, S. (1992) Life expectancy after total hip arthroplasty. *J. Arthroplasty*, **7**, 183–186

Holmstrup, P. (1991) Reactions of the oral mucosa related to silver amalgam: a review. *J. oral Pathol. Med.*, **20**, 1–7

Holmstrup, P. (1999) Oral lichen planus. *Dtsch. Zahnärztl. Z.*, **54**, 10–14

Homma, Y. & Oyasu, R. (1986) Transient and persistent hyperplasia in heterotopically transplanted rat urinary bladders induced by formalin and foreign bodies. *J. Urol.*, **136**, 136–140

Hoopes, J.E., Edgerton, M.T., Jr & Sheeley, W. (1967) Organic synthetics for augmentation mammaplasty: their relation to breast cancer. *Plast. reconstr. Surg.*, **39**, 263–270

Horowitz, S.M., Luchetti, W.T., Gonzales, J.B. & Ritchie, C.K. (1998) The effects of cobalt chromium upon macrophages. *J. biomed. Mater. Res.*, **41**, 468–473

Hörsted, P.B., Simonsen, A.-M. & Larsen, M.J. (1986) Monkey pulp reactions to restorative materials. *Scand. J. dent. Res.*, **94**, 154–163

Hörsted-Bindslev, P. (1987) Monkey pulp reactions to cavities treated with Gluma Dentin Bond and restored with a microfilled composite. *Scand. J. dent. Res.*, **95**, 347–355

Hsieh, C.-C. & Trichopoulos, D. (1991) Breast size, handedness and breast cancer risk. *Eur. J. Cancer.*, **27**, 131–135

Huaux, F., Louahed, J., Hudspith, B., Meredith, C., Delos, M., Renauld, J.-C. & Lison, D. (1998) Role of interleukin-10 in the lung response to silica in mice. *Am. J. respir. Cell mol. Biol.*, **18**, 51–59

Hudson, L.D. (1987) Phototoxic reaction triggered by a new dental instrument. *Am. Acad. Dermatol.*, **17**, 508–509

Hueper, H.C. (1952) Experimental studies in metal cancerigenesis. I. Nickel cancers in rats. *Texas Rep. Biol. Med.*, **16**, 167–186

Hueper, H.C. (1955a) Experimental studies in metal cancerigenesis. VII. Tissue reactions to parenterally introduced powdered metallic chromium and chromite ore. *J. natl Cancer Inst.*, **16**, 447–462

Hueper, H.C. (1955b) Experimental studies in metal cancerigenesis. IV. Cancer produced by parenterally introduced metallic nickel. *J. natl Cancer Inst.*, **16**, 55–67

Hueper, H.C. (1958) Experimental studies in metal cancerigenesis. IV. Pulmonary lesions in guinea pigs and rats exposed to prolonged inhalation of powdered metallic nickel. *Arch. Pathol.*, **65**, 600–607

Hueper, W.C. (1959) Carcinogenic studies on water-soluble and insoluble macromolecules. *Arch. Pathol.*, **67**, 589–617

Hueper, W.C. (1960) Experimental production of cancer by means of implanted polyurethane plastic. *Am. J. clin. Pathol.*, **34**, 328–333

Hueper, W.C. (1961) Carcinogenic studies on water-insoluble polymers. *Pathol. Microbiol.*, **24**, 77–106

Hueper, W.C. (1964) Cancer induction by polyurethane and polysilicone plastics. *J. natl Cancer Inst.*, **33**, 1005–1027

Hueper, H.C. & Payne, W.W. (1962) Experimental studies in metal cancerigenesis. Chromium, nickel, iron, arsenic. *Arch. environ. Health*, **5**, 445–462

Hughes, A.W., Sherlock, D.A., Hamblen, D.L. & Reid, R. (1987) Sarcoma at the site of a single hip screw. A case report. *J. Bone Joint Surg.*, **69B**, 470–472

Husgafvel-Pursiainen, K., Hackman, P., Ridanpää, M., Anttila, S., Karjalainen, A., Partanen, T., Taikina-aho, O., Heikkilä, L. & Vainio, H. (1993) K-*ras* mutations in human adenocarcinoma of the lung: association with smoking and occupational exposure to asbestos. *Int. J. Cancer*, **53**, 250–256

Husgafvel-Pursiainen, K., Kannio, A., Oksa, P., Suitiala, T., Koskinen, H., Partanen, T., Hemminki, K., Smith, S., Rosenstock-Leibu, R. & Brandt-Rauf, P.W. (1997) Mutations, tissue accumulation, and serum levels of p53 in patients with occupational cancers from asbestos and silica exposure. *Environ. mol. Mutagen.*, **30**, 224–230

IARC (1977) *IARC Monographs on the Evaluation of Carcinogenic Risk of Chemicals to Man*, Vol. 14, *Asbestos*, Lyon

IARC (1979a) *IARC Monographs on the Evaluation of the Carcinogenic Risk of Chemicals to Humans*, Vol. 19, *Some Monomers, Plastics and Synthetic Elastomers, and Acrolein*, Lyon, pp. 377–438

IARC (1979b) *IARC Monographs on the Evaluation of the Carcinogenic Risk of Chemicals to Humans*, Vol. 19, *Some Monomers, Plastics and Synthetic Elastomers, and Acrolein*, Lyon, pp. 187–211

IARC (1979c) *IARC Monographs on the Evaluation of the Carcinogenic Risk of Chemicals to Humans*, Vol. 19, *Some Monomers, Plastics and Synthetic Elastomers, and Acrolein*, Lyon, pp. 41–71

IARC (1980) *IARC Monographs on the Evaluation of the Carcinogenic Risk of Chemicals to Humans*, Vol. 23, *Some Metals and Metallic Compounds*, Lyon, pp. 325–415

IARC (1986) *IARC Monographs on the Evaluation of the Carcinogenic Risk of Chemicals to Humans*, Vol. 39, *Some Chemicals Used in Plastics and Elastomers*, Lyon

IARC (1987a) *IARC Monographs on the Evaluation of Carcinogenic Risks to Humans*, Suppl. 7, *Overall Evaluations of Carcinogenicity: An Update of IARC Monographs Volumes 1 to 42*, Lyon, pp. 106–116

IARC (1987b) *IARC Monographs on the Evaluation of the Carcinogenic Risks of Chemicals to Humans*, Suppl. 7, *Overall Evaluations of Carcinogenicity: An Update of IARC Monographs Volumes 1 to 42*, Lyon, pp. 373–376

IARC (1987c) *IARC Monographs on the Evaluation of Carcinogenic Risks to Humans*, Suppl. 7, *Overall Evaluations of Carcinogenicity: An Update of IARC Monographs Volumes 1 to 42*, Lyon, pp. 230–232

IARC (1987d) *IARC Monographs on the Evaluation of Carcinogenic Risks to Humans*, Suppl. 6, *Genetic and Related Effects: An Update of Selected IARC Monographs Volumes 1 to 42*, Lyon, p. 203

IARC (1988) *IARC Monographs on the Evaluation of Carcinogenic Risks to Humans*, Vol. 43, *Man-Made Mineral Fibres and Radon*, Lyon, pp. 39–171

IARC (1990a) *IARC Monographs on the Evaluation of Carcinogenic Risks to Humans*, Vol. 49, *Chromium, Nickel and Welding*, Lyon, pp. 49–256

IARC (1990b) *IARC Monographs on the Evaluation of Carcinogenic Risks to Humans*, Vol. 49, *Chromium, Nickel and Welding*, Lyon, pp. 257–445

IARC (1991) *IARC Monographs on the Evaluation of Carcinogenic Risks to Humans*, Vol. 52, *Chlorinated Drinking-Water; Chlorination By-products; Some other Halogenated Compounds; Cobalt and Cobalt Compounds*, Lyon, pp. 363–472

IARC (1993a) *IARC Monographs in the Evaluation of Carcinogenic Risks to Humans*, Vol. 58, *Beryllium, Cadmium, Mercury and Exposures in the Glass Manufacturing Industry*, Lyon, pp. 239–345

IARC (1993b) *IARC Monographs in the Evaluation of Carcinogenic Risks to Humans*, Vol. 58, *Beryllium, Cadmium, Mercury and Exposures in the Glass Manufacturing Industry*, Lyon, pp. 119–237

IARC (1993c) *IARC Monographs in the Evaluation of Carcinogenic Risks to Humans*, Vol. 58, *Beryllium, Cadmium, Mercury and Exposures in the Glass Manufacturing Industry*, Lyon, pp. 41–117

IARC (1994a) *IARC Monographs on the Evaluation of Carcinogenic Risks to Humans*, Vol. 60, *Some Industrial Chemicals*, Lyon, pp. 45–159

IARC (1994b) *IARC Monographs on the Evaluation of Carcinogenic Risks to Humans*, Vol. 60, *Some Industrial Chemicals*, Lyon, pp. 445–474

IARC (1994c) *IARC Monographs on the Evaluation of Carcinogenic Risks to Humans*, Vol. 59, *Hepatitis Viruses*, Lyon

IARC (1994d) *IARC Monographs on the Evaluation of Carcinogenic Risks to Humans*, Vol. 61, *Schistosomes, Liver Flukes and* Helicobacter pylori, Lyon, pp. 177–240

IARC (1996) *IARC Monographs on the Evaluation of Carcinogenic Risks to Humans*, Vol. 67, *Human Immunodeficiency Viruses and Human T-cell Lymphootrophic Viruses*, Lyon, pp. 31–257

IARC (1997a) *IARC Monographs on the Evaluation of Carcinogenic Risks to Humans*, Vol. 68, *Silica, Some Silicates, Coal Dust and para-Aramid Fibrils*, Lyon, pp. 41–242

IARC (1997b) *IARC Monographs on the Evaluation of Carcinogenic Risks to Humans*, Vol. 69, *Polychlorinated Dibenzo-dioxins and Polychlorinated Dibenzofurans*, Lyon, pp. 33–243, 525–630

IARC (1997c) *IARC Monographs on the Evaluation of Carcinogenic Risks to Humans*, Vol. 70, *Epstein-Barr Virus and Kaposi's Sarcoma Herpesvirus/Human Herpesvirus*, Lyon, pp. 375–492

IARC (1997d) *IARC Monographs on the Evaluation of Carcinogenic Risks to Humans*, Vol. 68, *Silica, Some Silicates, Coal Dust and para-Aramid Fibrils*, Lyon, pp. 337–406

IARC (1999a) *IARC Monographs on the Evaluation of Carcinogenic Risks to Humans*, Vol. 71, *Re-evaluation of Some Organic Chemicals, Hydrazine and Hydrogen Peroxide*, Lyon, pp. 1181–1187

IARC (1999b) *IARC Monographs on the Evaluation of Carcinogenic Risks to Humans*, Vol. 71, *Re-evaluation of Some Organic Chemicals, Hydrazine and Hydrogen Peroxide*, Lyon, pp. 345–358

IARC (2000) *IARC Monographs on the Evaluation of Carcinogenic Risks to Humans*, Vol. 75, *X- and γ-Radiation and Neutrons*, Lyon (in press)

Iglesias, M.E., Vázques Doval, F.J., Idoate, F., Valentí, J.R. & Quintanilla, E. (1994) Malignant fibrous histiocytoma at the site of total knee replacement (Letter to the Editor). *J. dermatol. Surg. Oncol.*, **20**, 846–849

ILSI Risk Science Institute Workshop Consensus Report (2000) The relevance of the rat lung response to particle overload for human risk assessment: a workshop consensus report. *Inhal. Toxicol.*, **12** (in press)

Imai, Y. & Masuhara, E. (1982) Long-term *in vivo* studies of poly(2-hydroxyethyl methacrylate). *J. biomed. Mater. Res.*, **16**, 609–617

Imai, Y. & Watanabe, A. (1987) Tumorigenesis from polyurethane materials. *Jpn. J. artif. Organs*, **16**, 1329–1332

Imai, Y., Watanabe, M., Lee, H.E., Kojima, K. & Kadoma, Y. (1988) Cytotoxicity of monomers used in dental resins. *Reports of the Institute for Medical & Dental Engineering*, **22**, 87–90 (in Japanese)

Imai, K., Nakamura, M., Matsumoto, R. & Kokita, K. (1992) Cytotoxicity test using cell recovery test method—comparison with the conventional cell growth method. *Med. Biol.*, **125**, 109–112 (in Japanese)

Inokoshi, S., Shimada, Y., Fujitani, M., Otsuki, M., Shono, T., Onoe, N., Morigami, M. & Takatsu, T. (1995) Monkey pulpal response to adhesively luted indirect resin composite inlays. *Oper. Dent.*, **20**, 111–118

ISO (1998) *Annual Report of ISO/TC 194 for 1997* (Doc. ISO/TC 194 N 267), Pforzheim, International Organization for Standardization

Ivankovic, S., Seller, W.J., Lehmann, E., Komitowski, D. & Frölich, N (1987) Different carcinogenicity of two nickel alloys following intratracheal administration in the hamster (Abstract No. 103). *Naunyn-Schmiedeberg Arch. Pharmacol.*, **335**, R26

Ivankovic, S., Zeller, W.J., Komitowski, D., Edler, L., Lehmann, E. & Frölich, N. (1988) Carcinogenese von Nickellegierungen beim Hamster nach intratrachealer Applikation (Schriftenreihe der Bundesanstalt für Arbeitsschutz), Bremerhaven, Wirtschaftsverlag, p. 81

Jackman, L.A. (1981) Metal treatments. In: Mark, H.F., Othmer, D.F., Overberger, C.G. & Seaborg, G.T., eds, *Kirk-Othmer Encyclopedia of Chemical Technology*, Vol. 15, 3rd Ed., New York, John Wiley, pp. 325–345

Jacobs, A.M. & Oloff, L.M. (1985) Podiatric metallurgy and the effects of implanted metals on living tissues. *Clin. Pediatr.*, **2**, 121–141

Jacobs, J.J., Rosenbaum, D.H., Hay, R.M., Gitelis, J.S. & Black, J. (1992) Early sarcomatous degeneration near a cementless hip replacement. A case report and review. *J. Bone Joint Surg.*, **74B**, 740–744

Jacobs, J.J., Skipor, A.K., Doorn, P.F., Campbell, P., Schmalzried, T.P., Black, J. & Amstutz, H. (1996) Cobalt and chromium concentrations in patients with metal on metal total hip replacements. *Clin. Orthop. rel. Res.*, **329** (Suppl.), S256–S263

Jacobsen, N., Åsenden, R. & Hensten-Pettersen, A. (1991) Occupational health complaints and adverse patient reactions as perceived by personnel in public dentistry. *Comm. Dent. oral Epidemiol.*, **19**, 155–159

James, S.J., Pogribna, M., Miller, B.J., Bolon, B. & Muskhelishvili, L. (1997) Characterization of cellular response to silicone implants in rats: implications for foreign-body carcinogenesis. *Biomaterials*, **18**, 667–675

Janssen, Y.M.W., Marsh, J.P., Absher, M.P., Hemenway, D., Vacek, P.M., Leslie, K.O., Borm, P.J.A. & Mossman, B.T. (1992) Expression of antioxidant enzymes in rat lungs after inhalation of asbestos or silica. *J. biol. Chem.*, **267**, 10625–10630

Janssen, Y.M.W., Driscoll, K.E., Howard, B., Quinlan, T.R., Treadwell, M., Barchowsky, A. & Mossman, B.T. (1997) Asbestos causes translocation of p65 protein and increases NF-κB DNA binding activity in rat lung epithelial and pleural mesothelial cells. *Am. J. Pathol.*, **151**, 389–401

Jasmin, G. & Riopelle, J.L. (1976) Renal carcinomas and erythrocytosis in rats following intrarenal injection of nickel subsulfide. *Lab. Invest.*, **35**, 71–78

Jaurand, M.-C. (1996) Use of in-vitro genotoxicity and cell transformation assays to evaluate the potential carcinogenicity of fibres. In: Kane, A.B., Boffetta, P., Saracci, R. & Wilbourn, J.D., eds, *Mechanisms of Fibre Carcinogenesis* (IARC Scientific Publications No. 140), Lyon, IARC, pp. 55–72

Jeffery, J.A. & McCullough, C.J. (1995) Metastasis as a cause of pain following total hip arthroplasty. A case report. *Today's O.R. Nurse*, **17**, 41–42

Jennings, T.A., Peterson, L., Axiotis, C.A., Friedlaender, G.E., Cooke, R.A. & Rosai, J. (1988) Angiosarcoma associated with foreign body material. A report of three cases. *Cancer*, **62**, 2436–2444

Jensen, C.G., Jensen, L.C.W., Reider, C.L., Cole, R.W. & Ault, J.G. (1996) Long crocidolite asbestos fibers cause polyploidy by sterically blocking cytokinesis. *Carcinogenesis*, **17**, 2013–2021

Jesch, N.K., Dörger, M., Enders, G., Reider, G., Vogelmeier, C., Messmer, K. & Krombach, F. (1997) Expression of inducible nitric oxide synthase and formation of nitric oxide by alveolar macrophages: an interspecies comparison. *Environ. Health Perspect.*, **105** (Suppl. 4), 1297–1300

Johnson, N.F. & Hahn, F.F. (1996) Induction of mesothelioma after intrapleural inoculation of F344 rats with silicon carbide whiskers or continuous ceramic filaments. *Occup. environ. Med.*, **53**, 813–816

Johnson, K.H., Ghobrial, H.K.G., Buoen, L.C., Brand, I. & Brand, K.G. (1973a) Nonfibroblastic origin of foreign body sarcomas implicated by histological and electron microscopic studies. *Cancer Res.*, **33**, 3139–3154

Johnson, K.H., Ghobrial, H.K.G., Buoen, L.C., Brand, I. & Brand, K.G. (1973b) Intracisternal type A particles occuring in foreign body-induced sarcomas. *Cancer Res.*, **33**, 1165–1168

Johnson, K.H., Buoen, L.C., Brand, I. & Brand, K.G. (1977) Light-microscopic morphology of cell types cultured during preneoplasia from foreign body-reactive tissues and films. *Cancer Res.*, **37**, 3228–3237

Johnson, K.H., Ghobrial, H.K.G., Buoen, L.C., Brand, I. & Brand, K.G. (1980) Ultrastructure of cell types cultured during preneoplasia from implant surfaces and foreign-body-reactive tissues in mice. *J. natl Cancer Inst.*, **64**, 1383–1392

Johnston, R.B., Jr & Kitagawa, S. (1985) Molecular basis for the enhanced respiratory burst of activated macrophages. *Fed. Proc.*, **44**, 2927–2932

Jones, A.J., Denning, N.T. & Sharp, D.J. (1991) *Biomaterials: Materials for Medical Devices*, Canberra, Department of Industry, Technology and Commerce, pp. 13–20, 174–177

Jontell, M., Hanks, C.T., Bratel, J. & Bergenholtz, G. (1995) Effects of unpolymerized resin components on the function of accessory cells derived from the rat incisor pulp. *J. dent. Res.*, **74**, 1162–1167

Jorgenson, D.S., Centeno, J.A., Mayer, M.H., Topper, M.J., Nossov, P.C., Mullick, F.G. & Manson, P.N. (1999) Biologic response to passive dissolution of titanium craniofacial microplates. *Biomaterials*, **20**, 675–682

Ju, D.M.C. (1966) Fibrosarcoma arising in surgical scars. *Plast. reconstr. Surg.*, **38**, 429–437

Judde, J.G., Breillout, F., Clemenceau, C., Poupon, M.F. & Jasmin, C. (1987) Inhibition of rat natural killer cell function by carcinogenic nickel compounds: preventive action of manganese. *J. natl Cancer Inst.*, **78**, 1185–1190

Kahn, D.G. & Blazina, M.E. (1993) Incidental metastatic mammary carcinoma in a total knee arthroplasty patient. *Clin. Orthop. rel. Res.*, **295**, 142–145

Kala, S.V., Lykissa, E.D. & Lebovitz, R.M. (1997) Detection and characterization of poly(dimethylsiloxane)s in biological tissues by GA/AED and GC/MS. *Anal. Chem.*, **69**, 1267–1272

Kallus, T. (1984) Evaluation of the toxicity of denture base polymers after subcutaneous implantation in guinea pigs. *J. prosthet. Dent.*, **52**, 126–134

Kallus, T. & Mjör, I.A. (1991) Incidence of adverse effects of dental materials. *Scand. J. dent. Res.*, **99**, 236–240

Kanaar, P. & Oort, J. (1969) Fibrosarcomas developing in scar-tissue. *Dermatologica*, **138**, 312–319

Kane, A.B. (1996a) Mechanisms of mineral fibre carcinogenesis. In: Kane, A.B., Boffetta, P., Saracci, R. & Wilbourn, J.D., eds, *Mechanisms of Fibre Carcinogenesis* (IARC Scientific Publications No. 140), Lyon, IARC, pp. 11–34

Kane, A.B. (1996b) Questions and controversies about the pathogenesis of silicosis. In: Castranova, V., Vallyathan, V. & Wallace, W.E., eds, *Silica and Silica-induced Lung Diseases*, Boca Raton, FL, CRC Press, pp. 121–136

Kane, A.B. (1998) Animal models of malignant mesothelioma. In: Rom, W.N., ed., *Environmental and Occupational Medicine*, 3rd Ed., Philadelphia, Lippincott-Raven, pp. 377–387

Kane, A.B., Boffetta, P., Saracci, R. & Wilbourn, J.D., eds (1996) *Mechanisms of Fibre Carcinogenesis* (IARC Scientific Publications No. 140), Lyon, IARC

Kane, A.B., Macdonald, J.L. & Vaslet, C.A. (1997) Regulation of mesothelial cell proliferation in vitro and in vivo. In: Dungworth, D.L., Adler, K.B., Harris, C.C. & Plopper, C.G., eds, *Correlations Between In Vitro and In Vivo Investigations in Inhalation Toxicology*, Washington DC, ILSI Press, pp. 163–171

Kanerva, L., Estlander, T. & Jolanki, R. (1995) Dental problems. In: Guin, J.D., ed., *Practical Contact Dermatitis*, New York, McGraw-Hill, pp. 397–432

Kang, H., Enziger, F., Breslin, P., Feil, M., Lee, Y. & Shepard, B. (1987) Soft tissue sarcoma and military service in Vietnam: a case–control study. *J. natl Cancer Inst.*, **79**, 693–699

Kaplan, R.P. (1987) Cancer complicating chronic ulcerative and scarifying mucocutaneous disorders. *Adv. Dermatol.*, **2**, 19–46

Kappert, H.F., Mau, J., Pfeiffer, P., Richter, G., Schneider, S., Schwickerath, H. & Siebert, G.K. (1998) *Verträglichheit von Dentallegieriungen unter besonderer Berücksichtigung 'alternativer' Verfahren zur Diagnostik*, Institut der Deutschen Zahnärzte, Köln, Deutscher Ärzte-Verlag

Karp, R.D., Johnson, K.H., Buoen, L.C., Ghobrial, H.K.G., Brand, I. & Brand, K.G. (1973) Tumorigenesis by Millipore filters in mice: histology and ultrastructure of tissue reactions as related to pore size. *J. natl Cancer Inst.*, **51**, 1275–1285

Kass, P., Barnes, W., Spangler, W., Chomel, B. & Culbertson, M. (1993) Epidemiologic evidence for a causal relation between vaccination and fibrosarcoma tumorigenesis in cats. *J. Am. vet. Med. Assoc.*, **203**, 396–405

Katabami, M., Dosaka-Akita, H., Honma, K., Kimura, K., Fujino, M., Uchida, Y., Mikami, H., Ohsaki, Y., Kawakami, Y. & Kikuchi, K. (1998) p53 and Bcl-2 expression in pneumoconiosis-related pre-cancerous lesions and lung cancers: frequent and preferential p53 expression in pneumoconiotic bronchiolar dysplasias. *Int. J. Cancer*, **75**, 504–511

Kathren, R.L., McInroy, J.F., Moore, R.H. & Dietert, S.E., (1989) Uranium in the tissues of an occupationally exposed individual. *Health Phys.*, **57**, 17–21

Katzner, M. & Schvingt, E. (1983) Complications of a total hip prosthesis revealing a renal cell carcinoma. *Arch. orthop. Trauma Surg.*, **102**, 126–127

Kawai, K., Yamamoto, M., Kameyama, S., Kawamata, H., Rademaker, A. & Oyasu, R. (1993) Enhancement of rat urinary bladder tumorigenesis by lipopolysaccharide-induced inflammation. *Cancer Res.*, **53**, 5172–5175

Kawai, A., Woodruff, J., Healey, J.H., Brennan, M.F., Antonescu, C.R. & Ladanyi, M. (1998) SYT–SSX gene fusion as a determinant of morphology and prognosis in synovial sarcoma. *New Engl. J. Med.*, **338**, 153–160

Keller (1938) *Haemangioendotheliom*, Thesis, Tübingen

Kelly, E.J. (1982) Electrochemical behavior of titanium. *Mod. Aspect. Electrochem.*, **14**, 319–424

Kelly, K.M., Womer, R.B., Sorensen, P.H.B., Xiong, Q.-B. & Barr, F.G. (1997) Common and variant gene fusions predict distinct clinical phenotypes in rhabdomyosarcoma. *J. clin. Oncol.*, **15**, 1831–1836

Kennedy, A.L., Wilson, T.R., Stock, M.F., Alarie, Y. & Brown, W.E. (1994) Distribution and reactivity of inhaled ^{14}C-labelled toluene diisocyanate (TDI) in rats. *Arch. Toxicol.*, **68**, 434–443

Kern, K.A., Flannery, J.T. & Kuehn, P.G. (1997) Carcinogenic potential of silicone breast implants: a Connecticut statewide study. *Plast. reconstr. Surg.*, **100**, 737–747

Kernohan, J. & Hall, A.J. (1985) Case report 297. *Skeletal Radiol.*, **13**, 77–79

Keruso, H., Moe, G. & Hensten-Pettersen, A. (1997) Salivary nickel and chromium in subjects with different types of fixed orthodontic appliances. *Am. J. Orthod. Dentofac. Orthop.*, **111**, 595–598

Khurana, J.S., Rosenberg, A.E., Kattapuram, S.V., Fernandez, O.S. & Ehara, S. (1991) Malignancy supervening on an intramedullary nail. *Clin. Orthop. rel. Res.*, **267**, 251–254

Kilpatrick, S.E., Koplay, P., Pope, T.L., Jr & Ward, W.G. (1997) Clinical radiologic and pathologic spectrum of myositis ossificans and related lesions: a unifying concept. *Adv. Anat. Pathol.*, **4**, 277–286

Kim, Y.-H. & Yun, Y.-H. (1986) Metastasis of lung carcinoma to proximal femur after hip implant. *Orthop. Rev.*, **15**, 91–96

Kine, B.B. (1981) Methacrylic polymers. In: Mark, H.F., Othmer, D.F., Overberger, C.G. & Seaborg, G.T., eds, *Kirk-Othmer Encyclopedia of Chemical Technology,* Vol. 15, 3rd Ed., New York, John Wiley, pp. 377–398

Kinoshita, Y., Kuzuhara, T., Kirigakubo, M., Kobayashi, M., Shimura, K. & Ikada, Y. (1993) Reduction in tumour formation on porous polyethylene by collagen immobilization. *Biomaterials*, **14**, 546–550

Kitchen, S.B., Paletta, C.E., Shehadi, S.I. & Bauer, W.C. (1994) Epithelialization of the lining of a breast implant capsule. Possible origin of squamous cell carcinoma associated with a breast implant capsule. *Cancer*, **73**, 1449–1452

Klärner, P. (1962) Production of sarcomas by foreign bodies made of polymethacrylates and additives. *Z. Krebsforsch.*, **65**, 99–100 (in German)

Knecht, C.D. & Priester, W.A. (1978) Osteosarcoma in dogs: a study of previous trauma, fracture, and fracture fixation. *J. Am. anim. Hosp. Assoc.*, **14**, 82–84

Knittel, D. (1983) Titanium and titanium alloys. In: Mark, H.F., Othmer, D.F., Overberger, C.G. & Seaborg, G.T., eds, *Kirk-Othmer Encyclopedia of Chemical Technology*, Vol. 23, 3rd Ed., New York, John Wiley, pp. 98–130

Knutson, K., Lewold, S., Robertsson, O. & Lidgren, L. (1994) The Swedish knee arthroplasty register. A nation-wide study of 30,003 knees 1976–1992. *Acta orthop. scand.*, **65**, 375–386

Ko, C., Ahn, C.Y. & Markowitz, B.L. (1995) Injected liquid silicone, chronic mastitis, and undetected breast cancer. *Ann. plast. Surg.*, **34**, 176–179

Kochhar, R.K. & Kissin, Y.V. (1981) Polymers of higher olefins. In: Mark, H.F., Othmer, D.F., Overberger, C.G. & Seaborg, G.T., eds, *Kirk-Othmer Encyclopedia of Chemical Technology*, Vol. 16, 3rd Ed., New York, John Wiley, pp. 470–479

Koda, T., Tsuchiya, H., Yamauchi, M., Ohtani, S., Takagi, N. & Kawano, J. (1990) Leachability of denture-base acrylic resins in artificial saliva. *Dent. Mater.*, **6**, 13–16

Kogan, A.H. & Tugarinova, V.N. (1959) On the blastomogenic action of polyvinyl chloride. *Vop. Onkol.*, **5**, 540–545 (in Russian)

Kohn, H. & Langer, R. (1996) Bioresorbable and bioerodible materials. In: Ratner, B.D., Hoffman, A.S., Schoen, F.J. & Lemons, J.E., eds, *Biomaterials Science: An Introduction to Materials in Medicine*, San Diego, Academic Press, pp. 64–73

Kolstadt, K. & Högstorp, H. (1990) Gastric carcinoma metastasis to a knee with a newly inserted prosthesis. A case report. *Acta orthop. scand.*, **61**, 369–370

Kopas, Mr (1929) Testicular sarcoma after trauma. *Zentralblatt. Chir.*, **56**, 83–84 (in German)

Korhonen, A., Hemminki, K. & Vainio, H. (1984) Embryotoxic effects of eight organic peroxides and hydrogen peroxide on three-day chicken embryos. *Environ. Res.*, **33**, 54–61

Krevet, Dr (1888) New sarcomatous growth in fistula 15 years after gunshot injury with retention of the bullet. *Dtsch. Militärärtz. Z.*, **17**, 241–248 (in German)

Krutenat, R.C. (1981) Metallic coatings. In: Mark, H.F., Othmer, D.F., Overberger, C.G. & Seaborg, G.T., eds, *Kirk-Othmer Encyclopedia of Chemical Technology*, Vol. 15, 3rd Ed., New York, John Wiley, pp. 241–274

Kulesh, D.A. & Greene, J.J. (1986) Shape-dependent regulation of proliferation in normal and malignant human cells and its alteration by interferon. *Cancer Res.*, **46**, 2793–2797

Kumar, K. (1996) Osteosarcoma associated with a metal implant. *Int. Orthop. (SICOT)*, **20**, 335–336

Kunze, P. (1965) Carcinogenesis after war injuries. *Arch. Geschwulstforsch.*, **25**, 97–117 (in German)

Kuo, T.T., Hu, S., Huang, C.L., Chan, H.L., Chang, M.J., Dunn, P. & Chen, Y.J. (1997) Cutaneous involvement in polyvinylpyrrolidone storage disease: a clinicopathologic study of five patients, including two patients with severe anemia. *Am. J. surg. Pathol.*, **21**, 1361–1367

Kurpat, D. & Baudrexl, A. (1971) Bullet foreign-body in the lung and scirrhous carcinoma. *Z. Chir.*, **18**, 608–617 (in German)

Kydd, W.L. & Sreebny, L.M. (1960) Potential oncogenic properties of high polymers in mice. *J. natl Cancer Inst.*, **25**, 749–751

Lai, F.M.-M. & Lam, W.Y. (1993) Nodular fasciitis of the dermis. *J. cutan. Pathol.*, **20**, 66–69

Lamovec, J., Zidar, A. & Cucek-Plenicar, M. (1988) Synovial sarcoma associated with total hip replacement. A case report. *J. Bone Joint Surg.*, **70A**, 1558–1560

Lanam, R.D. & Zysk, E.D. (1982) Platinum-group metals. In: Mark, H.F., Othmer, D.F., Overberger, C.G. & Seaborg, G.T., eds, *Kirk-Othmer Encyclopedia of Chemical Technology*, Vol. 18, 3rd Ed., New York, John Wiley, pp. 228–253

Langkamer, V.G., Case, C.P., Collins, C., Watt, I., Dixon, J., Kemp, A.J. & Atkins, R.M. (1997) Tumors around implants. *J. Arthroplasty*, **12**, 812–818

Laskin, D.M., Robinson, I.B. & Weinman, J.P. (1954) Experimental production of sarcomas by methylmethacrylate implants. *Proc. Soc. exp. Biol. Med.*, **87**, 329–332

Laskin, S., Drew, R.T., Cappiello, V.P. & Kuschner, M. (1972) Inhalation studies with freshly generated polyurethane foam dust. In: Mercer, T.T., ed., *Assessment of Airborne Particles, Fundamentals, Applications and Implications to Inhalation Toxicity*, Springfield, IL, C.C. Thomas, pp. 382–404

Laskin, W.B., Silverman, T.A. & Enzinger, F.M. (1988) Postradiation soft tissue sarcomas. An analysis of 53 cases. *Cancer*, **62**, 2330–2340

Lauer, D.H. & Enzinger, F.M. (1980) Cranial fasciitis of childhood. *Cancer*, **45**, 401–406

Lavorgna, J.J., Burstein, N.A., Schiller, A.L. & Harris, W.H. (1972) The carcinogenesis of plastics used in orthopedic surgery. *Clin. Ortho. rel. Res.*, **88**, 223–227

Lechner, J.F., Tesfaigzi, J. & Gerwin, B.I. (1997) Oncogenes and tumor-suppressor genes in mesothelioma—a synopsis. *Environ. Health Perspect.*, **105** (Suppl. 5), 1061–1067

Lee, Y.-S., Pho, R.W.H. & Nather, A. (1984) Malignant fibrous histiocytoma at site of metal implant. *Cancer*, **54**, 2286–2289

Lee, E.S., Locker, J., Nalesnik, M., Reyes, J., Jaffe, R., Alashari, M., Nour, B., Tzakis, A. & Dickman, P.S. (1995) The association of Epstein–Barr virus with smooth–muscle tumors occurring after organ transplantation. *New Engl. J. Med.*, **332**, 19–25

Lee, B.W., Wain, J.C., Kelsey, K.T., Wiencke, J.K. & Christiani, D.C. (1998) Association of cigarette smoking and asbestos exposure with location and histology of lung cancer. *Am. J. respir. crit. Care Med.*, **157**, 748–755

Lehmann, F., Leyhausen, G., Spahl, W. & Geurtsen, W. (1993) Comparative cell culture studies of the cytotoxicity of composite resin components. *Dtsch. Zahnärztl. Z.*, **48**, 651–653 (in German)

Leicher, H. (1950) Development of a malignant tumour with a long latency. *Z. Laryngol. Rhinol. Otol.*, **29**, 557–564 (in German)

Leinfelder, K.F. (1988) Posterior composit resins. *J. Am. dent. Assoc.*, **117**, 21–26

Lenz, R.W. (1989) Polymerization mechanisms and processes. In: Grayson, M., Mark, H.F., Othmer, D.F. & Othmer, D.F., eds, *Kirk-Othmer Concise Encyclopedia of Chemical Technology*, Vol. 18, 3rd Ed., New York, John Wiley, pp. 933–934

Lester, S., Clemett, T.Y. & Burt, A. (1996) Vaccine site-associated sarcomas in cats: clinical experience and a laboratory review (1982–1993). *J. Am. anim. Hosp. Assoc.*, **32**, 91–95

Levresse, V., Renier, A., Fleury-Feith, J., Levy, F., Moritz, S., Vivo, C., Pilatte, Y. & Jaurand, M.-C. (1997) Analysis of cell cycle disruptions in cultures of rat pleural mesothelial cells exposed to asbestos fibers. *Am. J. respir. Cell mol. Biol.*, **17**, 660–671

Lewis, C.M. (1980) Inflammatory carcinoma of the breast following silicone injections. *Plast. reconstr. Surg.*, **66**, 134–136

Lewis, C.G., Belniak, R.M., Plowman, M.C., Hopfer, S.M., Knight, J.A. & Sunderman, F.W., Jr (1995) Intraarticular carcinogenesis bioassays of CoCrMo and TiAlV alloys in rats. *J. Arthroplasty*, **10**, 75–82

Lewold, S., Olsson, H., Gustafson, P., Rydholm, A. & Lidgren, L. (1996) Overall cancer incidence not increased after prosthetic knee replacement: 14,551 patients followed for 66,622 person-years. *Int. J. Cancer*, **68**, 30–33

Leyhausen, G., Heil, J., Reifferscheid, G. & Geurtsen, W. (1995) The genotoxic potential of resin components. *Dtsch. Zahnärztl. Z.*, **50**, 134–136 (in German)

Li, Y., Noblitt, T.W., Dunipace, A.J. & Stookey, G.K. (1990) Evaluation of mutagenicity of restorative dental materials using the Ames Salmonella/microsome test. *J. dent. Res.*, **69**, 1188–1192

Li, X.Q., Hom, D.L., Black, J. & Stevenson, S. (1993) Relationship between metallic implants and cancer: A case-control study in a canine population. *Vet. comp. Orthop. Traumatol.*, **6**, 70–74

Liczkowski, B. & Barnbeck, F. (1984) Breast carcinoma in pacemaker patients. *Zentralbl. Chir.*, **109**, 880–881 (in German)

Lilla, J.A. & Vistnes, L.M. (1976) Long-term study of reactions to various silicone breast implants in rabbits. *Plastic reconstr. Surg.*, **57**, 637–649

Lind, P.O. (1988) Oral lichenoid reactions related to composite restorations. *Acta odontol. scand.*, **46**, 63–65

Lindeman, G., McKay, M.J., Taubman, L.K. & Bilous, A.M. (1990) Malignant fibrous histiocytoma developing in bone 44 years after shrapnel trauma. *Cancer*, **66**, 2229–2232

Linden, M.A., Marton, W.I., Stewart, R.M., Thal, E.R. & Feit, W. (1982) Lead poisoning from retained bullets. Pathogenesis, diagnosis, and management. *Ann. Surg.*, **195**, 305–313

Liu, J.-Y., Morris, G.F., Lei, W.-H., Corti, M. & Brody, A.R. (1996) Up-regulated expression of transforming growth factor-α in the bronchiolar-alveolar duct regions of asbestos-exposed rats. *Am. J. Pathol.*, **149**, 205–217

Liu, C., Wang, W., Shen, W., Chen, T., Hu, L. & Chen, Z. (1997) Evaluation of the biocompatibility of a nonceramic hydroxyapatite. *J. Endodontics*, **23**, 490–493

Lloyd, T.B. & Showak, W. (1984) Zinc and zinc alloys. In: Mark, H.F., Othmer, D.F., Overberger, C.G. & Seaborg, G.T., eds, *Kirk-Othmer Encyclopedia of Chemical Technology*, Vol. 24, 3rd Ed., New York, John Wiley, pp. 807–851

Löwenthal, C. (1895) Traumatic origin of a tumour. *Langenbecks Arch. klin. Chir.*, **49**, 335–352 (in German)

Lucas, D.R., Shroyer, K.R., McCarthy, P.J., Markham, N.E., Fujita, M. & Enomoto, T.E. (1997) Desmoid tumor is a clonal cellular proliferation: PCR amplification of HUMARA for analysis of patterns of X-chromosome inactivation. *Am. J. surg. Pathol.*, **21**, 306–311

Luckow, Dr (1933) Lung carcinoma following fragment in the lung 14 years after injury. *Z. ärtzl. Fortbild.*, **30**, 702–703 (in German)

Luke, J.L., Kalasinsky, V.F., Turnicky, R.P., Centeno, J.A., Johnson, F.B. & Mullick, F.G. (1997) Pathological and biophysical findings associated with silicone breast implants: A study of capsular tissues from 86 cases. *Plast. reconstr. Surg.*, **100**, 1558–1565

Luster, M.I. (1993) *Immunotoxicity of Silicone in Female B6C3F1 Mice—180 Day Exposure* (Report to NTP, Protocol SIL-180-1-SC), Washington DC, US Department of Health and Human Services

Luu, H.-M., Hutter, J.C. & Bushar, H.F. (1998) A physiologically based pharmacokinetic model for 2,4-toluenediamine leached from polyurethane foam-covered breast implants. *Environ. Health Perspect.*, **106**, 393–400

Lykissa, E.D., Kala, S.V., Hurley, J. & Lebovitz, R.M. (1997) Release of low molecular weight silicones and platinum from breast gel implants. *Anal. Chem.*, 69, 4912–4916

Macdonald, J.L. & Kane, A.B. (1997) Mesothelial cell proliferation and biopersistence of wollastonite and crocidolite asbestos fibers. *Fundam. appl. Toxicol.*, **38**, 173–183

Macdonald, P., Plavac, N., Peters, W., Lugowski, S. & Smith, D. (1995) Failure of ^{29}Si NMR to detect increased blood silicon levels in silicone gel breast implant recipients. *Anal. Chem.*, **67**, 3799–3801

Machle, W. (1940) Lead absorption from bullets lodged in tissues. *J. Am. med. Assoc.*, **115**, 1536–1541

Maddox, A., Schoenfeld, A., Sinnett, H.D. & Shousha, S. (1993) Breast carcinoma occurring in association with silicone augmentation. *Histopathology*, **23**, 379–382

Madewell, B.R., Pool, R.R. & Leighton, R.L. (1977) Osteogenic sarcoma at the site of a chronic nonunion fracture and internal fixation device in a dog. *J. Am. vet. Med. Assoc.*, **171**, 187–189

Maekawa, A., Ogiu, T., Onodera, H., Furuta, K., Matsuoka, C., Ohno, Y., Tanigawa, H., Salmo, G.S., Matsuyama, M. & Hayashi, Y. (1984) Foreign-body tumorigenesis in rats by various kinds of plastics—induction of malignant fibrous histiocytomas. *J. toxicol. Sci.*, **9**, 263–272

Magilligan, D.J., Jr & Isshak, G. (1980) Carcinoma of the breast in a pacemaker pocket—simple recurrence or oncotaxis? *PACE*, **3**, 220–223

Magos, L. (1994) Lead poisoning from retained lead projectiles. A critical review of case reports. *Hum. exp. Toxicol.*, **13**, 735–742

Maier, W. & Beck, C. (1992) Laryngeal cancer following gunshot injury and paraffin injection. *Laryngo-Rhino-Otol.*, **71**, 83–85 (in German)

Malchau, H. & Herberts, P. (1998) Prognosis of total hip replacement. Revision and re-revision rate in THR. A revision-risk study of 148,359 primary operations. In: *61st annual meeting of the American Academy of Orthopaedic Surgeons, February 22–26, 1996, Altanta, USA*, Göteberg, The National Hip Arthroplasty Register

Malchau, H., Herberts, P. & Ahnfelt, L. (1993) Prognosis of total hip replacement. Follow-up on 92,675 operations performed 1978–1990. *Acta orthop. scand.*, **64**, 497–506

Malone, K.E., Stanford, J.L., Daling, J.R. & Voigt, L.F. (1992) Implants and breast cancer (Letter to the Editor). *Lancet*, **339**, 1365

Mannick, E.E., Bravo, L.E., Zarama, G., Realpe, J.L., Zhang, X.-J., Ruiz, B., Fontham, E.T.H., Mera, R., Miller, M.J.S. & Correa, P. (1996) Inducible nitric oxide synthase, nitrotyrosine, and apoptosis in *Helicobacter pylori* gastritis: effect of antibiotics and antioxidants. *Cancer Res.*, **56**, 3238–3243

Manton, W.I. & Thal, E.R. (1986) Lead poisoning from retained missiles. An experimental study. *Ann. Surg.*, **204**, 594–599

Marcus, D.M. (1996) An analytical review of silicone immunology. *Arthritis Rheum.*, **39**, 1619–1626

Mark, R.J., Poen, J., Tran, L.M., Fu, Y.S., Selch, M.T. & Parker, R.G. (1994) Postirradiation sarcomas. A single–institution study and review of the literature. *Cancer*, **73**, 2653–2662

Martin, A., Bauer, T.W., Manley, M.T. & Marks, K.E. (1988) Osteosarcoma at the site of total hip replacement. A case report. *J. Bone Joint Surg.*, **70A**, 1561–1567

Mathiesen, E.B., Ahlbom, A., Bermann, G. & Lindgren, J.U. (1995) Total hip replacement and cancer. A cohort study. *J. Bone Joint Surg.*, **77B**, 345–350

May, O. (1937) Sarcoma of the forearm after war injury. *Zentralbl. Chir.*, **64**, 1889–1894 (in German)

May, D.S. & Stroup, N.E. (1991) The incidence of sarcomas of the breast among women in the United States, 1973–1986. *Plast. reconstr. Surg.*, **87**, 193–194

Mayall, F.G., Goddard, H. & Gibbs, A.R. (1992) p53 immunostaining in the distinction between benign and malignant mesothelial proliferations using formalin-fixed paraffin sections. *J. Pathol.*, **168**, 377–381

Mazabraud, A., Florent, J. & Laurent, M. (1989) A case of epidermoid carcinoma developed in contact with a hip prosthesis. *Bull. Cancer*, **76**, 573–581 (in French)

McCarthy, T.J., Hayes, E.P., Schwartz, C.S. & Witz, G. (1994) The reactivity of selected acrylate esters toward glutathione and deoxyribonucleosides *in vitro*: structure–activity relationships. *Fund. appl. Toxicol.*, **22**, 543–548

McCarthy, P.E., Hedlund, C.S., Veazy, R.S., Prescott-Mathews, J. & Cho, D.Y. (1996) Liposarcoma associated with a glass foreign body in a dog. *J. Am. vet. med. Assoc.*, **209**, 612–614

McCarthy, S.J., Meijs, G.F., Mitchell, N., Gunatillake, P.A., Heath, G., Brandwood, A. & Schindhelm, K. (1997) In-vivo degradation of polyurethanes: transmission-FTIR microscopic characterisation of polyurethanes sectioned by cryomicrotomy. *Biomaterials*, **18**, 1387–1409

McClain, K.L., Leach, C.T., Jenson, H.B., Joshi, V.V., Pollock, B.H., Parmley, R.T., DiCarlo, F.J., Chadwick, E.G. & Murphy, S.B. (1995) Association of Epstein–Barr virus with leiomyosarcomas in children with AIDS. *New Engl. J. Med.*, **332**, 12–18

McDonald, I. (1981) Malignant lymphoma associated with internal fixation of a fractured tibia. *Cancer*, **48**, 1009–1011

McDougall, A. (1956) Malignant tumour at site of bone plating. *J. Bone Joint Surg.*, **38B**, 709–713

McElfresh, E. (1991) History of arthroplasty. In: Petty, W., ed., *Total Joint Replacement*, Philadelphia, W.B. Saunders, pp. 3–18

McInnes-Ledoux, P., Cleaton-Jones, P.E. & Austin, J.C. (1985) The pulpal response to dilute citric acid smear removers. *J. oral Rehabil.*, **12**, 215–228

McKellop, H., Park, S.-H., Chiesa, R., Doorn, P., Lu, B., Normand, P., Grigoris, P. & Amstutz, H. (1996) In vivo wear of 3 types of metal on metal hip prostheses during 2 decades of use. *Clin. Orthop. rel. Res.*, **329** (Suppl.), S128–S140

McLaughlin, J.K., Fraumeni, J.F., Jr, Olsen, J. & Mellemkjaer, L. (1994) Re: Breast implants, cancer and systemic sclerosis (Letter to the Editor). *J. natl Cancer Inst.*, **86**, 1424

McLaughlin, J.K., Olsen, J.H., Friis, S., Mellemkjaer, L. & Fraumeni, J.F., Jr (1995a) Re: Breast implants, cancer, and systemic sclerosis (Letter to the Editor). *J. natl Cancer Inst.*, **87**, 1415–1416

McLaughlin, J.K., Fraumeni, J.F., Jr, Nyren, O. & Adami, H.-O. (1995b) Silicone breast implants and risk of cancer? (Letter to the Editor). *J. Am. Med. Assoc.*, **273**, 116

McLaughlin, J.K., Nyrén, O., Blot, W.J., Yin, L., Josefsson, S., Fraumeni, J.F., Jr & Adami, H.-O. (1998) Cancer risk among women with cosmetic breast implants: a population-based cohort study in Sweden. *J. natl Cancer Inst.*, **90**, 156–158

McQueen, D., Sundgren, J.-E., Ivarsson, B., Lundström, I., af Ekenstrom B., Svensson, A., Brånemark, P.-I., & Albrektsson, T. (1982) Auger electroscopic studies of titanium implants. In: Lee, A.I.C., Albrektsson, T. & Brånemark, P.-I., eds, *Clinical Application of Biomaterials*, New York, John Wiley, pp. 179–185

Meachim, G., Pedley, R.B. & Williams, D.F. (1982) A study of sarcogenicity associated with Co-Cr-Mo particles implanted in animal muscle. *J. biomed. Mat. Res.*, **16**, 407–416

Meis, J.M. & Enzinger, F.M. (1991) Inflammatory fibrosarcoma of the mesentery and retroperitoneum. A tumor closely simulating inflammatory pseudotumor. *Am. J. surg. Pathol.*, **15**, 1146–1156

Meis, J.M. & Enzinger, F.M. (1992) Proliferative fasciitis and myositis of childhood. *Am. J. surg. Pathol.*, **16**, 364–372

Meister, P., Bückmann, F.W. & Konrad, E. (1978) Nodular fasciitis (analysis of 100 cases and review of the literature). *Pathol. Res. Pract.*, **162**, 133–165

Melzner, E. (1927) On sarcoma development following war injuries. *Langenbecks Arch. Klin.*, **147**, 153–161 (in German)

Memoli, V.A., Urban, R.M., Alroy, J. & Galante, J.O. (1986) Malignant neoplasms associated with orthopedic implant materials in rats. *J. orthoped. Res.*, **4**, 346–355

Menard, S. & Della Porta, G. (1976) Incidence, growth and antigenicity of fibrosarcomas induced by Teflon disc in mice. *Tumori*, **62**, 565–573

Mendez-Fernandez, M.A., Henly, W.S., Geis, R.C., Schoen, F.J. & Hausner, R.J. (1980) Paget's disease of the breast after subcutaneous mastectomy and reconstruction with a silicone prosthesis. *Plast. reconstr. Surg.*, **65**, 683–685

Meneses, M.F., Unni, K.K. & Swee, R.G. (1993) Bizarre parosteal osteochondromatous proliferation of bone (Nora's lesion). *Am. J. surg. Pathol.*, **17**, 691–697

Menon, A.G., Anderson, K.M., Riccardi, V.M., Chung, R.Y., Whaley, J.M., Yandell, D.W., Farmer, G.E., Freiman, R.N., Lee, J.K., Li, F.P., Barker, D.F., Ledbetter, D.H., Kleider, A., Martuza, R.L., Gusella, J.F. & Seizinger, B.R. (1990) Chromosome 17p deletions and p53 gene mutations associated with the formation of malignant neurofibrosarcomas in von Recklinghausen neurofibromatosis. *Proc. natl Acad. Sci. USA*, **87**, 5435–5439

Merritt, K. & Brown, S.A. (1995) Distribution of titanium and vanadium following repeated injection of high-dose salts. *J. biomed. Mater. Res.*, **29**, 1175–1178

Merritt, K. & Brown, S.A. (1996) Distribution of cobalt chromium wear and corrosion products and biologic reactions. *Clin. Orthop. rel. Res.*, **329** (Suppl.), S233–S243

Merritt, K., Brown, S.A. & Sharkey, N.A. (1984a) Blood distribution of nickel, cobalt, and chromium following intramuscular injection into hamsters. *J. biomed. Mater. Res.*, **18**, 991–1004

Merritt, K., Brown, S.A. & Sharkey, N.A. (1984b) The binding of metal salts and corrosion products to cells and proteins *in vitro*. *J. biomed. Mater. Res.*, **18**, 1005–1015

Merritt, K., Wenz, L. & Brown, S.A. (1991) Cell association of fretting corrosion products generated in a cell culture. *J. orthop. Res.*, **9**, 289–296

Merwin, R.M. & Redmon, L.W. (1963) Induction of plasma cell tumors and sarcomas in mice by diffusion chambers placed in the peritoneal cavity. *J. natl Cancer Inst.*, **31**, 997–1017

Meryon, S.D. & Brook, A.M. (1989) *In vitro* cytotoxicity of three dentine bonding agents. *J. Dent.*, **17**, 279–283

Mesnil, M. & Yamasaki, H. (1993) Cell-cell communication and growth of normal and cancer cells: evidence and hypothesis. *Mol. Carcinog.*, **7**, 14–17

Miller, E.G., Washington, V.H., Bowles, W.H. & Zimmermann, E.R. (1986) Mutagenic potential of some chemical components of dental materials. *Dent. Mater.*, **2**, 163–165

Miller, A.C., Fuciarelli, A.F., Jackson, W.E., Ejnik, E.J., Emond, C., Strocko, S., Hogan, J., Page, N. & Pellmar, T. (1998a) Urinary and serum mutagenicity studies with rats implanted with depleted uranium or tantalum pellets. *Mutagenesis*, **13**, 643–648

Miller, A.C., Blakely, W.F., Livengood, D., Whittaker, T., Xu, J., Ejnik, J.W., Hamilton, M.M., Parlette, E., St. John, T., Gerstenberg, H.M. & Hsu, H. (1998b) Transformation of human osteoblast cells to the tumorigenic phenotype by depleted uranium-uranyl chloride. *Environ. Health Perspect.*, **106**, 465–471

Mills, G. & Cusumano, J.A. (1979) Catalysis. In: Mark, H.F., Othmer, D.F., Overberger, C.G. & Seaborg, G.T., eds, *Kirk-Othmer Encyclopedia of Chemical Technology*, Vol. 5, 3rd Ed., New York, John Wiley, pp. 16–61

Mishra A., Liu, J.-Y., Brody, A.R. & Morris, G.F. (1997) Inhaled asbestos fibers induce p53 expression in the rat lung. *Am. J. respir. Cell mol. Biol.*, **16**, 479–485

Mitchell, D.F., Shankwalker, G.B. & Shazer, S. (1960) Determining the tumorigenicity of dental materials. *J. dent. Res.*, **39**, 1023–1028

Mitelman, F., Fregert, S., Hedner, K. & Hillbertz-Nilsson, K. (1980) Occupational exposure to epoxy resins has no cytogenetic effect. *Mutat. Res.*, **77**, 345–348

Mjör, I.A. & Moorhead, J.E. (1998) Selection of restorative materials, reasons for replacement and longevity of restorations in Florida. *J. Am. Coll. Dent.*, **65**, 27–33

Mohanan, P.V. & Rathinam, K. (1996) Effect of bone wax extract on the frequency of bone marrow erythrocyte micronuclei in mice. *Vet. hum. Toxicol.*, **38**, 427–428

Moizhess, T.G. & Vasiliev, J.M. (1989) Early and late stages of foreign-body carcinogenesis can be induced by implants of different shapes. *Int. J. Cancer*, **44**, 449–453

Monkman, G.R., Orwoll, G. & Ivins, J.C. (1974) Trauma and oncogenesis. *Mayo Clin. Proc.*, **49**, 157–163

Monsein, L.H. (1997a) Primer on medical device regulation: part I. History and background. *Radiology*, **205**, 1–9

Monsein, L.H. (1997b) Primer on medical device regulation: part II. Regulation of medical devices by the U.S. Food and Drug Administration. *Radiology*, **205**, 10–18

Montag, C. & Mondry, F. (1952) Ulcerations and fistular cancer following war injuries. *Strahlentherapie*, **87**, 104–112 (in German)

Monteny, E., Delespesse, G., Screyen, H. & Spiette, M. (1978) Methylmethacrylate hypersensitivity in orthopaedic surgery. *Acta orthop. scand.*, **49**, 186–191

Montgomery, E.A. & Meis, J.M. (1991) Nodular fasciitis. Its morphologic spectrum and immunohistochemical profile. *Am. J. surg. Pathol.*, **15**, 942–948

Montgomery, E.A., Meis, J.M., Mitchell, M.S. & Enzinger, F.M. (1992) Atypical decubital fibroplasia. A distinctive fibroblastic pseudotumor occurring in debilitated patients. *Am. J. surg. Pathol.*, **16**, 708–715

Moore, R.M., Jr, Hamburger, S., Jeng, L.L. & Hamilton, P.M. (1991) Orthopedic implant devices: prevalence and sociodemographic findings from the 1988 National Health Interview Survey. *J. appl. Biomat.*, **2**, 127–131

Morgan, R.W. & Elcock, M.E. (1995) Artificial implants and soft tissue sarcomas. *J. clin. Epidemiol.*, **48**, 545–549

Morgenstern, L., Gleischman, S.H., Michel, S.L., Rosenberg, J.E., Knight, I. & Goodman, D. (1985) Relation of free silicone to human breast carcinoma. *Arch. Surg.*, **120**, 573–577

Morrissey, R.E., George, J.D., Price, C.J., Tyl, R.W., Marr, M.C. & Kimmel, C.A. (1987) The developmental toxicity of bisphenol A in rats and mice. *Fundam. appl. Toxicol.*, **8**, 571–582

Morrow, P.E., Haseman, J.K., Hobbs, C.H., Driscoll, K.E., Vu, V. & Oberdörster, G. (1996) The maximum tolerated dose for inhalation bioassays: toxicity vs overload. *Fundam. appl. Toxicol.*, **29**, 155–167

Morse, D. & Steiner, R.M. (1985) Cardiac valve identification atlas and guide. In: Morse, D., Steiner, R.M. & Fernandez, J., eds, *Guide to Prosthetic Cardiac Valves*, New York, Springer-Verlag, pp. 257–346

Mossman, B.T., Faux, S., Janssen, Y., Jimenez, L.A., Timblin, C., Zanella, C., Goldberg, J., Walsh, E., Barchowsky, A. & Driscoll, K. (1997) Cell signaling pathways elicited by asbestos. *Environ. Health Perspect.*, **105** (Suppl. 5), 1121–1125

Mrksich, M. & Whitesides, G.M. (1996) Using self-assembled monolayers to understand the interactions of man-made surfaces with proteins and cells. *Annu. Rev. Biophys. Biomol. Struct.*, **25**, 55–78

Muhle, H., Bellman, B., Takenaka, S., Fuhst, R., Mohr, U. & Pott, F. (1992) Chronic effects of intratracheally instilled nickel-containing particles in hamsters. In: Nieboer, E. & Nriagu, J.O., eds, *Nickel and Human Health: Current Perspectives*, New York, John Wiley, pp. 467–479

Müller, H. R. (1939) Accident and brain tumour. *Zentralbl. Chir.*, **20**, 1164 (in German)

Munksgaard, E.C. (1992) Permeability of protective gloves to (di)methacrylates in resinous dental materials. *Scand. J. dent. Res.*, **100**, 189–192

Munksgaard, E.C. & Freund, M. (1990) Enzymatic hydrolysis of (di)methacrylates and their polymers. *Scand. J. dent. Res.*, **98**, 261–267

Murakata, L.A. & Rangwala, A.F. (1989) Silicone lymphadenopathy with concomitant malignant lymphoma. *J. Rheumatol.*, **16**, 1480–1482

Murphy, S.T., Parker, R.B. & Woodard, J.C. (1997) Osteosarcoma following total hip arthroplasty in a dog. *J. small Anim. Pract.*, **38**, 263–267

Murray, D.W., Carr, A.J. & Bulstrode, C.J. (1994) Which primary total hip replacement? *J. Bone Joint Surg.*, **77B**, 520–527

Nagamoto, T. & Eguchi, G. (1997) Morphologic compatibility of intraocular lens haptics and the lens capsule. *J. Cataract refract. Surg.*, **23**, 1254–1259

Naim, J.O., Lanzafame, R.J. & van Oss, C.J. (1993) The adjuvant effect of silicone-gel on antibody formation in rats. *Immunol. Invest.*, **22**, 151–161

Nakada, T., Higo, N., Iijima, M., Nakayama, H. & Maibach, H.I. (1997) Patch test materials for mercury allergic contact dermatitis. *Contact Derm.*, **36**, 237–239

Nakamoto, B., Guidotti, L.G., Kuhlen, C.V., Fowler, P. & Chisari, F.V. (1998) Immune pathogenesis of hepatocellular carcinomas. *J. exp. Med.*, **188**, 341–350

Nakamura, M., Imai, K., Oshima, H., Kudo, T., Yoshioka, S. & Kawahara, H. (1985) Biocompatibility test of light-cured composites in vitro. *Dental Mater. J.*, **4**, 231–237

Nakamura, A., Kawasaki, Y., Takada, K., Aida, Y., Kurokawa, Y., Kojima, S., Shintani, H., Matsui, M., Nohmi, T., Matsuoka, A., Sofuni, T., Kurihara, M., Miyata, N., Uchima, T. & Fujimaki, M. (1992) Difference in tumor incidence and other tissue responses to polyetherurethanes and polydimethylsiloxane in long-term subcutaneous implantation into rats. *J. biomed. Mater. Res.*, **26**, 631–650

Nakamura, T., Shimizu, Y., Okumura, N., Matsui, T., Hyon, S.-H. & Shimamoto, T. (1994) Tumorigenicity of poly-L-lactide (PLLA) plates compared with medical-grade polyethylene. *J. biomed. Mater. Res.*, **28**, 17–25

Nakamura, A., Kojima, S., Isama, K., Umemura, T., Kawasaki, Y., Takada, K., Tsuda, M. & Kurokawa, Y. (1995) The effects of oligomers content and surface morphology on foreign-body tumorigenesis with polyetherurethanes: two years subcutaneous implantation study in rats. *J. long-term Effects med. Implants*, **5**, 263–273

Nakamura, A., Tsuchiya, T., Nakaoka, R., Wang, C., Nakamura, T., Imai, K. & Inoue, H. (1997) Studies on the development of evaluation method for the material/tissue interaction. In: *Annual Report of Cooperative Research Projects between Governmental and Private Institutions*, Part IV, Tokyo, Japan Health Science Foundation, pp. 123–132

Nakamura, T., Shimizu, Y., Takimoto, Y., Tsuda, T., Li, Y.-H., Kiyotani, T., Teramachi, M., Hyon, S.-H., Ikada, Y. & Nishiya, K. (1998) Biodegradation and tumorigenicity of implanted plates made from a copolymer of ε-caprolactone and L-lactide in rats. *J. biomed. Mater. Res.*, **42**, 475–484

Nakaoka, R., Tsuchiya, T., Kato, K., Ikada, Y. & Nakamura, A. (1997) Studies on tumor-promoting activity of polyethylene: inhibitory activity of metabolic cooperation on polyethylene surfaces is markedly decreased by surface modification with collagen but not with RGDS peptide. *J. biomed. Mater. Res.*, **35**, 391–397

Nasjleti, C.E., Castelli, W.A. & Caffesse, R.G. (1983) Effects of composite restorations on the periodontal membrane in monkeys. *J. dent. Res.*, **62**, 75–78

Nassiri, M.R., Hanks, C.T., Cameron, M.J., Strawn, S.E. & Craig, R.G. (1994) Application of flow cytometry to determine the cytotoxicity of urethane dimethacrylate in human cells. *J. biomed. Mater. Res.*, **28**, 153–158

National Technical Program (1992) NTP Technical Report on Toxicity Studies of 2-Hydroxy-4-Methoxybenzophenone, Administered Topically and in Dosed Feed to F344/N Rats and B6C3F1 Mice (Report Tx-21), Washington DC, US Department of Health and Human Services

Nelson, J.P. & Phillips, P.H. (1990) Malignant fibrous histiocytoma associated with total hip replacement. A case report. *Orthop. Rev.*, **19**, 1078–1080

Nelson, H.H., Wiencke, J.K., Gunn, L., Wain, J.C., Christiani, D.C. & Kelsey, K.T. (1998) Chromosome 3p14 alterations in lung cancer: evidence that *FHIT* exon deletion is a target of tobacco carcinogens and asbestos. *Cancer Res.*, **58**, 1804–1807

Nishimoto, S., Matsushita, T., Matsumoto, K. & Adachi, S. (1996) A rare case of burn scar malignancy. *Burns*, **22**, 497–499

Nolte, D. (1966) On sarcoma development following war injuries. *Monatschr. Unfallheilk. Versicher. Versorg. Verkehrmed.*, **69**, 124–135 (in German)

Nora, F.E., Dahlin, D.C. & Beabout, J.W. (1983) Bizarre parosteal osteochondromatous proliferations of the hands and feet. *Am. J. Surg. Pathol.*, **7**, 245–250

Nothdurft, H. (1955) Experimental occurrence of sarcomas in rats and mice after implantation of round disks of gold, silver, platin or ivory. *Naturwissenschaften*, **42**, 75–76 (in German)

Nothdurft, H. (1956) Experimental induction of sarcomas by implants. *Strahlentherapie*, **100**, 192–210 (in German)

Nyrén, O., McLaughlin, J.K., Gridley, G., Ekbom, A., Johnell, O., Fraumeni, J.F., Jr & Adami, H.-O. (1995) Cancer risk after hip relacement with metal implants: a population based cohort study in Sweden. *J. natl Cancer Inst.*, **87**, 28–33

Oberdörster, G. (1997) Pulmonary carcinogenicity of inhaled particles and the maximum tolerated dose. *Environ. Health Perspect.*, **105** (Suppl. 5), 1347–1356

O'Connell, T.X., Fee, H.J. & Golding, A. (1976) Sarcoma associated with Dacron prosthetic material. Case report and review of the literature. *J. thorac. cardiovasc. Surg.*, **72**, 94–96

Ognibene, F.A. & Theodoulou, M.H. (1991) Long-standing reaction to a hemi-silastic implant. *J. Foot Surg.*, **30**, 156–159

Okada, T. & Ikada, Y. (1995) Surface modification of silicone for percutaneous implantation. *J. biomater. Sci. Polym. Ed.*, **7**, 171–180

Olea, N., Pulgar, R., Pérez, P., Olea-Serrano, F., Rivas, A., Novello-Fertrell, A., Pedrza, V., Soto, A.M. & Sonnenschein, C. (1996) Estrogenicity of resin-based composites and sealants used in dentistry. *Environ. Health Perspect.*, **104**, 298–305

Olsen, J.H., McLaughlin, J.K., Nyrén, O., Mellemkjaer, L., Lipworth, L., Blot, W.J. & Fraumeni, J.F., Jr (1999) Hip and knee implantations among patients with osteoarthritis and risk of cancer: a record-linkage study from Denmark. *Int. J. Cancer*, **81**, 719–722

Ol'shevskaya, L.V. (1962) Changes in rat connective tissue associated with the development of tumors caused by implantation of cellophane. *Bull. exp. Biol. Med. (USSR)*, **52**, 1419–1422

Oppenheimer, B.S., Oppenheimer, E.T. & Stout, A.P. (1948) Sarcomas induced in rats by implanting cellophane. *Proc. Soc. exp. Biol. Med.*, **67**, 33–34

Oppenheimer, B.S., Oppenheimer, E.T. & Stout, A.P. (1952) Sarcomas induced in rodents by imbedding various plastic films. *Proc. Soc. exp. Biol. Med.*, **79**, 366–369

Oppenheimer, B.S., Oppenheimer, E.T., Stout, A.P. & Danishefsky, I. (1953) Malignant tumors resulting from embedding plastics in rodents. *Science*, **118**, 305–306

Oppenheimer, B.S., Oppenheimer, E.T., Danishefsky, I., Stout, A.P. & Eirich, F.R. (1955) Further studies of polymers as carcinogenic agents in animals. *Cancer Res.*, **15**, 333–340

Oppenheimer, B.S., Oppenheimer, E.T., Danishefsky, I. & Stout, A.P. (1956) Carcinogenic effect of metals in rodent. *Cancer Res.*, **16**, 439–441

Oppenheimer, B.S., Oppenheimer, E.T., Stout, A.P., Willhite, M. & Danishefsky, I. (1958) The latent period in carcinogenesis by plastics in rats and its relation to the presarcomatous stage. *Cancer*, **11**, 204–213

Oppenheimer, E.T., Willhite, M., Danishefsky, I. & Stout, A.P. (1961) Observations on the effects of powdered polymer in the carcinogenic process. *Cancer Res.*, **21**, 132–137

Oppenheimer, E.T., Willhite, M., Stout, A.P., Danishefsky, I. & Fishman, M.M. (1964) A comparative study of the effects of imbedding cellophane and polystyrene films in rats. *Cancer Res.*, **24**, 379–387

Ørstavik, D. & Hongslo, J.K. (1985) Mutagenicity of endodontic sealers. *Biomaterials*, **6**, 129–132

Ousterhout, D.K. & Stelnicki, E.J. (1996) Plastic surgery's plastics. *Clin. Plast. Surg.*, **23**, 183–190

Øysæd, H., Ruyter, I.E. & Sjøvik Kleven, I.J. (1988) Release of formaldehyde from dental composites. *J. dent. Res.*, **67**, 1289–1294

Paavolainen, P., Pukkala, E., Pulkkinen, P. & Visuri, T. (1999) Cancer incidence in Finnish hip replacement patients from 1980 to 1995. A nationwide cohort study involving 31,651 patients. *J. Arthroplasty*, **14**, 272–280

Pache, J.-C., Janssen, Y.M.W., Walsh, E.S., Quinlan, T.R., Zanella, C.L., Low, R.B., Taatjes, D.J. & Mossman, B.T. (1998) Increased epidermal growth factor-receptor protein in a human mesothelial cell line in response to long asbestos fibers. *Am. J. Pathol.*, **152**, 333–340

Paletta, C., Paletta, F.X., Jr & Paletta, F.X., Sr (1992) Squamous cell carcinoma following breast augmentation. *Ann. plast. Surg.*, **29**, 425–429

Pande, G.S. (1983) Thermoplastic polyurethanes as insulating materials for long-life cardiac pacing leads. *Pacing clin. Electrophysiol.*, **6**, 858–867

Pardo, A.D., Adams, W.H., McCraken, D. & Legendre, A.M. (1990) Primary jejunal osteosarcoma associated with a surgical sponge in a dog. *J. Am. vet. med. Assoc.*, **196**, 935–938

Parham, D.M. & Fisher, C. (1997) Angiosarcomas of the breast developing post radiotherapy. *Histopathology*, **31**, 189–195

Park, S.-H. & Aust, A.E. (1998) Participation of iron and nitric oxide in the mutagenicity of asbestos in $hgprt^-$, gpt^+ Chinese hamster V79 cells. *Cancer Res.*, **58**, 1144–1148

Parkin, D.M., Whelan, S.L., Ferlay, J., Raymond, L. & Young, J., eds (1997) *Cancer Incidence in Five Continents,* Vol. VII (IARC Scientific Publications No. 143), Lyon, IARC

Paschke, E. (1981) Ziegler process polyethylene. In: Mark, H.F., Othmer, D.F., Overberger, C.G. & Seaborg, G.T., eds, *Kirk-Othmer Encyclopedia of Chemical Technology,* Vol. 16, 3rd Ed., New York, John Wiley, pp. 433–452

Patchefsky, A.S. & Enzinger, F.M. (1981) Intravascular fasciitis: a report of 17 cases. *Am. J. surg. Pathol.*, **5**, 29–36

Paterson, H.S., Meredith, D.J. & Craddock, D.R. (1989) Malignant fibrous histiocytoma associated with a Dacron vascular prosthesis. *Ann. thorac. Surg.*, **47**, 772–774

Paulini, K., Beneke, G., Körner, B. & Enders, R. (1975) The relationship between the latent period and animal age in the development of foreign body sarcomas. *Beitr. Pathol.*, **154**, 161–169

Pellengahr, C., Jansson, V., Hagena, H.J. & Refior, H.J. (1997) Loosening of total knee arthroplasty, initiated by non-Hodgkin lymphoma. *Z. Orthop.*, **135**, 171–173 (in German)

Pellmar, T.C., Hogan, J.B., Benson, K.A. & Landauer, M.R. (1998) *Toxicological Evaluation of Depleted Uranium in Rats: Six-Month Evaluation Point* (AFRRI Special Publication 98-1), Bethesda, MD, Armed Forces Radiobiological Research Institute

Pellmar, T.C., Fuciarelli, A.F., Ejnik, J.W., Hamilton, M., Hogan, J., Strocko, S., Emond, C., Mottaz, H.M. & Landauer, M.R. (1999) Distribution of uranium in rats implanted with depleted uranium pellets. *Toxicol. Sci.*, **49**, 29–39

Penman, H.G. & Ring, P.A. (1984) Osteosarcoma in association with total hip replacement. *J. Bone Joint Surg.*, **66B**, 632–634

Pennisi, V.R. (1984) Obscure carcinoma encountered in subcutaneous mastectomy in silicone- and paraffin-injected breasts: two patients. *Plast. reconstr. Surg.*, **74**, 535–538

Peppas, N.A. (1996) Hydrogels. In: Ratner, B.D., Hoffman, A.S., Schoen, F.J. & Lemons, J.E. eds, *Biomaterial Science: An Introduction to Materials in Medicine*, San Diego, Academic Press, pp. 60–64

Pereira, M.C., Pereira, M.L. & Sousa, J.P. (1998) Evaluation of nickel toxicity on liver, spleen, and kidney of mice after administration of high-dose metal ion. *J. biomed. Mater. Res.*, **40**, 40–47

Perera, F.P. (1996) Molecular epidemiology: insights into cancer susceptibility, risk assessment, and prevention. *J. natl Cancer Inst.*, **88**, 496–509

Perosio, P.M. & Weiss, S.W. (1993) Ischemic fasciitis: a juxta-skeletal fibroblastic proliferation with a predilection for elderly patients. *Mod. Pathol.*, **6**, 69–72

Peter, L. (1966) Lung carcinoma after shrapnell fragment in situ injury. *Z. allg. Pathol.*, **109**, 158–163 (in German)

Petit, J.-Y., Lê, M.G., Mouriesse, H., Rietjens, M., Gill, P., Contesso, G. & Lehmann, A. (1994) Can breast reconstruction with gel-filled silicone implants increase the risk of death and second primary cancer in patients treated by mastectomy for breast cancer? *Plast. reconstr. Surg.*, **94**, 115–119

Pfleiderer, B., Ackerman, J.L. & Garrido, L. (1993a) *In vivo* localized proton NMR spectroscopy of silicone. *Magn. Reson. Med.*, **30**, 149–154

Pfleiderer, B., Ackerman, J.L. & Garrido, L. (1993b) Migration and biodegradation of free silicone from silicone gel-filled implants after long-term implantation. *Magn. Reson. Med.*, **30**, 534–543

Philip, J. (1982) Squamous cell carcinoma arising at the site of an underlying bullet. *J. Roy. Coll. Surg. Edinb.*, **27**, 365–366

Philippsberg, K. (1922) The traumatic sarcoma. *Klin. Wochenschr.*, **48**, 2385–2386 (in German)

Picha, G.J. & Goldstein, J.A. (1991) Analysis of the soft-tissue response to components used in the manufacture of breast implants: rat animal model. *Plast. reconstr. Surg.*, **87**, 490–500

Piconi, C., Burger, W., Richter, H.G., Cittadini, A., Maccauro, G., Covacci, V., Bruzzese, N., Ricci, G.A. & Marmo, E. (1998) Y-TZP ceramics for artifical joint replacements. *Biomaterials*, **19**, 1489–1494

Piguet, P.F. & Vesin C. (1994) Treatment by human recombinant soluble TNF receptor of pulmonary fibrosis induced by bleomycin or silica in mice. *Eur. respir. J.*, **7**, 515–518

Pinchuk, L. (1994) A review of the biostability and carcinogenicity of polyurethanes in medicine and the new generation of 'biostable' polyurethanes. *J. biomater. Sci. Polymer Ed.*, **6**, 225–267

Piskin, E. (1994) Biodegradable polymers as biomaterials. *J. biomater. Sci. Polymer Ed.*, **6**, 775–795

Pitcher, M.E., Davidson, T.I., Fisher, C. & Thomas, J.M. (1994) Post irradiation sarcoma of soft tissue and bone. *Eur. J. surg. Oncol.*, **20**, 53–56

Planinsek, F. (1979) Cobalt and cobalt alloys. In: Mark, H.F., Othmer, D.F., Overberger, C.G. & Seaborg, G.T., eds, *Kirk-Othmer Encyclopedia of Chemical Technology*, Vol. 6, 3rd Ed., New York, John Wiley, pp. 481–494

Plant, C.G., Tobias, R.S. & Browne, R.M. (1986) Pulpal response to an experimental adhesion promoter. *J. oral Pathol.*, **15**, 196–200

Pogribna, M., Pogribny, I., Miller, B., Melnyk, S., Muskhelishvili, L. & James, J. (1997) Foreign body carcinogenesis is associated with p53 mutations (Abstract). *Proc. Am. Assoc. Cancer Res.*, **38**, 280

Polyzois, G.L., Dahl, J.E. & Hensten-Pettersen, A. (1995) Biological testing of dental materials: development of national and international standards. *J. biomater. Appl.*, **9**, 355–362

Pomplun, S. (1970) Carcinoma formation after intrapulmonary foreign body. *Z. Erkrank. Atmungsorg. Folia Bronchol.*, **132**, 257–262 (in German)

Pott, F., Ziem, U., Reiffer, F.-J., Huth, F., Ernst, H. & Mohr, U. (1987) Carcinogenicity studies on fibres, metal compounds, and some other dust in rats. *Exp. Pathol.*, **32**, 129–152

Pott, F., Rippe, R.M., Roller, M., Csicsaky, M., Rosenbruch, M. & Huth, F. (1989) Tumours in the abdominal cavity of rats after intraperitoneal injection of nickel compounds. In: Vernet, J.-P., ed., *Proceedings of the International Conference on Heavy Metals in the Environment, Geneva, 12–15 September 1989*, Vol. 2, Geneva, World Health Organization, pp. 127–129

Pott, F., Rippe, R.M., Roller, M., Csicsaky, M., Rosenbruch, M. & Huth, F. (1992) Carcinogenicity studies on nickel compounds and nickel alloys in rats by intraperitoneal injection. In: Nieboer, E. & Nriagu, J.O., eds, *Nickel and Human Health: Current Perspectives*, New York, John Wiley, pp. 491–502

Preston, R.J., Au, W., Bender, M.A., Brewen, J.G., Carrano, A.V., Heddle, J.A., McFee, A.F., Wolff, S. & Wassom, J.S. (1981) Mammalian in vivo and in vitro cytogenetic assays: a report of the U.S. EPA's gene-tox program. *Mutat. Res.*, **87**, 143–188

Price, S.K., Kahn, L.B. & Saxe, N. (1993) Dermal and intravascular fasciitis. Unusual variants of nodular fasciitis. *Am. J. Dermatopathol.*, **15**, 539–543

Proppe, K.H., Scully, R.E. & Rosai, J. (1984) Postoperative spindle cell nodules of genitourinary tract resembling sarcomas. A report of eight cases. *Am. J. surg. Pathol.*, **8**, 101–108

Prosinger, F. (1952) Contribution to bone sarcoma development after accident. *Langenbecks Arch. dtsch. Z. Chir.*, **272**, 392–407 (in German)

Putscher, R.E. (1982) Polyamides (general). In: Mark, H.F., Othmer, D.F., Overberger, C.G. & Seaborg, G.T., eds, *Kirk-Othmer Encyclopedia of Chemical Technology*, Vol. 18, 3rd Ed., New York, John Wiley, pp. 328–371

Puza, V., Novák, L. & Komárek S. (1990) *In vitro* studies on cytotoxicity of the dental composite Heliosit at different stages of polymerisation. *Dtsch. Stomatol.*, **40**, 423–425 (in German)

Quinlan, T.R., BeruBe, K.A., Hacker, M.P., Taatjes, D.J., Timblin, C.R., Goldberg, J., Kimberley, P., O'Shaughnessy, P., Hemenway, D., Torino, J., Jimenez, L.A. & Mossman, B.T. (1998) Mechanisms of asbestos-induced nitric oxide production by rat alveolar macrophages in inhalation and in vitro models. *Free Rad. Biol. Med.*, **24**, 778–788

Qvist, V., Stoltze, K. & Qvist, J. (1989) Human pulp reactions to resin restorations performed with different acid-etch restorative procedures. *Acta odontol. scand.*, **47**, 253–263

Rabkin, C.S., Silverman, S., Tricot, G., Garland, L.L., Ballester, O. & Potter, M. (1996) The National Cancer Institute Silicone Implant/Multiple Myeloma Registry. *Curr. Topics Microbiol. Immunol.*, **210**, 385–387

Rachko, D. & Brand, K.G. (1983) Chromosomal aberrations in foreign body tumorigenesis of mice. *Proc. Soc. exp. Biol. Med.*, **172**, 382–388

Radio, S.J. & McManus, B.M. (1996) Pathology of prosthetic materials and devices. In: Damjanov, I. & Linder, J., eds, *Anderson's Pathology*, 10th Ed., St. Louis, Mosby, pp. 685–711

Raikhlin, N.T. & Kogan, A.H. (1961) On the development and malignization of connective tissue capsules around plastic implants. *Vop. Onkol.*, **7**, 13–17 (in Russian)

Ramael, M., Lemmens, G., Eerdekens, C., Buysse, C., Deblier, I., Jacobs, W. & van Marck, E. (1992) Immunoreactivity for p53 protein in malignant mesothelioma and non-neoplastic mesothelium. *J. Pathol.*, **168**, 371–375

Rasmussen, P. (1997) Immediate allergic reaction to latex gloves in a child patient. *Nor. Tannlegefor. Tid.*, **107**, 16–17 (in Danish)

Rasmussen, K., Grimsgaard, C., Vik-Mo, H. & Stalsberg, H. (1985) Male breast cancer from pacemaker pocket. *PACE*, **8**, 761–763

Rasmusson, C.-G. & Lundin, S. (1995) Class II restorations in six different posterior composite resins; five year results. *Swed. dent. J.* **19**, 173–182

Raso, A.M., Rispoli, P., Castagno, P.L., Muncinelli, M., Maggio, D. & Sandrone, N. (1993) Malignant fibrohistiocytoma arising at a femoral Dacron vascular prosthesis. Case report and review of the literature. *Minerva Chir.*, **48**, 1227–1232 (in Italian)

Ratanasathien, S., Wataha, J.C., Hanks, C.T. & Dennison, J.B. (1995) Cytotoxic interactive effects of dentin bonding components on mouse fibroblasts. *J. dent. Res.*, **74**, 1602–1606

Rathbun, M.A., Craig, R.G., Hanks, C.T. & Filisko, F.E. (1991) Cytotoxicity of a BIS-GMA dental composite before and after leaching in organic solvents. *J. biomed. Mater. Res.*, **25**, 443–457

Ratner, B.D., Hoffman, A.S., Schoen, F.J. & Lemons, J.E., eds (1996) *Biomaterials Science: An Introduction to Materials in Medicine*, New York, Academic Press, pp. 3–4

Ravaglioli, A. & Krajewski, A. (1992) Maxillofacial implants. In: Ravaglioli, A. & Krajewski, A., eds, *Bioceramics, Materials, Properties, Applications*, London, Chapman & Hall, pp. 289–313

Reck, R. (1984) Bioactive glass-ceramics in ear surgery: animal studies and clinical results. *Laryngoscope*, **94**, 1–54

Reckling, F.W. & Dillon, W.L. (1977) The bone-cement interface temperature during total joint replacement. *J. Bone Joint Surg.*, **59**, 80–82

Rees, T.D., Ballantyne, D.L., Jr & Hawthorne, G.A. (1970) Silicone fluid research. A follow-up summary. *Plast. reconstr. Surg.*, **46**, 50–56

Reinhardt, G. (1928) Trauma–foreign body–brain tumour. *Münch. Med. Wochenschr.*, **75**, 399–401 (in German)

Richards Manufacturing Company (1980) *Biophase™ Implant Material Technical Information* (Technical Publication No. 3846), Memphis, TN

Richardson, P.N. (1982) Plastic processing. In: Mark, H.F., Othmer, D.F., Overberger, C.G. & Seaborg, G.T., eds, *Kirk-Othmer Encyclopedia of Chemical Technology*, Vol. 18, 3rd Ed., New York, John Wiley, pp. 184–206

Rigdon, R.H. (1975) Tissue reaction to foreign materials. *Crit. Rev. Food Sci. Nutr.*, **August**, 435–476

Rivière, M.R., Chouroulinkov, I. & Guerin, M. (1960) Sarcomas produced by implantation of polystyrene in rats: results appreciably different according to the strain of animals used. *C. R. Soc. Biol.*, **154**, 485–487 (in French)

Robertson, J.S. & Hussain, M. (1969) Metabolism of camphors and related compounds. *Biochem. J.*, **113**, 57–65

Rock, M.G. (1993) Toxicity oncogenesis. Case reports. In: Morrey, B.F., ed., *Biological, Material and Mechanical Considerations of Joint Replacement*, New York, Raven Press, pp. 339–351

Rodriguez-Bigas, M., Mahoney, M.C., Karakousis, C.P. & Petrelli, N.J. (1994) Desmoid tumors in patients with familial adenomatous polyposis. *Cancer*, **74**, 1270–1274

Roe, F.J., Dukes, C.E. & Mitchley, B.C. (1967) Sarcomas at the site of implantation of a poly-vinyl plastic sponge: incidence reduced by use of thin implants. *Biochem. Pharmacol.*, **16**, 647–650

Rogers, J.G., Greenaway, J.C., Mirkes, P.E. & Shepard, T.H. (1986) Methacrylic acid as a teratogen in rat embryo culture. *Teratology*, **33**, 113–117

Rosenthal, G.J., Germolec, D.R., Blazka, M.E., Corsini, E., Simeonova, P., Pollock, P., Kong, L.Y., Kwon, J. & Luster, M.I. (1994) Asbestos stimulates IL-8 production from human lung epithelial cells. *J. Immunol.*, **153**, 3237–3244

Rostoker, G., Robin, J., Binet, O. & Paupe, J. (1986) Dermatoses caused by intolerance to metals of osteosynthesis materials and protheses (nickel, chromium, cobalt). *Ann. Dermatol. Venereol.*, **113**, 1097–1108 (in French)

Rothenberger-Janzen, K., Flueckiger, A. & Bigler, R. (1998) Carcinoma of the breast and pacemaker generators. *PACE*, **21**, 769–771

Rowland, P.H., Moise, N.S. & Severson, D. (1991) Myxoma at the site of a subcutaneous pacemaker in a dog. *J. Am. anim. Hosp. Assoc.*, **27**, 649–651

Rudmann, D.G., Van Alstine, W.G., Doddy, A.F., Sandusky, G.E., Barkdull, T. & Janovitz, E.B. (1996) Pulmonary and mediastinal metastases of a vaccination site sarcoma in a cat. *Vet. Pathol.*, **33**, 466–469

Rushforth, G.F. (1974) Osteosarcoma of the pelvis following radiotherapy for carcinoma of the cervix. *Br. J. Radiol.*, **47**, 147–152

Russell, F.E., Simmers, M.H., Hirst, A.E. & Pudenz, R.H. (1959) Tumors associated with embedded polymers. *J. natl Cancer Inst.*, **23**, 305–315

Ruyter, I.E. (1995) Physical and chemical aspects related to substances released from polymer materials in an aqueous environment. *Adv. dent. Res.*, **9**, 344–347

Ryan, P.C., Newcomb, G.M., Seymour, G.J. & Powell, R.N. (1984) The pulpal response to citric acid in cats. *J. clin. Periodontol.*, **11**, 633–643

Ryan, P., Lee, M.W., North, B. & McMichael, A.J. (1992) Amalgam fillings, diagnostic dental X-rays and tumours of the brain and meninges. *Oral Oncol., Eur. J. Cancer*, **28B**, 91–95

Ryhänen, J., Niemi, E., Serlo, W., Niemelä, E., Sandvik, P., Pernu, H. & Salo, T. (1997) Biocompatability of nickel-titanium shape memory metal and its corrosion behavior in human cell cultures. *J. biomed. Mater. Res.*, **35**, 451–457

Ryu, R.K.N., Bovill, E.G, Jr, Skinner, H.B. & Murray, W.R. (1987) Soft tissue sarcoma associated with aluminum oxide ceramic total hip arthroplasty. A case report. *Clin. Orthop. rel. Res.*, **216**, 207–212

Salnikow, K., Wang, S. & Costa, M. (1997) Induction of activating transcription factor 1 by nickel and its role as a negative regulator of thrombospondin I gene expression. *Cancer Res.*, **57**, 5060–5066

Sandler, I., Teeger, M. & Best, S. (1997) Metastatic vaccine-associated fibrosarcoma in a 10-year-old cat. *Can. Vet. J.*, **38**, 374

Saunders, J.H. (1982) Polyamide fibers. In: Mark, H.F., Othmer, D.F., Overberger, C.G. & Seaborg, G.T., eds, *Kirk-Othmer Encyclopedia of Chemical Technology*, Vol. 18, 3rd Ed., New York, John Wiley, pp. 372–405

Schäfer, K. (1965) An accidental contribution to meningioma formation after a trauma. *Zentralbl. Allg. Pathol.*, **107**, 476–480 (in German)

Schaller, H.G., Klaiber, B., Götze, W. & Benz, M. (1985) *In vitro* cytotoxicity of dentine bonding, enamel bonding and cavity lining agents. *Dtsch. Zahnärztl. Z.*, **40**, 929–934 (in German)

Schapira, R.M., Ghio, A.J., Effros, R.M., Morrisey, J., Dawson, C.A. & Hacker, A.D. (1994) Hydroxyl radicals are formed in the rat lung after asbestos instillation *in vivo*. *Am. J. respir. Cell mol. Biol.*, **10**, 573–579

Schedle, A., Franz, A., Rausch-Fan, X., Samorapoompichit, P., Boltz-Nitulescu, G. & Slavicek, R. (1994) Cytotoxicity testing of dental materials: composite versus amalgam. *Z. Stomatol.*, **Suppl. 6**: 39-42 (in German)

Schedle, A., Samorapoompichit, P., Rausch-Fan, X.H., Franz, A., Füreder, W., Sperr, W.R., Sperr, W., Ellinger, A., Slavicek, R., Boltz-Nitulescu, G. & Valent, P. (1995) Response of L-929 fibroblasts, human gingival fibroblasts, and human tissue mast cells to various metal cations. *J. dent. Res.*, **74**, 1513–1520

Schedle, A., Samorapoompichit, P., Füreder, W., Rausch-Fan, X.H., Franz, A., Sperr, W.R., Sperr, W., Slavicek, R., Simak, S., Klepetko, W., Ellinger, A., Ghannadan, M., Baghestanian, M., & Valent, P. (1998a) Metal ion-induced toxic histamine release from human basophils and mast cells. *J. biomed. Mater. Res.*, **39**, 560–567

Schedle, A., Rausch-Fan, X.H., Samorapoompichit, P., Franz, A., Leutmezer, F., Spittler, A., Baghestanian, M., Lucas, T., Valent, P., Slavicek, R. & Boltz-Nitulescu, G. (1998b) Effects of dental amalgam and heavy metal cations on cytokine production by peripheral blood mononuclear cells *in vitro*. *J. biomed. Mater. Res.*, **42**, 76–84

Schedle, A., Franz, A., Rausch-Fan, X.H., Spittler, A., Lucas, T., Samorapoompichit, P., Sperr, W. & Boltz-Nitulescu, G. (1999) Cytotoxic effects of dental composites, adhesive substances, compomers and cements. *Dental Mater.*, (in press)

Scheid, P. (1938) Tumour formation after bullet injury. *Frankfurt Z. Pathol.*, **51**, 446–478 (in German)

Schinz, H.R. & Uehlinger, E. (1942) Metals: a new principle of carcinogenesis. *Z. Krebsforsch.*, **52**, 425–437

Schmalz, G., Langer, H. & Schweikl, H. (1998a) Cytotoxicity of dental alloy extracts and corresponding metal salt solutions. *J. dent. Res.*, **77**, 1772–1778

Schmalz, G., Schuster, U. & Schweikl, H. (1998b) Influence of metals on IL-6 release in vitro. *Biomaterials*, **19**, 1689–1694

Schmidt, H. & Jaquet, G.-H. (1963) Meningioma formation and foreign body. *Z. Neurochir.*, **24**, 65–73 (in German)

Schmidt, M., Weber, H. & Schön, R. (1996) Cobalt chromium molybdenum metal combination for modular hip prostheses. *Clin. Orthop.*, **329S**, S35–S47

Schneberger, G.L. (1981) Metal surface treatments (cleaning). In: Mark, H.F., Othmer, D.F., Overberger, C.G. & Seaborg, G.T., eds, *Kirk-Othmer Encyclopedia of Chemical Technology*, Vol. 15, 3rd Ed., New York, John Wiley, pp. 296–312

Schneider, T., Renney, J. & Hayman, J. (1997) Angiosarcoma occurring with chronic osteomyelitis and residual foreign material: Case report of a late World War II wound complication. *Aust. N.Z. J. Surg.*, **67**, 576–578

Schoen, F.J. (1987) Biomaterial-associated infection, neoplasia, and calcification. Clinicopathologic features and pathophysiologic concepts. *Trans. Am. Soc. Artif. Intern. Organs*, **33**, 8–18

Schuh, M.E. & Radford, D.M. (1994) Desmoid tumor of the breast following augmentation mammaplasty. *Plast. reconstr. Surg.*, **93**, 603–605

Schultze, A. & Bingas, B. (1968) Meningioma formation induced by foreign body. *Beitr. Neurochir.*, **15**, 297–301 (in German)

Schürch, W. (1997) Myofibroblast. In: Sternberg, S.S., ed., *Histology for Pathologists*, 2nd Ed., New York, Raven Press, pp. 129–165

Schweikl, H. & Schmalz, G. (1997) Glutaraldehyde-containing dentin bonding agents are mutagens in mammalian cells *in vitro*. *J. biomed. Mater. Res.*, **36**, 284–288

Schweikl, H. & Schmalz, G. (1999) Triethylene glycol dimethacrylate induces large deletions in the *hprt* gene of V79 cells. *Mutat. Res.*, **438**, 71–78

Schweikl, H., Schmalz, G. & Bey, B. (1994) Mutagenicity of dentin bonding agents. *J. biomed. Mater. Res.*, **28**, 1061–1067

Schweikl, H., Schmalz, G. & Göttke, C. (1996) Mutagenic activity of various dentine bonding agents. *Biomaterials*, **17**, 1451–1456

Schweikl, H., Schmalz, G. & Rackebrandt, K. (1998) The mutagenic activity of unpolymerized resin monomers in *Salmonella typhimurium* and V79 cells. *Mutat. Res.*, **415**, 119–130

Scully, R.E., Mark, E.J., McNeely, W.F. & McNeely, B.U. (1991) Case records of the Massachusetts General Hospital. Weekly clinicopathological exercises. Case 4-1991. *New Engl. J. Med.*, **324**, 251–259

Scully, C., Beyli, M., Ferreiro, M.C., Ficarra, G., Gill, Y., Griffiths, M., Holmstrup, P., Mutlu, S., Porter, S. & Wray, D. (1998) Update on oral lichen planus: etiopathogenesis and management. *Crit. Rev. oral Biol. Med.*, **9**, 86–122

Sears, J.K. & Touchette, N.W. (1989) Plasticizers. In: Grayson, M., Mark, H.F., Othmer, D.F. & Othmer, D.F. eds, *Kirk-Othmer Concise Encyclopedia of Chemical Technology*, Vol. 18, 3rd Ed., New York, John Wiley, pp. 902–906

Semlitsch, M. (1992) 25 years Sulzer development of implant materials for total hip prostheses. *Medicajournal*, **Spring**, 1–7

Semlitsch, M. & Willert, H.G. (1980) Properties of implant alloys for artificial hip joints. *Med. biol. Eng. Comp.*, **18**, 511–520

Seppäläinen, A.M. & Rajaniemi, R. (1984) Local neurotoxicity of methyl methacrylate among dental technicians. *Am. J. ind. Med.*, **5**, 471–477

Sever, C.E., Leith, C.P., Appenzeller, J. & Foucar, K. (1996) Kikuchi's histiocytic necrotizing lymphadenitis associated with ruptured silicone breast implant. *Arch. Pathol. Lab. Med.*, **120**, 380–385

Seydel, M.H. (1892) Medical Association of Munich. Demonstrations. *Münch. Med. Wochenschr.*, **8**, 787 (in German)

Shanklin, D.R. & Smalley, D.L. (1995) Quantitative aspects of cellular responses to silicone. *Int. J. occup. Med. Toxicol.*, **4**, 99–111

Shearman, C.P. & Watts, G.T. (1986) Paget's disease of the nipple after subcutaneous mastectomy for cancer with primary reconstruction. *Ann. Roy. Coll. Surg. Engl.*, **68**, 17–18

Sherlock, D.J., Rickards, H., Gardecki, T.I.M. & Hamer, J.D. (1987) Development of a sarcoma in a surgical scar. *Postgrad. med. J.*, **63**, 1097–1098

Shulman, J., Wiznitzer, T. & Neuman, Z. (1963) Comparative study of sarcoma formation by implanted polyethylene film and mesh in white rats. *Br. J. plast. Surg.*, **16**, 336–340

Siddons, A.H.M. & MacArthur, A.M. (1952) Carcinomata developing at the site of foreign bodies in the lung. *Br. J. Surg.*, **39**, 542–545

Silicosis and Silicate Disease Committee (1988) Diseases associated with exposure to silica and nonfibrous silicate minerals. *Arch. Pathol. Lab. Med.*, **112**, 673–720

Silverman, B.G., Gross, T.P., Kaczmarek, R.G., Hamilton, P. & Hamburger, S. (1995) The epidemiology of pacemaker implantation in the United States. *Public Health Rep.*, **110**, 42–46

Silverstein, M.J., Gamagami, P. & Handel, N. (1990) Missed breast cancer in an augmented woman using implant displacement mammography. *Ann. plast. Surg.*, **25**, 210–213

Simeonova, P.P., Toriumi, W., Kommineni, C., Erkan, M., Munson, A.E., Rom, W.N. & Luster, M.I. (1997) Molecular regulation of IL-6 activation by asbestos in lung epithelial cells: role of reactive oxygen species. *J. Immunol.*, **159**, 3921–3928

Simmers, M.H., Agnew, W.F. & Pudenz, R.H. (1963) Effects of plastic polymers within the rat's peritoneal cavity. *Bol. Inst. Estud. med. biol. Mex.*, **21**, 1–13

Sinclair, T.M., Kerrigan, C.L., Buntic, R. & Szycher, M. (1993) Biodegradation of the polyurethane foam covering of breast implants. *Plast. reconstr. Surg.*, **92**, 1003–1014

Sinibaldi, K., Rosen, H., Liu, S. & DeAngelis, M. (1976) Tumors associated with metallic implants in animals. *Clin. Orthop.*, **118**, 257–266

Solomon, M.I. & Sekel, R. (1992) Total hip arthroplasty complicated by a malignant fibrous histiocytoma. A case report. *J. Arthroplasty*, **7**, 549–550

SOU (1989) To prevent allergy/hypersensitivity. In: *Att förebygga ALLERGI/överkänslighet* (Statens offentliga utredningar 1989:76), Stockholm, Social Department (in Swedish)

Stambolis, C., Fischer, P., Doppl, W. & Hocke, M. (1982) Lung scirrhous carcinoma after shrapnel fragment injury. *Med. Welt*, **33**, 177–181 (in German)

Stanley, H.R., Bowen, R.L. & Folio, J. (1979) Compatibility of various materials with oral tissues. II: Pulp responses to composite ingredients. *J. dent. Res.*, **58**, 1507–1517

Stea, S., Visentin, M., Cervellati, M., Verri, E., Cenni, E., Savarino, L., Stea, S. & Pizzoferrato, A. (1998) In vitro sister chromatid exchange induced by glass ionomer cements. *J. biomed. Mater. Res.*, **40**, 545–550

Steinbrunner, R.L., Setcos, J.C. & Kafrawy, A.H. (1991) Connective tissue reactions to glass ionomer cements and resin composites. *Am. J. Dent.*, **4**, 281–284

Stemmer, K.L., Bingham, E. & Barkley, W. (1975) Pulmonary response to polyurethane dust. *Environ. Health Perspect.*, **11**, 109–113

Stevenson, S. (1991) Fracture-associated sarcomas. *Vet. Clin. North Am. small Anim. Pract.*, **21**, 859–872

Stevenson, S., Hohn, R.B., Pohler, O.E., Fetter, A.W., Olmstead, M.L. & Wind, A.P. (1982) Fracture-associated sarcoma in the dog. *J. Am. vet. Med. Assoc.*, **180**, 1189–1196

Stinson, N.E. (1960) Tissue reaction to polymethylmethacrylate in rats and guinea pigs. *Nature*, **188**, 678

Stinson, N.E. (1964) The tissue reaction induced in rats and guinea pigs by polymethylmethacrylate (acrylic) and stainless steel (18/18/Mo). *Br. J. exp. Pathol.*, **45**, 21–29

Stone, J.W. & Arnold, G.E. (1967) Human larynx injected with Teflon paste. Histological study of innervation and tissue reaction. *Arch. Otolaryngol.*, **86**, 550–561

Stratton, M.R., Williams, S., Fisher, C., Ball, A., Westbury, G., Gusterson, B.A., Fletcher, C.D., Knight, J.C., Fung, Y.K. & Reeves, B.R. (1989) Structural alterations of the RB1 gene in human soft tissue tumours. *Br. J. Cancer*, **60**, 202–205

Strong, L.C., Williams, W.R. & Tainsky, M.A. (1992) The Li–Fraumeni syndrome: from clinical epidemiology to molecular genetics. *Am. J. Epidemiol.*, **135**, 190–199

Suda, M. & Kawase, T. (1991) Cytobiochemical study of composite resins. Effect of triethylene glycol dimethacrylate (TEGDMA) on the growth and differentiation of osteoblasts. *Kanagawa Shigaku*, **26**, 11–24 (in Japanese)

Sun, Z.L., Wataha, J.C. & Hanks, C.T. (1997) Effects of metal ions on osteoblast-like cell metabolism and differentiation. *J. Biomed. Mater. Res.*, **34**, 29–37

Sunderman, F.W., Jr (1984) Carcinogenicity of nickel compounds in animals. In: Sunderman, F.W., Jr, ed., *Nickel in the Human Environment* (IARC Scientific Publications No. 53), Lyon, IARC, pp. 127–142

Sunderman, F.W., Jr & Maenza, R.M. (1976) Comparisons of carcinogenicities of nickel compounds in rats. *Res. Commun. chem. Pathol. Pharmacol.*, **14**, 319–330

Sunderman, F.W., Jr, McCully, K.S. & Hopfer, S.M. (1984) Association between erythrocytosis and renal cancers in rats following intrarenal injection of nickel compounds. *Carcinogenesis*, **5**, 1511–1517

Sundgren, J.E., Bodo, P., Lundstrom, I., Berggren, A. & Hellem, S. (1985) Auger electron spectroscopic studies of stainless-steel implants. *J. biomed. Mater. Res.*, **19**, 663–671

Süry, P. & Semlitsch, M. (1978) Corrosion behavior of cast and forged cobalt-based alloys for double alloy joint endoprostheses. *J. biomed. Mater. Res.*, **12**, 723–741

Swafford, D.S., Nikula, K.J., Mitchell, C.E. & Belinsky, S.A. (1995) Low frequency of alterations in *p53*, K-*ras*, and *mdm*2 in rat lung neoplasms induced by diesel exhaust or carbon black. *Carcinogenesis*, **16**, 1215–1221

Swann, M. (1984) Malignant soft-tissue tumour at the site of a total hip replacement. *J. Bone Joint Surg.*, **B66**, 629–631

Swanson, S.A., Freeman, M.A. & Heath, J.C. (1973) Laboratory tests on total joint replacement prosthesis. *J. Bone Joint Surg.*, **55B**, 759–773

Swierenga, S.H. & Yamasaki, H. (1992) Performance of tests for cell transformation and gap-junction intercellular communication for detecting nongenotoxic carcinogenic activity. In: Vainio, H., Magee, P., McGregor, D. & McMichael, A., eds, *Mechanisms of Carcinogenesis in Risk Identification*, Lyon, IARC, pp. 165–193

Szycher, M. & Siciliano, A.A. (1991) Polyurethane-covered mammary prosthesis: a nine-year follow-up assessment. *J. Biomater. Appl.*, **5**, 282–322

Szycher, M., Lee, S.J. & Siciliano, A.A. (1991) Breast prostheses: A critical review. *J. Biomater. Appl.*, **5**, 256–281

Tait, N.P., Hacking, P.M. & Malcolm, A.J. (1988) Malignant fibrous histiocytoma occurring at the site of a previous total hip replacement. *Br. J. Radiol.*, **61**, 73–76

Takagi, M., Konttinen, Y.T., Santavirta, S., Kangaspunta, P., Suda, A. & Rokkanen, P. (1995) Cathepsin G and alpha 1-antichymotrypsin in the local host reaction to loosening of total hip prostheses. *J. Bone Joint Surg.*, **77A**, 16–25

Takahara, A., Coury, A.J., Hergenrother, R.W. & Cooper, S.L. (1991) Effect of soft segment chemistry on the biostability of segmented polyurethanes: I. In vitro oxidation. *J. biomed. Mater. Res.*, **25**, 342–356

Takami, Y., Nakazawa, T., Makinouchi, K., Glueck, J. & Nosé, Y. (1997) Biocompatibility of alumina ceramic and polyethylene as materials for pivot bearings of a centrifugal blood pump. *J. biomed. Mater. Res.*, **36**, 381–386

Takeda, S., Kakiuchi, H., Doi, H. & Nakamura, M. (1989) Cytotoxicity of pure metals. *Dent. Mater. Instrum.*, **8**, 648–652 (in Japanese)

Talmor, M., Rothaus, K.O., Shannahan, E., Cortese, A.F. & Hoffman, L.A. (1995) Squamous cell carcinoma of the breast after augmentation with liquid silicone injection. *Ann. plast. Surg.*, **34**, 619–623

Tang, L., Lucas, A.H. & Eaton, J.W. (1993) Inflammatory responses to implanted polymeric biomaterials: role of surface-adsorbed immunoglobin G. *J. Lab. clin. Med.*, **122**, 292–300

Tang, L., Ugarova, T.P., Plow, E.F. & Eaton, J.W. (1996) Molecular determinants of acute inflammatory responses to biomaterials. *J. clin. Invest.*, **97**, 1329–1334

Taningher, M., Pasquini, R., Tanzi, M.C. & Bonatti, S. (1992) Genotoxicity of *N*-acryloyl-*N'*-phenylpiperazine, a redox activator for acrylic resin polymerization. *Mutat. Res.*, **282**, 99–105

Taningher, M., Pasquini, R. & Bonatti, S. (1993) Genotoxicity analysis of *N,N*-dimethylaniline and *N,N*-dimethyl-*p*-toluidine. *Environ. mol. Mutagen.*, **21**, 349–356

Taylor, R.B. & Kennan, J.J. (1996) ^{29}Si NMR and blood silicon levels in silicone gel breast implant recipients. *Magn. Reson. Med.*, **36**, 498–499

Tayton, K.J.J. (1980) Ewing's sarcoma at the site of a metal plate. *Cancer*, **45**, 413–415

Tengvall, P., Lundström, I., Sjöqvist, L., Elwing, H. & Bjursten, L.M. (1989) Titanium-hydrogen peroxide interaction: model studies of the influence of the inflammatory response on titanium implants. *Biomaterials*, **10**, 166–175

Terry, M.B., Skovron, M.L., Garbers, S., Sonnenschein, E. & Toniolo, P. (1995) The estimated frequency of cosmetic breast augmentation among US women, 1963 through 1988. *Am. J. public Health*, **85**, 1122–1124

Testa, J.R., Carbone, M., Hirvonen, A., Khalili, K., Krynska, B., Linnainmaa, K., Pooley, F.D., Rizzo, P., Rusch, V. & Xiao, G.-H. (1998) A multi-institutional study confirms the presence and expression of simian virus 40 in human malignant mesotheliomas. *Cancer Res.*, **58**, 4505–4509

Theegarten, D., Sardisong, F. & Philippou, S. (1995) Malignant fibrous histiocytoma associated with total hip replacement. *Chirurg.*, **66**, 158–161 (in German)

Therapeutic Goods Administration (1998) *Australian Medical Device Requirements Version 4 under the Therapeutic Goods Act 1989*, Canberra, Commonwealth Department of Health and Family Series

Thies, O. (1936) Sarcoma after war injury. *Z. Chir.*, **63**, 1763–1770 (in German)

Thomassen, M.J., Buoen, L.C. & Brand, K.G. (1975) Foreign-body tumorigenesis: number, distribution, and cell density of preneoplastic clones. *J. natl Cancer Inst.*, **54**, 203–207

Thompson, J.R. & Entin, S.D. (1969) Primary extraskeletal chondrosarcoma. Report of a case arising in conjunction with extrapleural Lucite ball plombage. *Cancer*, **23**, 936–939

Thompson, G.J. & Puleo, D.A. (1996) Ti-6Al-4V ion solution inhibition of osteogenic cell phenotype as a function of differentiation timecourse *in vitro*. *Biomaterials*, **17**, 1949–1954

Thun, M.J., Baker, D.B., Steenland, K., Smith, A.B., Halperin, W. & Berl, T. (1985) Renal toxicity in uranium mill workers. *Scand. J. Work Environ. Health*, **11**, 83–90

Thyssen, J., Kimmerle, G., Dickhaus, S., Emminger, E. & Mohr, U. (1978) Inhalation studies with polyurethane foam dust in relation to respiratory tract carcinogenesis. *J. environ. Pathol. Toxicol.*, **1**, 501–508

Tien, J.K. & Howson, T.E. (1981) Nickel and nickel alloys. In: Mark, H.F., Othmer, D.F., Overberger, C.G. & Seaborg, G.T., eds, *Kirk-Othmer Encyclopedia of Chemical Technology*, Vol. 15, 3rd Ed., New York, John Wiley, pp. 787–801

Tigges, S., Stiles, R.G. & Roberson, J.R. (1994) Case report—aggressive granulomatosis complicating knee arthoplasty. *Can. Assoc. Radiol. J.*, **45**, 310–313

Timberlake, G.A. & Looney, G.R. (1986) Adenocarcinoma of the breast associated with silicone injections. *J. surg. Oncol.*, **32**, 79–81

Timchalk, C., Smith, F.A. & Bartels, M.J. (1994) Route-dependent comparative metabolism of [^{14}C]toluene 2,4-diisocyanate and [^{14}C]toluene 2,4-diamine in Fischer 344 rats. *Toxicol. appl. Pharmacol.*, **124**, 181–190

Tinkelman, D.C. & Tinkelman, C.L. (1979) An unusual etiology of contact urticaria. *Pediatrics*, **63**, 339

Tinkler, J. (1995) The impact of European directives. *J. Heart Valve Dis.*, **4**, S10–S12

Tinkler, J.J.B., Campbell, H.J., Senior, J.M. & Ludgate, S.M. (1993) *Evidence for an Association between the Implantation of Silicones and Connective Tissue Disease* (MDD Report MDD/92/42), London, Department of Health

Tomás, H., Carvalho, G.S., Fernandes, M.H., Freire, A.P. & Abrantes, L.M. (1997) The use of rat, rabbit or human bone marrow derived cells for cytocompatibility evaluation of metallic elements. *J. Mater. Sci.: Materials in Medicine*, **8**, 233–238

Tomatis, L. (1963) Studies in subcutaneous carcinogenesis with implants of glass and Teflon in mice. *Acta unio. int. contra Cancrum*, **19**, 607–611

Tomatis L. (1966a) Subcutaneous carcinogenesis by ^{14}C and ^{3}H labelled polymethylmethacrylate films. *Tumori*, **52**, 165–172

Tomatis, L. (1966b) Subcutaneous carcinogenesis by implants and by 7,12-dimethylbenz[a]anthracene. *Tumori*, **52**, 1–16

Tomatis, L. & Parmi, L. (1971) Effect of perinatal administration of 7,12-dimethylbenz(a)anthracene on the later response to a subcutaneous Teflon implant. *Tumori*, **57**, 55–62

Tomatis, L. & Shubik, P. (1963) Influence of urethane on subcutaneous carcinogenesis by 'Teflon' implants. *Nature*, **198**, 600–601

Trampnau, Dr (1922) Contribution to knowledge of carcinoma of nose and pharyngeal cavity with particular consideration of their aetiology. *Passow-Schäfer Beitr. Anat. Physiol. Pathol. Ther.*, **18**, 268–276 (in German)

Tricot, G.J.K., Naucke, S., Vaught, L., Vesole, D., Jagannath, S. & Barlogie, B. (1996) Is the risk of multiple myeloma increased in patients with silicone implants? *Curr. Topics Microbiol. Immunol.*, **210**, 357–359

Troop, J.K., Mallory, T.H., Fisher, D.A. & Vaughn, B.K. (1990) Malignant fibrous histiocytoma after total hip arthroplasty. A case report. *Clin. Orthop. rel. Res.*, **253**, 297–300

Trosko, J.E., Chang, C.-C. & Netzloff, M. (1982) The role of inhibited cell-cell communication in teratogenesis. *Teratog. Carcinog. Mutag.*, **2**, 31–45

Tsuchiya, T. (1998) Detection of tumor-promoting activities in biomaterials using *in vitro* cell culture methods. *Kobunshi Ronbunshu*, **55**, 314–322 (in Japanese)

Tsuchiya, T. & Nakamura, A. (1995) A new hypothesis of tumorigenesis induced by biomaterials: inhibitory potentials of intercellular communication play an important role on the tumor-promotion stage. *J. long-term Effects med. Implants*, **5**, 233–242

Tsuchiya, T., Hata, H. & Nakamura, A. (1995a) Studies on the tumor-promoting activity of biomaterials: inhibition of metabolic cooperation by polyetherurethane and silicone. *J. biomed. Mater. Res.*, **29**, 113–119

Tsuchiya, T., Takahara, A. & Cooper, S.L. & Nakamura, A. (1995b) Studies on the tumor-promoting activity of polyurethanes: depletion of inhibitory action of metabolic cooperation on the surface of a polyalkyleneurethane but not a polyetherurethane. *J. biomed. Mater. Res.*, **29**, 835–841

Tsuchiya, T., Nakaoka, R., Degawa, H. & Nakamura, A. (1996) Studies on the mechanisms of tumorigenesis induced by polyetherurethanes in rats: leachable and biodegradable oligomers involving the diphenylcarbamate structure acted as an initiator on the transformation of Balb 3T3 cells. *J. biomed. Mater. Res.*, **31**, 299–303

Tsuchiya, T., Wang, C., Nakaoka, R. & Nakamura, A. (1998) A molecular mechanism of tumorigenesis of polyurethanes in vivo and in vitro (Abstract). *Proc. Am. Assoc. Cancer Res.*, **39**, 200

Tsuchiya, T., Sayed M.A. & Nakamura, A. (1999) Tumor promoting mechanism of biomaterials: no involvement of mutation in cx43 gene in the tumorigenesis induced by polyurethanes in vitro. In: Ikura, K., Nagao, M., Masuda, S. & Sasalki, R., eds, *Proceedings of The JAACT/ESACT'98, Animal Cell Technology: Challenges for the 21st Century*, Dordrecht, Kluwer Academic Publishers, pp. 181–185

Ulrich, H. (1983) Urethane polymers. In: Mark, H.F., Othmer, D.F., Overberger, C.G. & Seaborg, G.T., eds, *Kirk-Othmer Encyclopedia of Chemical Technology*, Vol. 23, 3rd Ed., New York, John Wiley, pp. 576–608

Unfried, K., Kociok, N., Roller, M., Friedmann, J., Pott, F. & Dehnen, W. (1997) P53 mutations in tumours induced by intraperitoneal injection of crocidolite asbestos and benz[a]pyrene in rats. *Exp. Toxicol. Pathol.*, **49**, 181–187

United States Fish & Wildlife Services (1989) Non-toxic Shot, Federal Register 50, Code of Federal Regulations 20.134, Washington DC, US Government Printing Office, pp. 289–293

Vallyathan, V. & Shi, X. (1997) The role of oxygen free radicals in occupational and environmental lung disease. *Environ. Health Perspect.*, **105** (Suppl. 1), 165–177

Vallyathan, V., Castranova, V., Pack, D., Leonard, S., Shumaker, J., Hubbs, A.F., Shoemaker, D.A., Ramsey, D.M., Pretty, J.R., McLaurin, J.L., Khan, A. & Teass A. (1995) Freshly fractured quartz inhalation leads to enhanced lung injury and inflammation. *Am. J. respir. crit. Care Med.*, **152**, 1003–1009

Van Bree, H., Verschooten, F., Hoorens, J. & Mattheeuws, D. (1980) Internal fixation of a fractured humerus in a dog and late osteosarcoma development. *Vet. Rec.*, **107**, 501–502

van de Rijn, M., Barr, F.G., Xiong, Q.-B., Salhany, K.E., Fraker, D.L. & Fisher, C. (1997) Radiation-associated synovial sarcoma. *Hum. Pathol.*, **28**, 1325–1328

van der List, J.J.J., van Horn, J.R., Slooff, T.J.J.H. & Naudin ten Cate, L. (1988) Malignant epithelioid hemangioendothelioma at the site of a hip prosthesis. *Acta orthop. scand.*, **59**, 328–330

van Diest, P.J., Beekman, W.H. & Hage, J.J. (1998) Pathology of silicone leakage from breast implants. *J. clin. Pathol.*, **51**, 493–497

van Dijken, J.W.V., Sjöström, S. & Wing, K. (1987) Development of gingivitis around different types of composite resin. *J. clin. Periodontol.*, **14**, 257–260

Varpio, M., Warfvinge, J. & Norén, J.G. (1990) Proximo-occlusal composite restorations in primary molars: Marginal adaptation, bacterial penetration, and pulpal reactions. *Acta odontol. scand.*, **48**, 161–167

Vasiliev, J.M., Olshevskaja, L.V., Raikhlin, N.T. & Ivanova, O.J. (1962) Comparative study of alterations induced by 7,12-dimethylbenz[a]anthracene and polymer films in the subcutaneous connective tissue of rats. *J. natl Cancer Inst.*, **28**, 515–589

Visser, S.A., Hergenrother, R.W. & Cooper, S.L. (1996) Polymers. In: Ratner, B.D., Hoffman, A.S., Schoen, F.J. & Lemons, J.E., eds, *Biomaterials Science: An Introduction to Materials in Medicine*, San Diego, Academic Press, pp. 50–60

Visuri, T. & Koskenvuo, M. (1991) Cancer risk after McKee-Farrar total hip replacement. *Orthopedics*, **14**, 137–142

Visuri, T., Pulkkinen, P., Turula, K.B., Paavolainen, P. & Koskenvuo, M. (1994) Life expectancy after hip arthroplasty: case–control study of 1018 cases of primary arthrosis. *Acta orthop. scand.*, **65**, 9–11

Visuri, T., Pukkala, E., Paavolainen, P., Pulkkinen, P. & Riska, E.B. (1996) Cancer risk after metal on metal and polyethylene on metal total hip arthroplasty. *Clin. Orthop. rel. Res.*, **329** (Suppl.), S280–S289

Vives, P., Sevestre, H., Grodet, H. & Marie, F. (1987) Case report on malignant fibrous histiocytoma after total hip arthroplasty. *Rev. Chir. orthop.*, **73**, 407–409 (in French)

Vollmann, J. (1938) Animal experiments with intraosseous arsenic, chromium and cobalt implants. *Schweiz. Z. Allg. Pathol. Bakteriol.*, **1**, 440–443 (in German)

Vollmar, J. & Ott, G. (1961) Experimental tumour formation by surgical plastics. *Langenbecks Arch. klin. Chir.*, **298**, 729–736 (in German)

Waalkes, M.P., Rehm, S., Kasprzak, K.S. & Issaq, H.J. (1987) Inflammatory, proliferative, and neoplastic lesions at the site of metallic identification ear tags in Wistar [Crl:(WI)BR] rats. *Cancer Res.*, **47**, 2445–2450

Waegemaekers, T.H.J.M. & Bensink, M.P.M. (1984) Non-mutagenicity of 27 aliphatic acrylate esters in the Salmonella-microsome test. *Mutat. Res.*, **137**, 95–102

Wagner, M., Klein, C.L., van Kooten, T.G. & Kirkpatrick, C.J. (1998) Mechanisms of cell activation by heavy metal ions. *J. biomed. Mater. Res.*, **42**, 443–452

Walter, J.B. & Chiaramonte, L.G. (1965) Tissue responses of the rat to implanted Ivalon, Etheron and Polyfoam plastic sponges. *Br. J. Surg.*, **52**, 49–54

Wang, X., Christiani, D.C., Wiencke, J.K., Fischbein, M., Xu, X., Cheng, T.J., Mark, E., Wain, J.C. & Kelsey, K.T. (1995) Mutations in the p53 gene in lung cancer are associated with cigarette smoking and asbestos exposure. *Cancer Epidemiol. Biomarkers Prev.*, **4**, 543–548

Wang, B.H., Chang, B.W., Sargeant, R. & Manson, P.N. (1998) Late capsular hematoma after breast reconstruction with polyurethane-covered implants. *Plast. reconstr. Surg.*, **102**, 450–452

Wanivenhaus, A., Lintner, F., Wurnig, C. & Missaghi-Schinzl, M. (1991) Long-term reaction of the osseous bed around silicone implants. *Arch. orthop. Trauma Surg.*, **110**, 146–150

Wapner, K.L. (1991) Implications of metallic corrosion in total knee arthroplasty. *Clin. Orthop. rel. Res.*, **271**, 12–20

Ward, J.J., Thornbury, D.D., Lemons, J.E. & Dunham, W.K. (1990) Metal-induced sarcoma. A case report and literature review. *Clin. Orthop. rel. Res.*, **252**, 299–306

Warheit, D.B., Hansen, J.F., Yuen, I.S., Kelly, D.P., Snajdr, S.I. & Hartsky, M.A. (1997) Inhalation of high concentrations of low toxicity dusts in rats results in impaired pulmonary clearance mechanisms and persistent inflammation. *Toxicol. appl. Pharmacol.*, **145**, 10–22

Waring, R.H. & Pheasant, A.E. (1976) Some phenolic metabolites of 2,4-diaminotoluene in the rabbit, rat and guinea-pig. *Xenobiotica*, **6**, 257–262

Wataha, J.C., Hanks, C.T. & Craig, R.G. (1991) The *in vitro* effects of metal cations on eukaryotic cell metabolism. *J. biomed. Mater. Res.*, **25**, 1133–1149

Wataha, J.C., Hanks, C.T., Strawn, S.E. & Fat, J.C. (1994) Cytotoxicity of components of resins and other dental restorative materials. *J. oral Rehabilitation*, **21**, 453–462

Weber, P.C. (1986) Epitheloid sarcoma in association with total knee replacement. A case report. *J. Bone Joint Surg.*, **68**, 824–826

Weinberg, D.S. & Maini, B.S. (1980) Primary sarcoma of the aorta associated with a vascular prosthesis: a case report. *Cancer*, **46**, 398–402

Weiss, S.W., ed. (1994) *Histological Typing of Soft Tissue Tumours. International Histological Classification of Tumours*, 2nd Ed., Berlin, Springer–Verlag

Weiss, S.W. (1996) Lipomatous tumors. *Monogr. Pathol.*, **38**, 207–239

Weiss, S.W. & Enzinger, F.M. (1978) Malignant fibrous histiocytoma: an analysis of 200 cases. *Cancer*, **41**, 2250–2266

Weiss, E. & Krusen, F.H. (1922) Foreign body in the lung for forty-five years complicated by abscess and tumor formation. *J. Am. med. Assoc.*, **78**, 506–507

Weiss, W.M., Riles, T.S., Gouge, T.H. & Mizrachi, H.H. (1991) Angiosarcoma at the site of a Dacron vascular prosthesis: a case report and literature review. *J. vasc. Surg.*, **14**, 87–91

Welgos, R.J. (1982) Polyamide plastics. In: Mark, H.F., Othmer, D.F., Overberger, C.G. & Seaborg, G.T., eds, *Kirk-Othmer Encyclopedia of Chemical Technology*, Vol. 18, 3rd Ed., New York, John Wiley, pp. 406–425

Wenig, B.M., Heffner, D.K., Oertel, Y.C. & Johnson, F.B. (1990) Teflonomas of the larynx and neck. *Hum. Pathol.*, **21**, 617–623

Wening, J.V., Marquardt, H., Katzer, A., Jungbluth, K.H. & Marquardt, H. (1995) Cytotoxicity and mutagenicity of Kevlar®: an *in vitro* evaluation. *Biomaterials*, **16**, 337–340

Wennberg, A., Mjör, I.A. & Hensten-Pettersen, A. (1983) Biological evaluation of dental restorative materials—a comparison of different test methods. *J. biomed. Mater. Res.*, **17**, 23–36

Wever, D.J., Veldhuizen, A.G., Sanders, M.M., Schakenraad, J.M. & van Horn, J.R. (1997) Cytotoxic, allergic and genotoxic activity of a nickel–titanium alloy. *Biomaterials*, **18**, 1115–1120

Wiklund, T.A., Blomqvist, C.P., Raty, J., Elomaa, I., Rissanen, P. & Miettinen, M. (1991) Postirradiation sarcoma. Analysis of a nationwide cancer registry material. *Cancer*, **68**, 524–531

Wilkinson, J.D. (1989) Nickel allergy and orthopedic prostheses. In: Maibach, H.I. & Menne, T., eds, *Nickel and the Skin: Immunology and Toxicology*, Boca Raton, FL, CRC Press, pp. 187–193

Willert, H.G., Buchhorn, G.H.H., Göbel, D., Köster, G., Schaffner, S., Schenk, R. & Semlitsch, M. (1996) Wear behavior and histopathology of classic cemented metal on metal hip endoprostheses. *Clin. Orthop. rel. Res.*, **329** (Suppl.), S160–S186

Williams, D.F. & Roaf, R. (1973) *Implants in Surgery*, London, W.B. Saunders, pp. 5–23, 309–310, 416–417, 460–467

Wines, R.D. (1973) Possible hazard of polymethyl methacrylate (Letter to the Editor). *Br. med. J.*, **iii**, 409

Wink, D.A., Vodovotz, Y., Laval, J., Laval, F., Dewhirst, M.W. & Mitchell, J.B. (1998) The multifaceted roles of nitric oxide in cancer. *Carcinogenesis*, **19**, 711–721

Working Group on Dental Amalgam (1997) *Dental Amalgam and Alternative Restorative Material: An Update Report to the Environmental Health Policy Committee*, Washington DC, US Department of Health and Human Services

Wrangsjö, K., Wahlberg, J.E. & Axelsson, I.G.K. (1988) IgE-mediated allergy to natural rubber in 30 patients with contact urticaria. *Contact Derm.*, **19**, 264–271

Wroblewski, B.M. (1997) Wear of the high-density polyethylene socket in total hip arthroplasty and its role in endosteal cavitation. *Proc. Instn. Mech. Engrs.*, **211**, 109–118

Yamamoto, A., Honma, R. & Sumita, M. (1998) Cytotoxicity evaluation of 43 metal salts using murine fibroblasts and osteoblastic cells. *J. biomed. Mater. Res.*, **39**, 331–340

Yoda, R. (1998) Elastomers for biomedical applications. *J. biomater. Sci. Polymer Ed.*, **9**, 561–626

Younkin, C.N. (1974) Multiphase MP35N alloy for medical implants. *J. biomed. Mater. Res.*, **5**, 219–226

Yourtee, D.M., Tong, P.Y., Rose, L.A., Eick, J.D., Chappelow, C.C. & Bean, T.A. (1994) The effect of spiroorthocarbonate volume modifier co-monomers on the in vitro toxicology of trial non-shrinking dental epoxy co-polymers. *Res. Comm. mol. Pathol. Pharmacol.*, **86**, 347–360

Zafiracopoulos, P. & Rouskas, A. (1974) Breast cancer at site of implantation of pace maker generator (Letter to the Editor). *Lancet*, **i**, 1114

Zajdela, F. (1966) Production of subcutaneous sarcomas in the rat by cellulose membranes of known porosity. *Bull. Cancer*, **53**, 401–408 (in French)

Zanella, C.L., Posada, J., Tritton, T.R. & Mossman, B.T. (1996) Asbestos causes stimulation of the extracellular signal-regulated kinase 1 mitogen-activated protein kinase cascade after phosphorylation of the epidermal growth factor receptor. *Cancer Res.*, **56**, 5334–5338

Zeiger, E., Anderson, B., Haworth, S., Lawlor, T., Mortelmans, K. & Speck, W. (1987) *Salmonella* mutagenicity tests: III Results from the testing of 225 chemicals. *Environ. Mol. Mutagen.*, **9** (Suppl 9), 1–110

Zhang, Z., King, M.W., Guidoin, R., Therrien, M., Doillon, C., Diehl-Jones, W.L. & Huebner, E. (1994a) *In vitro* exposure of a novel polyesterurethane graft to enzymes: a study of the biostability of the Vasugraft® arterial prosthesis. *Biomaterials*, **15**, 1129–1144

Zhang, Z., King, M.W., Marois, Y., Marois, M. & Guidoin, R. (1994b) *In vivo* performance of the polyesterurethane Vasugraft® prosthesis implanted as a thoracoabdominal bypass in dogs: an exploratory study. *Biomaterials*, **15**, 1099–1112

Zhang, G., Latour, R.A., Jr, Kennedy, J.M., Del Schutte, H., Jr & Friedman, R.J. (1996) Long-term compressive property durability of carbon fibre-reinforced polyetheretherketone composite in physiological saline. *Biomaterials*, **17**, 781–789

CUMULATIVE CROSS INDEX TO *IARC MONOGRAPHS ON THE EVALUATION OF CARCINOGENIC RISKS TO HUMANS*

The volume, page and year of publication are given. References to corrigenda are given in parentheses.

A

A-α-C	*40*, 245 (1986); *Suppl. 7*, 56 (1987)
Acetaldehyde	*36*, 101 (1985) (*corr. 42*, 263); *Suppl. 7*, 77 (1987); *71*, 319 (1999)
Acetaldehyde formylmethylhydrazone (*see* Gyromitrin)	
Acetamide	*7*, 197 (1974); *Suppl. 7*, 389 (1987); *71*, 1211 (1999)
Acetaminophen (*see* Paracetamol)	
Acridine orange	*16*, 145 (1978); *Suppl. 7*, 56 (1987)
Acriflavinium chloride	*13*, 31 (1977); *Suppl. 7*, 56 (1987)
Acrolein	*19*, 479 (1979); *36*, 133 (1985); *Suppl. 7*, 78 (1987); *63*, 337 (1995) (*corr. 65*, 549)
Acrylamide	*39*, 41 (1986); *Suppl. 7*, 56 (1987); *60*, 389 (1994)
Acrylic acid	*19*, 47 (1979); *Suppl. 7*, 56 (1987); *71*, 1223 (1999)
Acrylic fibres	*19*, 86 (1979); *Suppl. 7*, 56 (1987)
Acrylonitrile	*19*, 73 (1979); *Suppl. 7*, 79 (1987); *71*, 43 (1999)
Acrylonitrile-butadiene-styrene copolymers	*19*, 91 (1979); *Suppl. 7*, 56 (1987)
Actinolite (*see* Asbestos)	
Actinomycin D (*see also* Actinomycins)	*Suppl. 7*, 80 (1987)
Actinomycins	*10*, 29 (1976) (*corr. 42*, 255)
Adriamycin	*10*, 43 (1976); *Suppl. 7*, 82 (1987)
AF-2	*31*, 47 (1983); *Suppl. 7*, 56 (1987)
Aflatoxins	*1*, 145 (1972) (*corr. 42*, 251); *10*, 51 (1976); *Suppl. 7*, 83 (1987); *56*, 245 (1993)
Aflatoxin B$_1$ (*see* Aflatoxins)	
Aflatoxin B$_2$ (*see* Aflatoxins)	
Aflatoxin G$_1$ (*see* Aflatoxins)	
Aflatoxin G$_2$ (*see* Aflatoxins)	
Aflatoxin M$_1$ (*see* Aflatoxins)	
Agaritine	*31*, 63 (1983); *Suppl. 7*, 56 (1987)
Alcohol drinking	*44* (1988)
Aldicarb	*53*, 93 (1991)
Aldrin	*5*, 25 (1974); *Suppl. 7*, 88 (1987)
Allyl chloride	*36*, 39 (1985); *Suppl. 7*, 56 (1987); *71*, 1231 (1999)

Allyl isothiocyanate	36, 55 (1985); *Suppl. 7*, 56 (1987); 73, 37 (1999)
Allyl isovalerate	36, 69 (1985); *Suppl. 7*, 56 (1987); 71, 1241 (1999)
Aluminium production	34, 37 (1984); *Suppl. 7*, 89 (1987)
Amaranth	8, 41 (1975); *Suppl. 7*, 56 (1987)
5-Aminoacenaphthene	16, 243 (1978); *Suppl. 7*, 56 (1987)
2-Aminoanthraquinone	27, 191 (1982); *Suppl. 7*, 56 (1987)
para-Aminoazobenzene	8, 53 (1975); *Suppl. 7*, 390 (1987)
ortho-Aminoazotoluene	8, 61 (1975) (*corr.* 42, 254); *Suppl. 7*, 56 (1987)
para-Aminobenzoic acid	16, 249 (1978); *Suppl. 7*, 56 (1987)
4-Aminobiphenyl	1, 74 (1972) (*corr.* 42, 251); *Suppl. 7*, 91 (1987)
2-Amino-3,4-dimethylimidazo[4,5-*f*]quinoline (*see* MeIQ)	
2-Amino-3,8-dimethylimidazo[4,5-*f*]quinoxaline (*see* MeIQx)	
3-Amino-1,4-dimethyl-5*H*-pyrido[4,3-*b*]indole (*see* Trp-P-1)	
2-Aminodipyrido[1,2-*a*:3′,2′-*d*]imidazole (*see* Glu-P-2)	
1-Amino-2-methylanthraquinone	27, 199 (1982); *Suppl. 7*, 57 (1987)
2-Amino-3-methylimidazo[4,5-*f*]quinoline (*see* IQ)	
2-Amino-6-methyldipyrido[1,2-*a*:3′,2′-*d*]imidazole (*see* Glu-P-1)	
2-Amino-1-methyl-6-phenylimidazo[4,5-*b*]pyridine (*see* PhIP)	
2-Amino-3-methyl-9*H*-pyrido[2,3-*b*]indole (*see* MeA-α-C)	
3-Amino-1-methyl-5*H*-pyrido[4,3-*b*]indole (*see* Trp-P-2)	
2-Amino-5-(5-nitro-2-furyl)-1,3,4-thiadiazole	7, 143 (1974); *Suppl. 7*, 57 (1987)
2-Amino-4-nitrophenol	57, 167 (1993)
2-Amino-5-nitrophenol	57, 177 (1993)
4-Amino-2-nitrophenol	16, 43 (1978); *Suppl. 7*, 57 (1987)
2-Amino-5-nitrothiazole	31, 71 (1983); *Suppl. 7*, 57 (1987)
2-Amino-9*H*-pyrido[2,3-*b*]indole (*see* A-α-C)	
11-Aminoundecanoic acid	39, 239 (1986); *Suppl. 7*, 57 (1987)
Amitrole	7, 31 (1974); 41, 293 (1986) (*corr.* 52, 513; *Suppl. 7*, 92 (1987)
Ammonium potassium selenide (*see* Selenium and selenium compounds)	
Amorphous silica (*see also* Silica)	42, 39 (1987); *Suppl. 7*, 341 (1987); 68, 41 (1997)
Amosite (*see* Asbestos)	
Ampicillin	50, 153 (1990)
Anabolic steroids (*see* Androgenic (anabolic) steroids)	
Anaesthetics, volatile	11, 285 (1976); *Suppl. 7*, 93 (1987)
Analgesic mixtures containing phenacetin (*see also* Phenacetin)	*Suppl. 7*, 310 (1987)
Androgenic (anabolic) steroids	*Suppl. 7*, 96 (1987)
Angelicin and some synthetic derivatives (*see also* Angelicins)	40, 291 (1986)
Angelicin plus ultraviolet radiation (*see also* Angelicin and some synthetic derivatives)	*Suppl. 7*, 57 (1987)
Angelicins	*Suppl. 7*, 57 (1987)
Aniline	4, 27 (1974) (*corr.* 42, 252); 27, 39 (1982); *Suppl. 7*, 99 (1987)
ortho-Anisidine	27, 63 (1982); *Suppl. 7*, 57 (1987); 73, 49 (1999)
para-Anisidine	27, 65 (1982); *Suppl. 7*, 57 (1987)
Anthanthrene	32, 95 (1983); *Suppl. 7*, 57 (1987)
Anthophyllite (*see* Asbestos)	
Anthracene	32, 105 (1983); *Suppl. 7*, 57 (1987)

Anthranilic acid	*16*, 265 (1978); *Suppl. 7*, 57 (1987)
Antimony trioxide	*47*, 291 (1989)
Antimony trisulfide	*47*, 291 (1989)
ANTU (*see* 1-Naphthylthiourea)	
Apholate	*9*, 31 (1975); *Suppl. 7*, 57 (1987)
para-Aramid fibrils	*68*, 409 (1997)
Aramite®	*5*, 39 (1974); *Suppl. 7*, 57 (1987)
Areca nut (*see* Betel quid)	
Arsanilic acid (*see* Arsenic and arsenic compounds)	
Arsenic and arsenic compounds	*1*, 41 (1972); *2*, 48 (1973); *23*, 39 (1980); *Suppl. 7*, 100 (1987)
Arsenic pentoxide (*see* Arsenic and arsenic compounds)	
Arsenic sulfide (*see* Arsenic and arsenic compounds)	
Arsenic trioxide (*see* Arsenic and arsenic compounds)	
Arsine (*see* Arsenic and arsenic compounds)	
Asbestos	*2*, 17 (1973) (*corr. 42*, 252); *14* (1977) (*corr. 42*, 256); *Suppl. 7*, 106 (1987) (*corr. 45*, 283)
Atrazine	*53*, 441 (1991); *73*, 59 (1999)
Attapulgite (*see* Palygorskite)	
Auramine (technical-grade)	*1*, 69 (1972) (*corr. 42*, 251); *Suppl. 7*, 118 (1987)
Auramine, manufacture of (*see also* Auramine, technical-grade)	*Suppl. 7*, 118 (1987)
Aurothioglucose	*13*, 39 (1977); *Suppl. 7*, 57 (1987)
Azacitidine	*26*, 37 (1981); *Suppl. 7*, 57 (1987); *50*, 47 (1990)
5-Azacytidine (*see* Azacitidine)	
Azaserine	*10*, 73 (1976) (*corr. 42*, 255); *Suppl. 7*, 57 (1987)
Azathioprine	*26*, 47 (1981); *Suppl. 7*, 119 (1987)
Aziridine	*9*, 37 (1975); *Suppl. 7*, 58 (1987); *71*, 337 (1999)
2-(1-Aziridinyl)ethanol	*9*, 47 (1975); *Suppl. 7*, 58 (1987)
Aziridyl benzoquinone	*9*, 51 (1975); *Suppl. 7*, 58 (1987)
Azobenzene	*8*, 75 (1975); *Suppl. 7*, 58 (1987)

B

Barium chromate (*see* Chromium and chromium compounds)	
Basic chromic sulfate (*see* Chromium and chromium compounds)	
BCNU (*see* Bischloroethyl nitrosourea)	
Benz[*a*]acridine	*32*, 123 (1983); *Suppl. 7*, 58 (1987)
Benz[*c*]acridine	*3*, 241 (1973); *32*, 129 (1983); *Suppl. 7*, 58 (1987)
Benzal chloride (*see also* α-Chlorinated toluenes and benzoyl chloride)	*29*, 65 (1982); *Suppl. 7*, 148 (1987); *71*, 453 (1999)
Benz[*a*]anthracene	*3*, 45 (1973); *32*, 135 (1983); *Suppl. 7*, 58 (1987)
Benzene	*7*, 203 (1974) (*corr. 42*, 254); *29*, 93, 391 (1982); *Suppl. 7*, 120 (1987)
Benzidine	*1*, 80 (1972); *29*, 149, 391 (1982); *Suppl. 7*, 123 (1987)

Benzidine-based dyes	Suppl. 7, 125 (1987)
Benzo[b]fluoranthene	3, 69 (1973); 32, 147 (1983); Suppl. 7, 58 (1987)
Benzo[j]fluoranthene	3, 82 (1973); 32, 155 (1983); Suppl. 7, 58 (1987)
Benzo[k]fluoranthene	32, 163 (1983); Suppl. 7, 58 (1987)
Benzo[ghi]fluoranthene	32, 171 (1983); Suppl. 7, 58 (1987)
Benzo[a]fluorene	32, 177 (1983); Suppl. 7, 58 (1987)
Benzo[b]fluorene	32, 183 (1983); Suppl. 7, 58 (1987)
Benzo[c]fluorene	32, 189 (1983); Suppl. 7, 58 (1987)
Benzofuran	63, 431 (1995)
Benzo[ghi]perylene	32, 195 (1983); Suppl. 7, 58 (1987)
Benzo[c]phenanthrene	32, 205 (1983); Suppl. 7, 58 (1987)
Benzo[a]pyrene	3, 91 (1973); 32, 211 (1983) (corr. 68, 477); Suppl. 7, 58 (1987)
Benzo[e]pyrene	3, 137 (1973); 32, 225 (1983); Suppl. 7, 58 (1987)
1,4-Benzoquinone (see para-Quinone)	
1,4-Benzoquinone dioxime	29, 185 (1982); Suppl. 7, 58 (1987); 71, 1251 (1999)
Benzotrichloride (see also α-Chlorinated toluenes and benzoyl chloride)	29, 73 (1982); Suppl. 7, 148 (1987); 71, 453 (1999)
Benzoyl chloride (see also α-Chlorinated toluenes and benzoyl chloride)	29, 83 (1982) (corr. 42, 261); Suppl. 7, 126 (1987); 71, 453 (1999)
Benzoyl peroxide	36, 267 (1985); Suppl. 7, 58 (1987); 71, 345 (1999)
Benzyl acetate	40, 109 (1986); Suppl. 7, 58 (1987); 71, 1255 (1999)
Benzyl chloride (see also α-Chlorinated toluenes and benzoyl chloride)	11, 217 (1976) (corr. 42, 256); 29, 49 (1982); Suppl. 7, 148 (1987); 71, 453 (1999)
Benzyl violet 4B	16, 153 (1978); Suppl. 7, 58 (1987)
Bertrandite (see Beryllium and beryllium compounds)	
Beryllium and beryllium compounds	1, 17 (1972); 23, 143 (1980) (corr. 42, 260); Suppl. 7, 127 (1987); 58, 41 (1993)
Beryllium acetate (see Beryllium and beryllium compounds)	
Beryllium acetate, basic (see Beryllium and beryllium compounds)	
Beryllium-aluminium alloy (see Beryllium and beryllium compounds)	
Beryllium carbonate (see Beryllium and beryllium compounds)	
Beryllium chloride (see Beryllium and beryllium compounds)	
Beryllium-copper alloy (see Beryllium and beryllium compounds)	
Beryllium-copper-cobalt alloy (see Beryllium and beryllium compounds)	
Beryllium fluoride (see Beryllium and beryllium compounds)	
Beryllium hydroxide (see Beryllium and beryllium compounds)	
Beryllium-nickel alloy (see Beryllium and beryllium compounds)	
Beryllium oxide (see Beryllium and beryllium compounds)	
Beryllium phosphate (see Beryllium and beryllium compounds)	
Beryllium silicate (see Beryllium and beryllium compounds)	
Beryllium sulfate (see Beryllium and beryllium compounds)	
Beryl ore (see Beryllium and beryllium compounds)	
Betel quid	37, 141 (1985); Suppl. 7, 128 (1987)
Betel-quid chewing (see Betel quid)	
BHA (see Butylated hydroxyanisole)	

BHT (see Butylated hydroxytoluene)
Bis(1-aziridinyl)morpholinophosphine sulfide   9, 55 (1975); Suppl. 7, 58 (1987)
Bis(2-chloroethyl)ether   9, 117 (1975); Suppl. 7, 58 (1987);
                                                      71, 1265 (1999)

N,N-Bis(2-chloroethyl)-2-naphthylamine   4, 119 (1974) (corr. 42, 253);
                                                      Suppl. 7, 130 (1987)
Bischloroethyl nitrosourea (see also Chloroethyl nitrosoureas)   26, 79 (1981); Suppl. 7, 150 (1987)
1,2-Bis(chloromethoxy)ethane   15, 31 (1977); Suppl. 7, 58 (1987);
                                                      71, 1271 (1999)
1,4-Bis(chloromethoxymethyl)benzene   15, 37 (1977); Suppl. 7, 58 (1987);
                                                      71, 1273 (1999)
Bis(chloromethyl)ether   4, 231 (1974) (corr. 42, 253);
                                                      Suppl. 7, 131 (1987)
Bis(2-chloro-1-methylethyl)ether   41, 149 (1986); Suppl. 7, 59 (1987);
                                                      71, 1275 (1999)
Bis(2,3-epoxycyclopentyl)ether   47, 231 (1989); 71, 1281 (1999)
Bisphenol A diglycidyl ether (see also Glycidyl ethers)   71, 1285 (1999)
Bisulfites (see Sulfur dioxide and some sulfites, bisulfites and
    metabisulfites)
Bitumens   35, 39 (1985); Suppl. 7, 133 (1987)
Bleomycins   26, 97 (1981); Suppl. 7, 134 (1987)
Blue VRS   16, 163 (1978); Suppl. 7, 59 (1987)
Boot and shoe manufacture and repair   25, 249 (1981); Suppl. 7, 232
                                                      (1987)
Bracken fern   40, 47 (1986); Suppl. 7, 135 (1987)
Brilliant Blue FCF, disodium salt   16, 171 (1978) (corr. 42, 257);
                                                      Suppl. 7, 59 (1987)
Bromochloroacetonitrile (see also Halogenated acetonitriles)   71, 1291 (1999)
Bromodichloromethane   52, 179 (1991); 71, 1295 (1999)
Bromoethane   52, 299 (1991); 71, 1305 (1999)
Bromoform   52, 213 (1991); 71, 1309 (1999)
1,3-Butadiene   39, 155 (1986) (corr. 42, 264
                                                      Suppl. 7, 136 (1987); 54, 237
                                                      (1992); 71, 109 (1999)
1,4-Butanediol dimethanesulfonate   4, 247 (1974); Suppl. 7, 137 (1987)
n-Butyl acrylate   39, 67 (1986); Suppl. 7, 59 (1987);
                                                      71, 359 (1999)
Butylated hydroxyanisole   40, 123 (1986); Suppl. 7, 59 (1987)
Butylated hydroxytoluene   40, 161 (1986); Suppl. 7, 59 (1987)
Butyl benzyl phthalate   29, 193 (1982) (corr. 42, 261);
                                                      Suppl. 7, 59 (1987); 73, 115 (1999)
β-Butyrolactone   11, 225 (1976); Suppl. 7, 59
                                                      (1987); 71, 1317 (1999)
γ-Butyrolactone   11, 231 (1976); Suppl. 7, 59
                                                      (1987); 71, 367 (1999)

C

Cabinet-making (see Furniture and cabinet-making)
Cadmium acetate (see Cadmium and cadmium compounds)

Cadmium and cadmium compounds　　　　　　　　2, 74 (1973); *11*, 39 (1976)
　　　　　　　　　　　　　　　　　　　　　　　　　　(*corr. 42*, 255); *Suppl. 7*, 139
　　　　　　　　　　　　　　　　　　　　　　　　　　(1987); *58*, 119 (1993)
Cadmium chloride (*see* Cadmium and cadmium compounds)
Cadmium oxide (*see* Cadmium and cadmium compounds)
Cadmium sulfate (*see* Cadmium and cadmium compounds)
Cadmium sulfide (*see* Cadmium and cadmium compounds)
Caffeic acid　　　　　　　　　　　　　　　　　　　　*56*, 115 (1993)
Caffeine　　　　　　　　　　　　　　　　　　　　　*51*, 291 (1991)
Calcium arsenate (*see* Arsenic and arsenic compounds)
Calcium chromate (see Chromium and chromium compounds)
Calcium cyclamate (*see* Cyclamates)
Calcium saccharin (*see* Saccharin)
Cantharidin　　　　　　　　　　　　　　　　　　　　*10*, 79 (1976); *Suppl. 7*, 59 (1987)
Caprolactam　　　　　　　　　　　　　　　　　　　　*19*, 115 (1979) (*corr. 42*, 258);
　　　　　　　　　　　　　　　　　　　　　　　　　　39, 247 (1986) (*corr. 42*, 264);
　　　　　　　　　　　　　　　　　　　　　　　　　　Suppl. 7, 390 (1987); *71*, 383
　　　　　　　　　　　　　　　　　　　　　　　　　　(1999)
Captafol　　　　　　　　　　　　　　　　　　　　　*53*, 353 (1991)
Captan　　　　　　　　　　　　　　　　　　　　　　*30*, 295 (1983); *Suppl. 7*, 59 (1987)
Carbaryl　　　　　　　　　　　　　　　　　　　　　*12*, 37 (1976); *Suppl. 7*, 59 (1987)
Carbazole　　　　　　　　　　　　　　　　　　　　　*32*, 239 (1983); *Suppl. 7*, 59
　　　　　　　　　　　　　　　　　　　　　　　　　　(1987); *71*, 1319 (1999)
3-Carbethoxypsoralen　　　　　　　　　　　　　　　*40*, 317 (1986); *Suppl. 7*, 59 (1987)
Carbon black　　　　　　　　　　　　　　　　　　　*3*, 22 (1973); *33*, 35 (1984);
　　　　　　　　　　　　　　　　　　　　　　　　　　Suppl. 7, 142 (1987); *65*, 149
　　　　　　　　　　　　　　　　　　　　　　　　　　(1996)
Carbon tetrachloride　　　　　　　　　　　　　　　　*1*, 53 (1972); *20*, 371 (1979);
　　　　　　　　　　　　　　　　　　　　　　　　　　Suppl. 7, 143 (1987); *71*, 401
　　　　　　　　　　　　　　　　　　　　　　　　　　(1999)
Carmoisine　　　　　　　　　　　　　　　　　　　　*8*, 83 (1975); *Suppl. 7*, 59 (1987)
Carpentry and joinery　　　　　　　　　　　　　　　*25*, 139 (1981); *Suppl. 7*, 378
　　　　　　　　　　　　　　　　　　　　　　　　　　(1987)
Carrageenan　　　　　　　　　　　　　　　　　　　　*10*, 181 (1976) (*corr. 42*, 255); *31*,
　　　　　　　　　　　　　　　　　　　　　　　　　　79 (1983); *Suppl. 7*, 59 (1987)
Catechol　　　　　　　　　　　　　　　　　　　　　*15*, 155 (1977); *Suppl. 7*, 59
　　　　　　　　　　　　　　　　　　　　　　　　　　(1987); *71*, 433 (1999)
CCNU (*see* 1-(2-Chloroethyl)-3-cyclohexyl-1-nitrosourea)
Ceramic fibres (see Man-made mineral fibres)
Chemotherapy, combined, including alkylating agents (*see* MOPP and
　　other combined chemotherapy including alkylating agents)
Chloral　　　　　　　　　　　　　　　　　　　　　*63*, 245 (1995)
Chloral hydrate　　　　　　　　　　　　　　　　　*63*, 245 (1995)
Chlorambucil　　　　　　　　　　　　　　　　　　*9*, 125 (1975); *26*, 115 (1981);
　　　　　　　　　　　　　　　　　　　　　　　　　　Suppl. 7, 144 (1987)
Chloramphenicol　　　　　　　　　　　　　　　　　*10*, 85 (1976); *Suppl. 7*, 145
　　　　　　　　　　　　　　　　　　　　　　　　　　(1987); *50*, 169 (1990)
Chlordane (*see also* Chlordane/Heptachlor)　　　　*20*, 45 (1979) (*corr. 42*, 258)
Chlordane/Heptachlor　　　　　　　　　　　　　　　*Suppl. 7*, 146 (1987); *53*, 115
　　　　　　　　　　　　　　　　　　　　　　　　　　(1991)
Chlordecone　　　　　　　　　　　　　　　　　　　*20*, 67 (1979); *Suppl. 7*, 59 (1987)
Chlordimeform　　　　　　　　　　　　　　　　　　*30*, 61 (1983); *Suppl. 7*, 59 (1987)
Chlorendic acid　　　　　　　　　　　　　　　　　　*48*, 45 (1990)

Chlorinated dibenzodioxins (other than TCDD) (*see also* Polychlorinated dibenzo-*para*-dioxins)	*15*, 41 (1977); *Suppl. 7*, 59 (1987)
Chlorinated drinking-water	*52*, 45 (1991)
Chlorinated paraffins	*48*, 55 (1990)
α-Chlorinated toluenes and benzoyl chloride	*Suppl. 7*, 148 (1987); *71*, 453 (1999)
Chlormadinone acetate	*6*, 149 (1974); *21*, 365 (1979); *Suppl. 7*, 291, 301 (1987); *72*, 49 (1999)
Chlornaphazine (*see* N,N-Bis(2-chloroethyl)-2-naphthylamine)	
Chloroacetonitrile (*see also* Halogenated acetonitriles)	*71*, 1325 (1999)
para-Chloroaniline	*57*, 305 (1993)
Chlorobenzilate	*5*, 75 (1974); *30*, 73 (1983); *Suppl. 7*, 60 (1987)
Chlorodibromomethane	*52*, 243 (1991); *71*, 1331 (1999)
Chlorodifluoromethane	*41*, 237 (1986) (*corr. 51*, 483); *Suppl. 7*, 149 (1987); *71*, 1339 (1999)
Chloroethane	*52*, 315 (1991); *71*, 1345 (1999)
1-(2-Chloroethyl)-3-cyclohexyl-1-nitrosourea (*see also* Chloroethyl nitrosoureas)	*26*, 137 (1981) (*corr. 42*, 260); *Suppl. 7*, 150 (1987)
1-(2-Chloroethyl)-3-(4-methylcyclohexyl)-1-nitrosourea (*see also* Chloroethyl nitrosoureas)	*Suppl. 7*, 150 (1987)
Chloroethyl nitrosoureas	*Suppl. 7*, 150 (1987)
Chlorofluoromethane	*41*, 229 (1986); *Suppl. 7*, 60 (1987); *71*, 1351 (1999)
Chloroform	*1*, 61 (1972); *20*, 401 (1979); *Suppl. 7*, 152 (1987); *73*, 131 (1999)
Chloromethyl methyl ether (technical-grade) (*see also* Bis(chloromethyl)ether)	*4*, 239 (1974); *Suppl. 7*, 131 (1987)
(4-Chloro-2-methylphenoxy)acetic acid (*see* MCPA)	
1-Chloro-2-methylpropene	*63*, 315 (1995)
3-Chloro-2-methylpropene	*63*, 325 (1995)
2-Chloronitrobenzene	*65*, 263 (1996)
3-Chloronitrobenzene	*65*, 263 (1996)
4-Chloronitrobenzene	*65*, 263 (1996)
Chlorophenols (*see also* Polychlorophenols and their sodium salts)	*Suppl. 7*, 154 (1987)
Chlorophenols (occupational exposures to)	*41*, 319 (1986)
Chlorophenoxy herbicides	*Suppl. 7*, 156 (1987)
Chlorophenoxy herbicides (occupational exposures to)	*41*, 357 (1986)
4-Chloro-*ortho*-phenylenediamine	*27*, 81 (1982); *Suppl. 7*, 60 (1987)
4-Chloro-*meta*-phenylenediamine	*27*, 82 (1982); *Suppl. 7*, 60 (1987)
Chloroprene	*19*, 131 (1979); *Suppl. 7*, 160 (1987); *71*, 227 (1999)
Chloropropham	*12*, 55 (1976); *Suppl. 7*, 60 (1987)
Chloroquine	*13*, 47 (1977); *Suppl. 7*, 60 (1987)
Chlorothalonil	*30*, 319 (1983); *Suppl. 7*, 60 (1987); *73*, 183 (1999)
para-Chloro-*ortho*-toluidine and its strong acid salts (*see also* Chlordimeform)	*16*, 277 (1978); *30*, 65 (1983); *Suppl. 7*, 60 (1987); *48*, 123 (1990)
Chlorotrianisene (*see also* Nonsteroidal oestrogens)	*21*, 139 (1979); *Suppl. 7*, 280 (1987)

2-Chloro-1,1,1-trifluoroethane	*41*, 253 (1986); *Suppl. 7*, 60 (1987); *71*, 1355 (1999)
Chlorozotocin	*50*, 65 (1990)
Cholesterol	*10*, 99 (1976); *31*, 95 (1983); *Suppl. 7*, 161 (1987)
Chromic acetate (*see* Chromium and chromium compounds)	
Chromic chloride (*see* Chromium and chromium compounds)	
Chromic oxide (*see* Chromium and chromium compounds)	
Chromic phosphate (*see* Chromium and chromium compounds)	
Chromite ore (*see* Chromium and chromium compounds)	
Chromium and chromium compounds (*see also* Implants, surgical)	*2*, 100 (1973); *23*, 205 (1980); *Suppl. 7*, 165 (1987); *49*, 49 (1990) (*corr. 51*, 483)
Chromium carbonyl (*see* Chromium and chromium compounds)	
Chromium potassium sulfate (*see* Chromium and chromium compounds)	
Chromium sulfate (*see* Chromium and chromium compounds)	
Chromium trioxide (*see* Chromium and chromium compounds)	
Chrysazin (*see* Dantron)	
Chrysene	*3*, 159 (1973); *32*, 247 (1983); *Suppl. 7*, 60 (1987)
Chrysoidine	*8*, 91 (1975); *Suppl. 7*, 169 (1987)
Chrysotile (*see* Asbestos)	
CI Acid Orange 3	*57*, 121 (1993)
CI Acid Red 114	*57*, 247 (1993)
CI Basic Red 9 (*see also* Magenta)	*57*, 215 (1993)
Ciclosporin	*50*, 77 (1990)
CI Direct Blue 15	*57*, 235 (1993)
CI Disperse Yellow 3 (see Disperse Yellow 3)	
Cimetidine	*50*, 235 (1990)
Cinnamyl anthranilate	*16*, 287 (1978); *31*, 133 (1983); *Suppl. 7*, 60 (1987)
CI Pigment Red 3	*57*, 259 (1993)
CI Pigment Red 53:1 (*see* D&C Red No. 9)	
Cisplatin	*26*, 151 (1981); *Suppl. 7*, 170 (1987)
Citrinin	*40*, 67 (1986); *Suppl. 7*, 60 (1987)
Citrus Red No. 2	*8*, 101 (1975) (*corr. 42*, 254); *Suppl. 7*, 60 (1987)
Clinoptilolite (*see* Zeolites)	
Clofibrate	*24*, 39 (1980); *Suppl. 7*, 171 (1987); *66*, 391 (1996)
Clomiphene citrate	*21*, 551 (1979); *Suppl. 7*, 172 (1987)
Clonorchis sinensis (infection with)	*61*, 121 (1994)
Coal dust	*68*, 337 (1997)
Coal gasification	*34*, 65 (1984); *Suppl. 7*, 173 (1987)
Coal-tar pitches (*see also* Coal-tars)	*35*, 83 (1985); *Suppl. 7*, 174 (1987)
Coal-tars	*35*, 83 (1985); *Suppl. 7*, 175 (1987)
Cobalt[III] acetate (*see* Cobalt and cobalt compounds)	
Cobalt-aluminium-chromium spinel (*see* Cobalt and cobalt compounds)	
Cobalt and cobalt compounds (*see also* Implants, surgical)	*52*, 363 (1991)
Cobalt[II] chloride (*see* Cobalt and cobalt compounds)	
Cobalt-chromium alloy (*see* Chromium and chromium compounds)	
Cobalt-chromium-molybdenum alloys (*see* Cobalt and cobalt compounds)	

Cobalt metal powder (*see* Cobalt and cobalt compounds)	
Cobalt naphthenate (*see* Cobalt and cobalt compounds)	
Cobalt[II] oxide (*see* Cobalt and cobalt compounds)	
Cobalt[II,III] oxide (*see* Cobalt and cobalt compounds)	
Cobalt[II] sulfide (*see* Cobalt and cobalt compounds)	
Coffee	*51*, 41 (1991) (*corr. 52*, 513)
Coke production	*34*, 101 (1984); *Suppl. 7*, 176 (1987)
Combined oral contraceptives (*see* Oral contraceptives, combined)	
Conjugated equine oestrogens	*72*, 399 (1999)
Conjugated oestrogens (*see also* Steroidal oestrogens)	*21*, 147 (1979); *Suppl. 7*, 283 (1987)
Contraceptives, oral (*see* Combined oral contraceptives; Sequential oral contraceptives)	
Copper 8-hydroxyquinoline	*15*, 103 (1977); *Suppl. 7*, 61 (1987)
Coronene	*32*, 263 (1983); *Suppl. 7*, 61 (1987)
Coumarin	*10*, 113 (1976); *Suppl. 7*, 61 (1987)
Creosotes (*see also* Coal-tars)	*35*, 83 (1985); *Suppl. 7*, 177 (1987)
meta-Cresidine	*27*, 91 (1982); *Suppl. 7*, 61 (1987)
para-Cresidine	*27*, 92 (1982); *Suppl. 7*, 61 (1987)
Cristobalite (*see* Crystalline silica)	
Crocidolite (*see* Asbestos)	
Crotonaldehyde	*63*, 373 (1995) (*corr. 65*, 549)
Crude oil	*45*, 119 (1989)
Crystalline silica (*see also* Silica)	*42*, 39 (1987); *Suppl. 7*, 341 (1987); *68*, 41 (1997)
Cycasin (*see also* Methylazoxymethanol)	*1*, 157 (1972) (*corr. 42*, 251); *10*, 121 (1976); *Suppl. 7*, 61 (1987)
Cyclamates	*22*, 55 (1980); *Suppl. 7*, 178 (1987); *73*, 195 (1999)
Cyclamic acid (*see* Cyclamates)	
Cyclochlorotine	*10*, 139 (1976); *Suppl. 7*, 61 (1987)
Cyclohexanone	*47*, 157 (1989); *71*, 1359 (1999)
Cyclohexylamine (*see* Cyclamates)	
Cyclopenta[*cd*]pyrene	*32*, 269 (1983); *Suppl. 7*, 61 (1987)
Cyclopropane (*see* Anaesthetics, volatile)	
Cyclophosphamide	*9*, 135 (1975); *26*, 165 (1981); *Suppl. 7*, 182 (1987)
Cyproterone acetate	*72*, 49 (1999)

D

2,4-D (*see also* Chlorophenoxy herbicides; Chlorophenoxy herbicides, occupational exposures to)	*15*, 111 (1977)
Dacarbazine	*26*, 203 (1981); *Suppl. 7*, 184 (1987)
Dantron	*50*, 265 (1990) (*corr. 59*, 257)
D&C Red No. 9	*8*, 107 (1975); *Suppl. 7*, 61 (1987); *57*, 203 (1993)
Dapsone	*24*, 59 (1980); *Suppl. 7*, 185 (1987)
Daunomycin	*10*, 145 (1976); *Suppl. 7*, 61 (1987)
DDD (*see* DDT)	
DDE (*see* DDT)	

DDT	5, 83 (1974) (corr. 42, 253); Suppl. 7, 186 (1987); 53, 179 (1991)
Decabromodiphenyl oxide	48, 73 (1990); 71, 1365 (1999)
Deltamethrin	53, 251 (1991)
Deoxynivalenol (see Toxins derived from *Fusarium graminearum, F. culmorum* and *F. crookwellense*)	
Diacetylaminoazotoluene	8, 113 (1975); Suppl. 7, 61 (1987)
N,N'-Diacetylbenzidine	16, 293 (1978); Suppl. 7, 61 (1987)
Diallate	12, 69 (1976); 30, 235 (1983); Suppl. 7, 61 (1987)
2,4-Diaminoanisole	16, 51 (1978); 27, 103 (1982); Suppl. 7, 61 (1987)
4,4'-Diaminodiphenyl ether	16, 301 (1978); 29, 203 (1982); Suppl. 7, 61 (1987)
1,2-Diamino-4-nitrobenzene	16, 63 (1978); Suppl. 7, 61 (1987)
1,4-Diamino-2-nitrobenzene	16, 73 (1978); Suppl. 7, 61 (1987); 57, 185 (1993)
2,6-Diamino-3-(phenylazo)pyridine (see Phenazopyridine hydrochloride)	
2,4-Diaminotoluene (see also Toluene diisocyanates)	16, 83 (1978); Suppl. 7, 61 (1987)
2,5-Diaminotoluene (see also Toluene diisocyanates)	16, 97 (1978); Suppl. 7, 61 (1987)
ortho-Dianisidine (see 3,3'-Dimethoxybenzidine)	
Diatomaceous earth, uncalcined (see Amorphous silica)	
Diazepam	13, 57 (1977); Suppl. 7, 189 (1987); 66, 37 (1996)
Diazomethane	7, 223 (1974); Suppl. 7, 61 (1987)
Dibenz[*a,h*]acridine	3, 247 (1973); 32, 277 (1983); Suppl. 7, 61 (1987)
Dibenz[*a,j*]acridine	3, 254 (1973); 32, 283 (1983); Suppl. 7, 61 (1987)
Dibenz[*a,c*]anthracene	32, 289 (1983) (corr. 42, 262); Suppl. 7, 61 (1987)
Dibenz[*a,h*]anthracene	3, 178 (1973) (corr. 43, 261); 32, 299 (1983); Suppl. 7, 61 (1987)
Dibenz[*a,j*]anthracene	32, 309 (1983); Suppl. 7, 61 (1987)
7*H*-Dibenzo[*c,g*]carbazole	3, 260 (1973); 32, 315 (1983); Suppl. 7, 61 (1987)
Dibenzodioxins, chlorinated (other than TCDD) (see Chlorinated dibenzodioxins (other than TCDD))	
Dibenzo[*a,e*]fluoranthene	32, 321 (1983); Suppl. 7, 61 (1987)
Dibenzo[*h,rst*]pentaphene	3, 197 (1973); Suppl. 7, 62 (1987)
Dibenzo[*a,e*]pyrene	3, 201 (1973); 32, 327 (1983); Suppl. 7, 62 (1987)
Dibenzo[*a,h*]pyrene	3, 207 (1973); 32, 331 (1983); Suppl. 7, 62 (1987)
Dibenzo[*a,i*]pyrene	3, 215 (1973); 32, 337 (1983); Suppl. 7, 62 (1987)
Dibenzo[*a,l*]pyrene	3, 224 (1973); 32, 343 (1983); Suppl. 7, 62 (1987)
Dibenzo-*para*-dioxin	69, 33 (1997)
Dibromoacetonitrile (see also Halogenated acetonitriles)	71, 1369 (1999)
1,2-Dibromo-3-chloropropane	15, 139 (1977); 20, 83 (1979); Suppl. 7, 191 (1987); 71, 479 (1999)

1,2-Dibromoethane (*see* Ethylene dibromide)
Dichloroacetic acid   *63*, 271 (1995)
Dichloroacetonitrile (*see also* Halogenated acetonitriles)   *71*, 1375 (1999)
Dichloroacetylene   *39*, 369 (1986); *Suppl. 7*, 62 (1987); *71*, 1381 (1999)
ortho-Dichlorobenzene   *7*, 231 (1974); *29*, 213 (1982); *Suppl. 7*, 192 (1987); *73*, 223 (1999)
meta-Dichlorobenzene   *73*, 223 (1999)
para-Dichlorobenzene   *7*, 231 (1974); *29*, 215 (1982); *Suppl. 7*, 192 (1987); *73*, 223 (1999)
3,3′-Dichlorobenzidine   *4*, 49 (1974); *29*, 239 (1982); *Suppl. 7*, 193 (1987)
trans-1,4-Dichlorobutene   *15*, 149 (1977); *Suppl. 7*, 62 (1987); *71*, 1389 (1999)
3,3′-Dichloro-4,4′-diaminodiphenyl ether   *16*, 309 (1978); *Suppl. 7*, 62 (1987)
1,2-Dichloroethane   *20*, 429 (1979); *Suppl. 7*, 62 (1987); *71*, 501 (1999)
Dichloromethane   *20*, 449 (1979); *41*, 43 (1986); *Suppl. 7*, 194 (1987); *71*, 251 (1999)

2,4-Dichlorophenol (*see* Chlorophenols; Chlorophenols, occupational exposures to; Polychlorophenols and their sodium salts)
(2,4-Dichlorophenoxy)acetic acid (*see* 2,4-D)
2,6-Dichloro-*para*-phenylenediamine   *39*, 325 (1986); *Suppl. 7*, 62 (1987)
1,2-Dichloropropane   *41*, 131 (1986); *Suppl. 7*, 62 (1987); *71*, 1393 (1999)
1,3-Dichloropropene (technical-grade)   *41*, 113 (1986); *Suppl. 7*, 195 (1987); *71*, 933 (1999)
Dichlorvos   *20*, 97 (1979); *Suppl. 7*, 62 (1987); *53*, 267 (1991)
Dicofol   *30*, 87 (1983); *Suppl. 7*, 62 (1987)
Dicyclohexylamine (*see* Cyclamates)
Dieldrin   *5*, 125 (1974); *Suppl. 7*, 196 (1987)
Dienoestrol (*see also* Nonsteroidal oestrogens)   *21*, 161 (1979); *Suppl. 7*, 278 (1987)
Diepoxybutane (*see also* 1,3-Butadiene)   *11*, 115 (1976) (*corr. 42*, 255); *Suppl. 7*, 62 (1987); *71*, 109 (1999)
Diesel and gasoline engine exhausts   *46*, 41 (1989)
Diesel fuels   *45*, 219 (1989) (*corr. 47*, 505)
Diethyl ether (*see* Anaesthetics, volatile)
Di(2-ethylhexyl)adipate   *29*, 257 (1982); *Suppl. 7*, 62 (1987)
Di(2-ethylhexyl)phthalate   *29*, 269 (1982) (*corr. 42*, 261); *Suppl. 7*, 62 (1987)
1,2-Diethylhydrazine   *4*, 153 (1974); *Suppl. 7*, 62 (1987); *71*, 1401 (1999)
Diethylstilboestrol   *6*, 55 (1974); *21*, 173 (1979) (*corr. 42*, 259); *Suppl. 7*, 273 (1987)

Diethylstilboestrol dipropionate (*see* Diethylstilboestrol)
Diethyl sulfate   *4*, 277 (1974); *Suppl. 7*, 198 (1987); *54*, 213 (1992); *71*, 1405 (1999)

Diglycidyl resorcinol ether	*11*, 125 (1976); *36*, 181 (1985); Suppl. 7, 62 (1987); *71*, 1417 (1999)
Dihydrosafrole	*1*, 170 (1972); *10*, 233 (1976) Suppl. 7, 62 (1987)
1,8-Dihydroxyanthraquinone (*see* Dantron)
Dihydroxybenzenes (*see* Catechol; Hydroquinone; Resorcinol)
Dihydroxymethylfuratrizine	*24*, 77 (1980); Suppl. 7, 62 (1987)
Diisopropyl sulfate	*54*, 229 (1992); *71*, 1421 (1999)
Dimethisterone (*see also* Progestins; Sequential oral contraceptives)	*6*, 167 (1974); *21*, 377 (1979))
Dimethoxane	*15*, 177 (1977); Suppl. 7, 62 (1987)
3,3′-Dimethoxybenzidine	*4*, 41 (1974); Suppl. 7, 198 (1987)
3,3′-Dimethoxybenzidine-4,4′-diisocyanate	*39*, 279 (1986); Suppl. 7, 62 (1987)
para-Dimethylaminoazobenzene	*8*, 125 (1975); Suppl. 7, 62 (1987)
para-Dimethylaminoazobenzenediazo sodium sulfonate	*8*, 147 (1975); Suppl. 7, 62 (1987)
trans-2-[(Dimethylamino)methylimino]-5-[2-(5-nitro-2-furyl)-vinyl]-1,3,4-oxadiazole	*7*, 147 (1974) (*corr. 42*, 253); Suppl. 7, 62 (1987)
4,4′-Dimethylangelicin plus ultraviolet radiation (*see also* Angelicin and some synthetic derivatives)	Suppl. 7, 57 (1987)
4,5′-Dimethylangelicin plus ultraviolet radiation (*see also* Angelicin and some synthetic derivatives)	Suppl. 7, 57 (1987)
2,6-Dimethylaniline	*57*, 323 (1993)
N,N-Dimethylaniline	*57*, 337 (1993)
Dimethylarsinic acid (*see* Arsenic and arsenic compounds)
3,3′-Dimethylbenzidine	*1*, 87 (1972); Suppl. 7, 62 (1987)
Dimethylcarbamoyl chloride	*12*, 77 (1976); Suppl. 7, 199 (1987); *71*, 531 (1999)
Dimethylformamide	*47*, 171 (1989); *71*, 545 (1999)
1,1-Dimethylhydrazine	*4*, 137 (1974); Suppl. 7, 62 (1987); *71*, 1425 (1999)
1,2-Dimethylhydrazine	*4*, 145 (1974) (*corr. 42*, 253); Suppl. 7, 62 (1987); *71*, 947 (1999)
Dimethyl hydrogen phosphite	*48*, 85 (1990); *71*, 1437 (1999)
1,4-Dimethylphenanthrene	*32*, 349 (1983); Suppl. 7, 62 (1987)
Dimethyl sulfate	*4*, 271 (1974); Suppl. 7, 200 (1987); *71*, 575 (1999)
3,7-Dinitrofluoranthene	*46*, 189 (1989); *65*, 297 (1996)
3,9-Dinitrofluoranthene	*46*, 195 (1989); *65*, 297 (1996)
1,3-Dinitropyrene	*46*, 201 (1989)
1,6-Dinitropyrene	*46*, 215 (1989)
1,8-Dinitropyrene	*33*, 171 (1984); Suppl. 7, 63 (1987); *46*, 231 (1989)
Dinitrosopentamethylenetetramine	*11*, 241 (1976); Suppl. 7, 63 (1987)
2,4-Dinitrotoluene	*65*, 309 (1996) (*corr. 66*, 485)
2,6-Dinitrotoluene	*65*, 309 (1996) (*corr. 66*, 485)
3,5-Dinitrotoluene	*65*, 309 (1996)
1,4-Dioxane	*11*, 247 (1976); Suppl. 7, 201 (1987); *71*, 589 (1999)
2,4′-Diphenyldiamine	*16*, 313 (1978); Suppl. 7, 63 (1987)
Direct Black 38 (*see also* Benzidine-based dyes)	*29*, 295 (1982) (*corr. 42*, 261)
Direct Blue 6 (*see also* Benzidine-based dyes)	*29*, 311 (1982)
Direct Brown 95 (*see also* Benzidine-based dyes)	*29*, 321 (1982)
Disperse Blue 1	*48*, 139 (1990)

Disperse Yellow 3	*8*, 97 (1975); *Suppl. 7*, 60 (1987); *48*, 149 (1990)
Disulfiram	*12*, 85 (1976); *Suppl. 7*, 63 (1987)
Dithranol	*13*, 75 (1977); *Suppl. 7*, 63 (1987)
Divinyl ether (*see* Anaesthetics, volatile)	
Doxefazepam	*66*, 97 (1996)
Droloxifene	*66*, 241 (1996)
Dry cleaning	*63*, 33 (1995)
Dulcin	*12*, 97 (1976); *Suppl. 7*, 63 (1987)

E

Endrin	*5*, 157 (1974); *Suppl. 7*, 63 (1987)
Enflurane (*see* Anaesthetics, volatile)	
Eosin	*15*, 183 (1977); *Suppl. 7*, 63 (1987)
Epichlorohydrin	*11*, 131 (1976) (*corr. 42*, 256); *Suppl. 7*, 202 (1987); *71*, 603 (1999)
1,2-Epoxybutane	*47*, 217 (1989); *71*, 629 (1999)
1-Epoxyethyl-3,4-epoxycyclohexane (*see* 4-Vinylcyclohexene diepoxide)	
3,4-Epoxy-6-methylcyclohexylmethyl 3,4-epoxy-6-methyl-cyclohexane carboxylate	*11*, 147 (1976); *Suppl. 7*, 63 (1987); *71*, 1441 (1999)
cis-9,10-Epoxystearic acid	*11*, 153 (1976); *Suppl. 7*, 63 (1987); *71*, 1443 (1999)
Epstein-Barr virus	*70*, 47 (1997)
d-Equilenin	*72*, 399 (1999)
Equilin	*72*, 399 (1999)
Erionite	*42*, 225 (1987); *Suppl. 7*, 203 (1987)
Estazolam	*66*, 105 (1996)
Ethinyloestradiol	*6*, 77 (1974); *21*, 233 (1979); *Suppl. 7*, 286 (1987); *72*, 49 (1999)
Ethionamide	*13*, 83 (1977); *Suppl. 7*, 63 (1987)
Ethyl acrylate	*19*, 57 (1979); *39*, 81 (1986); *Suppl. 7*, 63 (1987); *71*, 1447 (1999)
Ethylene	*19*, 157 (1979); *Suppl. 7*, 63 (1987); *60*, 45 (1994); *71*, 1447 (1999)
Ethylene dibromide	*15*, 195 (1977); *Suppl. 7*, 204 (1987); *71*, 641 (1999)
Ethylene oxide	*11*, 157 (1976); *36*, 189 (1985) (*corr. 42*, 263); *Suppl. 7*, 205 (1987); *60*, 73 (1994)
Ethylene sulfide	*11*, 257 (1976); *Suppl. 7*, 63 (1987)
Ethylene thiourea	*7*, 45 (1974); *Suppl. 7*, 207 (1987)
2-Ethylhexyl acrylate	*60*, 475 (1994)
Ethyl methanesulfonate	*7*, 245 (1974); *Suppl. 7*, 63 (1987)
N-Ethyl-*N*-nitrosourea	*1*, 135 (1972); *17*, 191 (1978); *Suppl. 7*, 63 (1987)
Ethyl selenac (*see also* Selenium and selenium compounds)	*12*, 107 (1976); *Suppl. 7*, 63 (1987)
Ethyl tellurac	*12*, 115 (1976); *Suppl. 7*, 63 (1987)

Ethynodiol diacetate   6, 173 (1974); 21, 387 (1979);
                                               Suppl. 7, 292 (1987); 72, 49
                                               (1999)
Eugenol   36, 75 (1985); Suppl. 7, 63 (1987)
Evans blue   8, 151 (1975); Suppl. 7, 63 (1987)

F

Fast Green FCF   16, 187 (1978); Suppl. 7, 63 (1987)
Fenvalerate   53, 309 (1991)
Ferbam   12, 121 (1976) (corr. 42, 256);
                                               Suppl. 7, 63 (1987)
Ferric oxide   1, 29 (1972); Suppl. 7, 216 (1987)
Ferrochromium (see Chromium and chromium compounds)
Fluometuron   30, 245 (1983); Suppl. 7, 63 (1987)
Fluoranthene   32, 355 (1983); Suppl. 7, 63 (1987)
Fluorene   32, 365 (1983); Suppl. 7, 63 (1987)
Fluorescent lighting (exposure to) (see Ultraviolet radiation)
Fluorides (inorganic, used in drinking-water) 27, 237 (1982); Suppl. 7, 208
                                               (1987)
5-Fluorouracil   26, 217 (1981); Suppl. 7, 210
                                               (1987)
Fluorspar (see Fluorides)
Fluosilicic acid (see Fluorides)
Fluroxene (see Anaesthetics, volatile)
Foreign bodies   74 (1999)
Formaldehyde   29, 345 (1982); Suppl. 7, 211
                                               (1987); 62, 217 (1995) (corr. 65,
                                               549; corr. 66, 485)
2-(2-Formylhydrazino)-4-(5-nitro-2-furyl)thiazole   7, 151 (1974) (corr. 42, 253);
                                               Suppl. 7, 63 (1987)
Frusemide (see Furosemide)
Fuel oils (heating oils)   45, 239 (1989) (corr. 47, 505)
Fumonisin B_1 (see Toxins derived from *Fusarium moniliforme*)
Fumonisin B_2 (see Toxins derived from *Fusarium moniliforme*)
Furan   63, 393 (1995)
Furazolidone   31, 141 (1983); Suppl. 7, 63 (1987)
Furfural   63, 409 (1995)
Furniture and cabinet-making   25, 99 (1981); Suppl. 7, 380 (1987)
Furosemide   50, 277 (1990)
2-(2-Furyl)-3-(5-nitro-2-furyl)acrylamide (see AF-2)
Fusarenon-X (see Toxins derived from *Fusarium graminearum*,
    F. culmorum and *F. crookwellense*)
Fusarenone-X (see Toxins derived from *Fusarium graminearum*,
    F. culmorum and *F. crookwellense*)
Fusarin C (see Toxins derived from *Fusarium moniliforme*)

G

Gasoline   45, 159 (1989) (corr. 47, 505)
Gasoline engine exhaust (see Diesel and gasoline engine exhausts)
Gemfibrozil   66, 427 (1996)

Glass fibres (see Man-made mineral fibres)
Glass manufacturing industry, occupational exposures in 58, 347 (1993)
Glasswool (see Man-made mineral fibres)
Glass filaments (see Man-made mineral fibres)
Glu-P-1 40, 223 (1986); Suppl. 7, 64 (1987)
Glu-P-2 40, 235 (1986); Suppl. 7, 64 (1987)
L-Glutamic acid, 5-[2-(4-hydroxymethyl)phenylhydrazide]
    (see Agaritine)
Glycidaldehyde 11, 175 (1976); Suppl. 7, 64 (1987); 71, 1459 (1999)
Glycidyl ethers 47, 237 (1989); 71, 1285, 1417, 1525, 1539 (1999)
Glycidyl oleate 11, 183 (1976); Suppl. 7, 64 (1987)
Glycidyl stearate 11, 187 (1976); Suppl. 7, 64 (1987)
Griseofulvin 10, 153 (1976); Suppl. 7, 391 (1987)
Guinea Green B 16, 199 (1978); Suppl. 7, 64 (1987)
Gyromitrin 31, 163 (1983); Suppl. 7, 391 (1987)

H

Haematite 1, 29 (1972); Suppl. 7, 216 (1987)
Haematite and ferric oxide Suppl. 7, 216 (1987)
Haematite mining, underground, with exposure to radon 1, 29 (1972); Suppl. 7, 216 (1987)
Hairdressers and barbers (occupational exposure as) 57, 43 (1993)
Hair dyes, epidemiology of 16, 29 (1978); 27, 307 (1982);
Halogenated acetonitriles 52, 269 (1991); 71, 1325, 1369, 1375, 1533 (1999)
Halothane (see Anaesthetics, volatile)
HC Blue No. 1 57, 129 (1993)
HC Blue No. 2 57, 143 (1993)
α-HCH (see Hexachlorocyclohexanes)
β-HCH (see Hexachlorocyclohexanes)
γ-HCH (see Hexachlorocyclohexanes)
HC Red No. 3 57, 153 (1993)
HC Yellow No. 4 57, 159 (1993)
Heating oils (see Fuel oils)
Helicobacter pylori (infection with) 61, 177 (1994)
Hepatitis B virus 59, 45 (1994)
Hepatitis C virus 59, 165 (1994)
Hepatitis D virus 59, 223 (1994)
Heptachlor (see also Chlordane/Heptachlor) 5, 173 (1974); 20, 129 (1979)
Hexachlorobenzene 20, 155 (1979); Suppl. 7, 219 (1987)
Hexachlorobutadiene 20, 179 (1979); Suppl. 7, 64 (1987); 73, 277 (1999)
Hexachlorocyclohexanes 5, 47 (1974); 20, 195 (1979) (corr. 42, 258); Suppl. 7, 220 (1987)
Hexachlorocyclohexane, technical-grade (see Hexachlorocyclohexanes)
Hexachloroethane 20, 467 (1979); Suppl. 7, 64 (1987); 73, 295 (1999)

Hexachlorophene	20, 241 (1979); *Suppl. 7*, 64 (1987)
Hexamethylphosphoramide	15, 211 (1977); *Suppl. 7*, 64 (1987); 71, 1465 (1999)
Hexoestrol (*see also* Nonsteroidal oestrogens)	*Suppl. 7*, 279 (1987)
Hormonal contraceptives, progestogens only	72, 339 (1999)
Human herpesvirus 8	70, 375 (1997)
Human immunodeficiency viruses	67, 31 (1996)
Human papillomaviruses	64 (1995) (*corr.* 66, 485)
Human T-cell lymphotropic viruses	67, 261 (1996)
Hycanthone mesylate	13, 91 (1977); *Suppl. 7*, 64 (1987)
Hydralazine	24, 85 (1980); *Suppl. 7*, 222 (1987)
Hydrazine	4, 127 (1974); *Suppl. 7*, 223 (1987); 71, 991 (1999)
Hydrochloric acid	54, 189 (1992)
Hydrochlorothiazide	50, 293 (1990)
Hydrogen peroxide	36, 285 (1985); *Suppl. 7*, 64 (1987); 71, 671 (1999)
Hydroquinone	15, 155 (1977); *Suppl. 7*, 64 (1987); 71, 691 (1999)
4-Hydroxyazobenzene	8, 157 (1975); *Suppl. 7*, 64 (1987)
17α-Hydroxyprogesterone caproate (*see also* Progestins)	21, 399 (1979) (*corr.* 42, 259)
8-Hydroxyquinoline	13, 101 (1977); *Suppl. 7*, 64 (1987)
8-Hydroxysenkirkine	10, 265 (1976); *Suppl. 7*, 64 (1987)
Hypochlorite salts	52, 159 (1991)

I

Implants, surgical	74, 1999
Indeno[1,2,3-*cd*]pyrene	3, 229 (1973); 32, 373 (1983); *Suppl. 7*, 64 (1987)
Inorganic acids (*see* Sulfuric acid and other strong inorganic acids, occupational exposures to mists and vapours from)	
Insecticides, occupational exposures in spraying and application of	53, 45 (1991)
IQ	40, 261 (1986); *Suppl. 7*, 64 (1987); 56, 165 (1993)
Iron and steel founding	34, 133 (1984); *Suppl. 7*, 224 (1987)
Iron-dextran complex	2, 161 (1973); *Suppl. 7*, 226 (1987)
Iron-dextrin complex	2, 161 (1973) (*corr.* 42, 252); *Suppl. 7*, 64 (1987)
Iron oxide (*see* Ferric oxide)	
Iron oxide, saccharated (*see* Saccharated iron oxide)	
Iron sorbitol-citric acid complex	2, 161 (1973); *Suppl. 7*, 64 (1987)
Isatidine	10, 269 (1976); *Suppl. 7*, 65 (1987)
Isoflurane (*see* Anaesthetics, volatile)	
Isoniazid (*see* Isonicotinic acid hydrazide)	
Isonicotinic acid hydrazide	4, 159 (1974); *Suppl. 7*, 227 (1987)
Isophosphamide	26, 237 (1981); *Suppl. 7*, 65 (1987)
Isoprene	60, 215 (1994); 71, 1015 (1999)
Isopropanol	15, 223 (1977); *Suppl. 7*, 229 (1987); 71, 1027 (1999)

Isopropanol manufacture (strong-acid process) *(see also* Isopropanol; Sulfuric acid and other strong inorganic acids, occupational exposures to mists and vapours from)	*Suppl. 7*, 229 (1987)
Isopropyl oils	*15*, 223 (1977); *Suppl. 7*, 229 (1987); *71*, 1483 (1999)
Isosafrole	*1*, 169 (1972); *10*, 232 (1976); *Suppl. 7*, 65 (1987)

J

Jacobine	*10*, 275 (1976); *Suppl. 7*, 65 (1987)
Jet fuel	*45*, 203 (1989)
Joinery *(see* Carpentry and joinery)	

K

Kaempferol	*31*, 171 (1983); *Suppl. 7*, 65 (1987)
Kaposi's sarcoma herpesvirus	*70*, 375 (1997)
Kepone *(see* Chlordecone)	

L

Lasiocarpine	*10*, 281 (1976); *Suppl. 7*, 65 (1987)
Lauroyl peroxide	*36*, 315 (1985); *Suppl. 7*, 65 (1987); *71*, 1485 (1999)
Lead acetate *(see* Lead and lead compounds)	
Lead and lead compounds *(see also* Foreign bodies)	*1*, 40 (1972) *(corr. 42*, 251); *2*, 52, 150 (1973); *12*, 131 (1976); *23*, 40, 208, 209, 325 (1980); *Suppl. 7*, 230 (1987)
Lead arsenate *(see* Arsenic and arsenic compounds)	
Lead carbonate *(see* Lead and lead compounds)	
Lead chloride *(see* Lead and lead compounds)	
Lead chromate *(see* Chromium and chromium compounds)	
Lead chromate oxide *(see* Chromium and chromium compounds)	
Lead naphthenate *(see* Lead and lead compounds)	
Lead nitrate *(see* Lead and lead compounds)	
Lead oxide *(see* Lead and lead compounds)	
Lead phosphate *(see* Lead and lead compounds)	
Lead subacetate *(see* Lead and lead compounds)	
Lead tetroxide *(see* Lead and lead compounds)	
Leather goods manufacture	*25*, 279 (1981); *Suppl. 7*, 235 (1987)
Leather industries	*25*, 199 (1981); *Suppl. 7*, 232 (1987)
Leather tanning and processing	*25*, 201 (1981); *Suppl. 7*, 236 (1987)
Ledate *(see also* Lead and lead compounds)	*12*, 131 (1976)
Levonorgestrel	*72*, 49 (1999)
Light Green SF	*16*, 209 (1978); *Suppl. 7*, 65 (1987)
d-Limonene	*56*, 135 (1993); *73*, 307 (1999)

Lindane (see Hexachlorocyclohexanes)
Liver flukes (see *Clonorchis sinensis*, *Opisthorchis felineus* and *Opisthorchis viverrini*)
Lumber and sawmill industries (including logging)   25, 49 (1981); *Suppl. 7*, 383 (1987)
Luteoskyrin   *10*, 163 (1976); *Suppl. 7*, 65 (1987)
Lynoestrenol   *21*, 407 (1979); *Suppl. 7*, 293 (1987); *72*, 49 (1999)

M

Magenta   *4*, 57 (1974) (*corr. 42*, 252); *Suppl. 7*, 238 (1987); *57*, 215 (1993)

Magenta, manufacture of (see also Magenta)   *Suppl. 7*, 238 (1987); *57*, 215 (1993)

Malathion   *30*, 103 (1983); *Suppl. 7*, 65 (1987)
Maleic hydrazide   *4*, 173 (1974) (*corr. 42*, 253); *Suppl. 7*, 65 (1987)

Malonaldehyde   *36*, 163 (1985); *Suppl. 7*, 65 (1987); *71*, 1037 (1999)

Malondialdehyde (see Malonaldehyde)
Maneb   *12*, 137 (1976); *Suppl. 7*, 65 (1987)
Man-made mineral fibres   *43*, 39 (1988)
Mannomustine   *9*, 157 (1975); *Suppl. 7*, 65 (1987)
Mate   *51*, 273 (1991)
MCPA (see also Chlorophenoxy herbicides; Chlorophenoxy herbicides, occupational exposures to)   *30*, 255 (1983)

MeA-α-C   *40*, 253 (1986); *Suppl. 7*, 65 (1987)
Medphalan   *9*, 168 (1975); *Suppl. 7*, 65 (1987)
Medroxyprogesterone acetate   *6*, 157 (1974); *21*, 417 (1979) (*corr. 42*, 259); *Suppl. 7*, 289 (1987); *72*, 339 (1999)

Megestrol acetate   *Suppl. 7*, 293 (1987); *72*, 49 (1999)
MeIQ   *40*, 275 (1986); *Suppl. 7*, 65 (1987); *56*, 197 (1993)

MeIQx   *40*, 283 (1986); *Suppl. 7*, 65 (1987); *56*, 211 (1993)

Melamine   *39*, 333 (1986); *Suppl. 7*, 65 (1987); *73*, 329 (1999)

Melphalan   *9*, 167 (1975); *Suppl. 7*, 239 (1987)
6-Mercaptopurine   *26*, 249 (1981); *Suppl. 7*, 240 (1987)

Mercuric chloride (see Mercury and mercury compounds)
Mercury and mercury compounds   *58*, 239 (1993)
Merphalan   *9*, 169 (1975); *Suppl. 7*, 65 (1987)
Mestranol   *6*, 87 (1974); *21*, 257 (1979) (*corr. 42*, 259); *Suppl. 7*, 288 (1987); *72*, 49 (1999)

Metabisulfites (see Sulfur dioxide and some sulfites, bisulfites and metabisulfites)
Metallic mercury (see Mercury and mercury compounds)
Methanearsonic acid, disodium salt (see Arsenic and arsenic compounds)

Methanearsonic acid, monosodium salt (*see* Arsenic and arsenic compounds
Methotrexate — 26, 267 (1981); *Suppl. 7*, 241 (1987)

Methoxsalen (*see* 8-Methoxypsoralen)
Methoxychlor — 5, 193 (1974); 20, 259 (1979); *Suppl. 7*, 66 (1987)

Methoxyflurane (*see* Anaesthetics, volatile)
5-Methoxypsoralen — 40, 327 (1986); *Suppl. 7*, 242 (1987)
8-Methoxypsoralen (*see also* 8-Methoxypsoralen plus ultraviolet radiation) — 24, 101 (1980)
8-Methoxypsoralen plus ultraviolet radiation — *Suppl. 7*, 243 (1987)
Methyl acrylate — 19, 52 (1979); 39, 99 (1986); *Suppl. 7*, 66 (1987); 71, 1489 (1999)

5-Methylangelicin plus ultraviolet radiation (*see also* Angelicin and some synthetic derivatives) — *Suppl. 7*, 57 (1987)
2-Methylaziridine — 9, 61 (1975); *Suppl. 7*, 66 (1987); 71, 1497 (1999)

Methylazoxymethanol acetate (*see also* Cycasin) — 1, 164 (1972); 10, 131 (1976); *Suppl. 7*, 66 (1987)

Methyl bromide — 41, 187 (1986) (*corr.* 45, 283); *Suppl. 7*, 245 (1987); 71, 721 (1999)

Methyl *tert*-butyl ether — 73, 339 (1999)
Methyl carbamate — 12, 151 (1976); *Suppl. 7*, 66 (1987)
Methyl-CCNU (*see* 1-(2-Chloroethyl)-3-(4-methylcyclohexyl)-1-nitrosourea)
Methyl chloride — 41, 161 (1986); *Suppl. 7*, 246 (1987); 71, 737 (1999)

1-, 2-, 3-, 4-, 5- and 6-Methylchrysenes — 32, 379 (1983); *Suppl. 7*, 66 (1987)
N-Methyl-*N*,4-dinitrosoaniline — 1, 141 (1972); *Suppl. 7*, 66 (1987)
4,4'-Methylene bis(2-chloroaniline) — 4, 65 (1974) (*corr.* 42, 252); *Suppl. 7*, 246 (1987); 57, 271 (1993)

4,4'-Methylene bis(*N*,*N*-dimethyl)benzenamine — 27, 119 (1982); *Suppl. 7*, 66 (1987)
4,4'-Methylene bis(2-methylaniline) — 4, 73 (1974); *Suppl. 7*, 248 (1987)
4,4'-Methylenedianiline — 4, 79 (1974) (*corr.* 42, 252); 39, 347 (1986); *Suppl. 7*, 66 (1987)

4,4'-Methylenediphenyl diisocyanate — 19, 314 (1979); *Suppl. 7*, 66 (1987); 71, 1049 (1999)

2-Methylfluoranthene — 32, 399 (1983); *Suppl. 7*, 66 (1987)
3-Methylfluoranthene — 32, 399 (1983); *Suppl. 7*, 66 (1987)
Methylglyoxal — 51, 443 (1991)
Methyl iodide — 15, 245 (1977); 41, 213 (1986); *Suppl. 7*, 66 (1987); 71, 1503 (1999)

Methylmercury chloride (*see* Mercury and mercury compounds)
Methylmercury compounds (*see* Mercury and mercury compounds)
Methyl methacrylate — 19, 187 (1979); *Suppl. 7*, 66 (1987); 60, 445 (1994)

Methyl methanesulfonate — 7, 253 (1974); *Suppl. 7*, 66 (1987); 71, 1059 (1999)

2-Methyl-1-nitroanthraquinone	27, 205 (1982); *Suppl. 7*, 66 (1987)
N-Methyl-N'-nitro-N-nitrosoguanidine	4, 183 (1974); *Suppl. 7*, 248 (1987)
3-Methylnitrosaminopropionaldehyde [*see* 3-(N-Nitrosomethylamino)-propionaldehyde]	
3-Methylnitrosaminopropionitrile [*see* 3-(N-Nitrosomethylamino)-propionitrile]	
4-(Methylnitrosamino)-4-(3-pyridyl)-1-butanal [*see* 4-(N-Nitrosomethylamino)-4-(3-pyridyl)-1-butanal]	
4-(Methylnitrosamino)-1-(3-pyridyl)-1-butanone [*see* 4-(-Nitrosomethylamino)-1-(3-pyridyl)-1-butanone]	
N-Methyl-N-nitrosourea	*1*, 125 (1972); *17*, 227 (1978); *Suppl. 7*, 66 (1987)
N-Methyl-N-nitrosourethane	4, 211 (1974); *Suppl. 7*, 66 (1987)
N-Methylolacrylamide	60, 435 (1994)
Methyl parathion	30, 131 (1983); *Suppl. 7*, 392 (1987)
1-Methylphenanthrene	32, 405 (1983); *Suppl. 7*, 66 (1987)
7-Methylpyrido[3,4-*c*]psoralen	40, 349 (1986); *Suppl. 7*, 71 (1987)
Methyl red	8, 161 (1975); *Suppl. 7*, 66 (1987)
Methyl selenac (*see also* Selenium and selenium compounds)	12, 161 (1976); *Suppl. 7*, 66 (1987)
Methylthiouracil	7, 53 (1974); *Suppl. 7*, 66 (1987)
Metronidazole	13, 113 (1977); *Suppl. 7*, 250 (1987)
Mineral oils	3, 30 (1973); *33*, 87 (1984) (*corr. 42*, 262); *Suppl. 7*, 252 (1987)
Mirex	5, 203 (1974); 20, 283 (1979) (*corr. 42*, 258); *Suppl. 7*, 66 (1987)
Mists and vapours from sulfuric acid and other strong inorganic acids	54, 41 (1992)
Mitomycin C	10, 171 (1976); *Suppl. 7*, 67 (1987)
MNNG (*see* N-Methyl-N'-nitro-N-nitrosoguanidine)	
MOCA (*see* 4,4'-Methylene bis(2-chloroaniline))	
Modacrylic fibres	19, 86 (1979); *Suppl. 7*, 67 (1987)
Monocrotaline	10, 291 (1976); *Suppl. 7*, 67 (1987)
Monuron	12, 167 (1976); *Suppl. 7*, 67 (1987); 53, 467 (1991)
MOPP and other combined chemotherapy including alkylating agents	*Suppl. 7*, 254 (1987)
Mordanite (*see* Zeolites)	
Morpholine	47, 199 (1989); *71*, 1511 (1999)
5-(Morpholinomethyl)-3-[(5-nitrofurfurylidene)amino]-2-oxazolidinone	7, 161 (1974); *Suppl. 7*, 67 (1987)
Musk ambrette	65, 477 (1996)
Musk xylene	65, 477 (1996)
Mustard gas	9, 181 (1975) (*corr. 42*, 254); *Suppl. 7*, 259 (1987)
Myleran (*see* 1,4-Butanediol dimethanesulfonate)	

N

Nafenopin	24, 125 (1980); *Suppl. 7*, 67 (1987)
1,5-Naphthalenediamine	27, 127 (1982); *Suppl. 7*, 67 (1987)

1,5-Naphthalene diisocyanate	*19*, 311 (1979); *Suppl. 7*, 67 (1987); *71*, 1515 (1999)
1-Naphthylamine	*4*, 87 (1974) (*corr. 42*, 253); *Suppl. 7*, 260 (1987)
2-Naphthylamine	*4*, 97 (1974); *Suppl. 7*, 261 (1987)
1-Naphthylthiourea	*30*, 347 (1983); *Suppl. 7*, 263 (1987)
Nickel acetate (*see* Nickel and nickel compounds)	
Nickel ammonium sulfate (*see* Nickel and nickel compounds)	
Nickel and nickel compounds (*see also* Implants, surgical)	*2*, 126 (1973) (*corr. 42*, 252); *11*, 75 (1976); *Suppl. 7*, 264 (1987) (*corr. 45*, 283); *49*, 257 (1990) (*corr. 67*, 395)
Nickel carbonate (*see* Nickel and nickel compounds)	
Nickel carbonyl (*see* Nickel and nickel compounds)	
Nickel chloride (*see* Nickel and nickel compounds)	
Nickel-gallium alloy (*see* Nickel and nickel compounds)	
Nickel hydroxide (*see* Nickel and nickel compounds)	
Nickelocene (*see* Nickel and nickel compounds)	
Nickel oxide (*see* Nickel and nickel compounds)	
Nickel subsulfide (*see* Nickel and nickel compounds)	
Nickel sulfate (*see* Nickel and nickel compounds)	
Niridazole	*13*, 123 (1977); *Suppl. 7*, 67 (1987)
Nithiazide	*31*, 179 (1983); *Suppl. 7*, 67 (1987)
Nitrilotriacetic acid and its salts	*48*, 181 (1990); *73*, 385 (1999)
5-Nitroacenaphthene	*16*, 319 (1978); *Suppl. 7*, 67 (1987)
5-Nitro-*ortho*-anisidine	*27*, 133 (1982); *Suppl. 7*, 67 (1987)
2-Nitroanisole	*65*, 369 (1996)
9-Nitroanthracene	*33*, 179 (1984); *Suppl. 7*, 67 (1987)
7-Nitrobenz[*a*]anthracene	*46*, 247 (1989)
Nitrobenzene	*65*, 381 (1996)
6-Nitrobenzo[*a*]pyrene	*33*, 187 (1984); *Suppl. 7*, 67 (1987); *46*, 255 (1989)
4-Nitrobiphenyl	*4*, 113 (1974); *Suppl. 7*, 67 (1987)
6-Nitrochrysene	*33*, 195 (1984); *Suppl. 7*, 67 (1987); *46*, 267 (1989)
Nitrofen (technical-grade)	*30*, 271 (1983); *Suppl. 7*, 67 (1987)
3-Nitrofluoranthene	*33*, 201 (1984); *Suppl. 7*, 67 (1987)
2-Nitrofluorene	*46*, 277 (1989)
Nitrofural	*7*, 171 (1974); *Suppl. 7*, 67 (1987); *50*, 195 (1990)
5-Nitro-2-furaldehyde semicarbazone (*see* Nitrofural)	
Nitrofurantoin	*50*, 211 (1990)
Nitrofurazone (*see* Nitrofural)	
1-[(5-Nitrofurfurylidene)amino]-2-imidazolidinone	*7*, 181 (1974); *Suppl. 7*, 67 (1987)
N-[4-(5-Nitro-2-furyl)-2-thiazolyl]acetamide	*1*, 181 (1972); *7*, 185 (1974); *Suppl. 7*, 67 (1987)
Nitrogen mustard	*9*, 193 (1975); *Suppl. 7*, 269 (1987)
Nitrogen mustard *N*-oxide	*9*, 209 (1975); *Suppl. 7*, 67 (1987)
1-Nitronaphthalene	*46*, 291 (1989)
2-Nitronaphthalene	*46*, 303 (1989)
3-Nitroperylene	*46*, 313 (1989)
2-Nitro-*para*-phenylenediamine (*see* 1,4-Diamino-2-nitrobenzene)	

2-Nitropropane	*29*, 331 (1982); *Suppl. 7*, 67 (1987); *71*, 1079 (1999)
1-Nitropyrene	*33*, 209 (1984); *Suppl. 7*, 67 (1987); *46*, 321 (1989)
2-Nitropyrene	*46*, 359 (1989)
4-Nitropyrene	*46*, 367 (1989)
N-Nitrosatable drugs	*24*, 297 (1980) (*corr. 42*, 260)
N-Nitrosatable pesticides	*30*, 359 (1983)
N'-Nitrosoanabasine	*37*, 225 (1985); *Suppl. 7*, 67 (1987)
N'-Nitrosoanatabine	*37*, 233 (1985); *Suppl. 7*, 67 (1987)
N-Nitrosodi-*n*-butylamine	*4*, 197 (1974); *17*, 51 (1978); *Suppl. 7*, 67 (1987)
N-Nitrosodiethanolamine	*17*, 77 (1978); *Suppl. 7*, 67 (1987)
N-Nitrosodiethylamine	*1*, 107 (1972) (*corr. 42*, 251); *17*, 83 (1978) (*corr. 42*, 257); *Suppl. 7*, 67 (1987)
N-Nitrosodimethylamine	*1*, 95 (1972); *17*, 125 (1978) (*corr. 42*, 257); *Suppl. 7*, 67 (1987)
N-Nitrosodiphenylamine	*27*, 213 (1982); *Suppl. 7*, 67 (1987)
para-Nitrosodiphenylamine	*27*, 227 (1982) (*corr. 42*, 261); *Suppl. 7*, 68 (1987)
N-Nitrosodi-*n*-propylamine	*17*, 177 (1978); *Suppl. 7*, 68 (1987)
N-Nitroso-*N*-ethylurea (*see N*-Ethyl-*N*-nitrosourea)	
N-Nitrosofolic acid	*17*, 217 (1978); *Suppl. 7*, 68 (1987)
N-Nitrosoguvacine	*37*, 263 (1985); *Suppl. 7*, 68 (1987)
N-Nitrosoguvacoline	*37*, 263 (1985); *Suppl. 7*, 68 (1987)
N-Nitrosohydroxyproline	*17*, 304 (1978); *Suppl. 7*, 68 (1987)
3-(*N*-Nitrosomethylamino)propionaldehyde	*37*, 263 (1985); *Suppl. 7*, 68 (1987)
3-(*N*-Nitrosomethylamino)propionitrile	*37*, 263 (1985); *Suppl. 7*, 68 (1987)
4-(*N*-Nitrosomethylamino)-4-(3-pyridyl)-1-butanal	*37*, 205 (1985); *Suppl. 7*, 68 (1987)
4-(*N*-Nitrosomethylamino)-1-(3-pyridyl)-1-butanone	*37*, 209 (1985); *Suppl. 7*, 68 (1987)
N-Nitrosomethylethylamine	*17*, 221 (1978); *Suppl. 7*, 68 (1987)
N-Nitroso-*N*-methylurea (*see N*-Methyl-*N*-nitrosourea)	
N-Nitroso-*N*-methylurethane (*see N*-Methyl-*N*-nitrosourethane)	
N-Nitrosomethylvinylamine	*17*, 257 (1978); *Suppl. 7*, 68 (1987)
N-Nitrosomorpholine	*17*, 263 (1978); *Suppl. 7*, 68 (1987)
N'-Nitrosonornicotine	*17*, 281 (1978); *37*, 241 (1985); *Suppl. 7*, 68 (1987)
N-Nitrosopiperidine	*17*, 287 (1978); *Suppl. 7*, 68 (1987)
N-Nitrosoproline	*17*, 303 (1978); *Suppl. 7*, 68 (1987)
N-Nitrosopyrrolidine	*17*, 313 (1978); *Suppl. 7*, 68 (1987)
N-Nitrososarcosine	*17*, 327 (1978); *Suppl. 7*, 68 (1987)
Nitrosoureas, chloroethyl (*see* Chloroethyl nitrosoureas)	
5-Nitro-*ortho*-toluidine	*48*, 169 (1990)
2-Nitrotoluene	*65*, 409 (1996)
3-Nitrotoluene	*65*, 409 (1996)
4-Nitrotoluene	*65*, 409 (1996)
Nitrous oxide (*see* Anaesthetics, volatile)	
Nitrovin	*31*, 185 (1983); *Suppl. 7*, 68 (1987)
Nivalenol (*see* Toxins derived from *Fusarium graminearum*, *F. culmorum* and *F. crookwellense*)	
NNA (*see* 4-(*N*-Nitrosomethylamino)-4-(3-pyridyl)-1-butanal)	
NNK (*see* 4-(*N*-Nitrosomethylamino)-1-(3-pyridyl)-1-butanone)	
Nonsteroidal oestrogens	*Suppl. 7*, 273 (1987)

Norethisterone	6, 179 (1974); 21, 461 (1979); Suppl. 7, 294 (1987); 72, 49 (1999)
Norethisterone acetate	72, 49 (1999)
Norethynodrel	6, 191 (1974); 21, 461 (1979) (corr. 42, 259); Suppl. 7, 295 (1987); 72, 49 (1999)
Norgestrel	6, 201 (1974); 21, 479 (1979); Suppl. 7, 295 (1987); 72, 49 (1999)
Nylon 6	19, 120 (1979); Suppl. 7, 68 (1987)

O

Ochratoxin A	10, 191 (1976); 31, 191 (1983) (corr. 42, 262); Suppl. 7, 271 (1987); 56, 489 (1993)
Oestradiol	6, 99 (1974); 21, 279 (1979); Suppl. 7, 284 (1987); 72, 399 (1999)
Oestradiol-17β (see Oestradiol)	
Oestradiol 3-benzoate (see Oestradiol)	
Oestradiol dipropionate (see Oestradiol)	
Oestradiol mustard	9, 217 (1975); Suppl. 7, 68 (1987)
Oestradiol valerate (see Oestradiol)	
Oestriol	6, 117 (1974); 21, 327 (1979); Suppl. 7, 285 (1987); 72, 399 (1999)
Oestrogen-progestin combinations (see Oestrogens, progestins (progestogens) and combinations)	
Oestrogen-progestin replacement therapy (see Post-menopausal oestrogen-progestogen therapy)	
Oestrogen replacement therapy (see Post-menopausal oestrogen therapy)	
Oestrogens (see Oestrogens, progestins and combinations)	
Oestrogens, conjugated (see Conjugated oestrogens)	
Oestrogens, nonsteroidal (see Nonsteroidal oestrogens)	
Oestrogens, progestins (progestogens) and combinations	6 (1974); 21 (1979); Suppl. 7, 272 (1987); 72, 49, 339, 399, 531 (1999)
Oestrogens, steroidal (see Steroidal oestrogens)	
Oestrone	6, 123 (1974); 21, 343 (1979) (corr. 42, 259); Suppl. 7, 286 (1987); 72, 399 (1999)
Oestrone benzoate (see Oestrone)	
Oil Orange SS	8, 165 (1975); Suppl. 7, 69 (1987)
Opisthorchis felineus (infection with)	61, 121 (1994)
Opisthorchis viverrini (infection with)	61, 121 (1994)
Oral contraceptives, combined	Suppl. 7, 297 (1987); 72, 49 (1999)
Oral contraceptives, investigational (see Combined oral contraceptives)	
Oral contraceptives, sequential (see Sequential oral contraceptives)	
Orange I	8, 173 (1975); Suppl. 7, 69 (1987)
Orange G	8, 181 (1975); Suppl. 7, 69 (1987)
Organolead compounds (see also Lead and lead compounds)	Suppl. 7, 230 (1987)

Oxazepam	13, 58 (1977); Suppl. 7, 69 (1987); 66, 115 (1996)
Oxymetholone (see also Androgenic (anabolic) steroids)	13, 131 (1977)
Oxyphenbutazone	13, 185 (1977); Suppl. 7, 69 (1987)

P

Paint manufacture and painting (occupational exposures in)	47, 329 (1989)
Palygorskite	42, 159 (1987); Suppl. 7, 117 (1987); 68, 245 (1997)
Panfuran S (see also Dihydroxymethylfuratrizine)	24, 77 (1980); Suppl. 7, 69 (1987)
Paper manufacture (see Pulp and paper manufacture)	
Paracetamol	50, 307 (1990); 73, 401 (1999)
Parasorbic acid	10, 199 (1976) (corr. 42, 255); Suppl. 7, 69 (1987)
Parathion	30, 153 (1983); Suppl. 7, 69 (1987)
Patulin	10, 205 (1976); 40, 83 (1986); Suppl. 7, 69 (1987)
Penicillic acid	10, 211 (1976); Suppl. 7, 69 (1987)
Pentachloroethane	41, 99 (1986); Suppl. 7, 69 (1987); 71, 1519 (1999)
Pentachloronitrobenzene (see Quintozene)	
Pentachlorophenol (see also Chlorophenols; Chlorophenols, occupational exposures to; Polychlorophenols and their sodium salts)	20, 303 (1979); 53, 371 (1991)
Permethrin	53, 329 (1991)
Perylene	32, 411 (1983); Suppl. 7, 69 (1987)
Petasitenine	31, 207 (1983); Suppl. 7, 69 (1987)
Petasites japonicus (see also Pyrrolizidine alkaloids)	10, 333 (1976)
Petroleum refining (occupational exposures in)	45, 39 (1989)
Petroleum solvents	47, 43 (1989)
Phenacetin	13, 141 (1977); 24, 135 (1980); Suppl. 7, 310 (1987)
Phenanthrene	32, 419 (1983); Suppl. 7, 69 (1987)
Phenazopyridine hydrochloride	8, 117 (1975); 24, 163 (1980) (corr. 42, 260); Suppl. 7, 312 (1987)
Phenelzine sulfate	24, 175 (1980); Suppl. 7, 312 (1987)
Phenicarbazide	12, 177 (1976); Suppl. 7, 70 (1987)
Phenobarbital	13, 157 (1977); Suppl. 7, 313 (1987)
Phenol	47, 263 (1989) (corr. 50, 385); 71, 749 (1999)
Phenoxyacetic acid herbicides (see Chlorophenoxy herbicides)	
Phenoxybenzamine hydrochloride	9, 223 (1975); 24, 185 (1980); Suppl. 7, 70 (1987)
Phenylbutazone	13, 183 (1977); Suppl. 7, 316 (1987)
meta-Phenylenediamine	16, 111 (1978); Suppl. 7, 70 (1987)
para-Phenylenediamine	16, 125 (1978); Suppl. 7, 70 (1987)
Phenyl glycidyl ether (see also Glycidyl ethers)	71, 1525 (1999)
N-Phenyl-2-naphthylamine	16, 325 (1978) (corr. 42, 257); Suppl. 7, 318 (1987)

ortho-Phenylphenol	30, 329 (1983); *Suppl. 7*, 70 (1987); 73, 451 (1999)
Phenytoin	13, 201 (1977); *Suppl. 7*, 319 (1987); 66, 175 (1996)
Phillipsite (*see* Zeolites)	
PhIP	56, 229 (1993)
Pickled vegetables	56, 83 (1993)
Picloram	53, 481 (1991)
Piperazine oestrone sulfate (*see* Conjugated oestrogens)	
Piperonyl butoxide	30, 183 (1983); *Suppl. 7*, 70 (1987)
Pitches, coal-tar (*see* Coal-tar pitches)	
Polyacrylic acid	19, 62 (1979); *Suppl. 7*, 70 (1987)
Polybrominated biphenyls	18, 107 (1978); 41, 261 (1986); *Suppl. 7*, 321 (1987)
Polychlorinated biphenyls	7, 261 (1974); 18, 43 (1978) (*corr.* 42, 258); *Suppl. 7*, 322 (1987)
Polychlorinated camphenes (*see* Toxaphene)	
Polychlorinated dibenzo-*para*-dioxins (other than 2,3,7,8-tetrachlorodibenzodioxin)	69, 33 (1997)
Polychlorinated dibenzofurans	69, 345 (1997)
Polychlorophenols and their sodium salts	71, 769 (1999)
Polychloroprene	19, 141 (1979); *Suppl. 7*, 70 (1987)
Polyethylene (*see also* Implants, surgical)	19, 164 (1979); *Suppl. 7*, 70 (1987)
Poly(glycolic acid) (*see* Implants, surgical)	
Polymethylene polyphenyl isocyanate (*see also* 4,4′-Methylenediphenyl diisocyanate)	19, 314 (1979); *Suppl. 7*, 70 (1987)
Polymethyl methacrylate (*see also* Implants, surgical)	19, 195 (1979); *Suppl. 7*, 70 (1987)
Polyoestradiol phosphate (*see* Oestradiol-17β)	
Polypropylene (*see also* Implants, surgical)	19, 218 (1979); *Suppl. 7*, 70 (1987)
Polystyrene (*see also* Implants, surgical)	19, 245 (1979); *Suppl. 7*, 70 (1987)
Polytetrafluoroethylene (*see also* Implants, surgical)	19, 288 (1979); *Suppl. 7*, 70 (1987)
Polyurethane foams (*see also* Implants, surgical)	19, 320 (1979); *Suppl. 7*, 70 (1987)
Polyvinyl acetate (*see also* Implants, surgical)	19, 346 (1979); *Suppl. 7*, 70 (1987)
Polyvinyl alcohol (*see also* Implants, surgical)	19, 351 (1979); *Suppl. 7*, 70 (1987)
Polyvinyl chloride (*see also* Implants, surgical)	7, 306 (1974); 19, 402 (1979); *Suppl. 7*, 70 (1987)
Polyvinyl pyrrolidone	19, 463 (1979); *Suppl. 7*, 70 (1987); 71, 1181 (1999)
Ponceau MX	8, 189 (1975); *Suppl. 7*, 70 (1987)
Ponceau 3R	8, 199 (1975); *Suppl. 7*, 70 (1987)
Ponceau SX	8, 207 (1975); *Suppl. 7*, 70 (1987)
Post-menopausal oestrogen therapy	*Suppl. 7*, 280 (1987); 72, 399 (1999)
Post-menopausal oestrogen-progestogen therapy	*Suppl. 7*, 308 (1987); 72, 531 (1999)
Potassium arsenate (*see* Arsenic and arsenic compounds)	
Potassium arsenite (*see* Arsenic and arsenic compounds)	
Potassium bis(2-hydroxyethyl)dithiocarbamate	12, 183 (1976); *Suppl. 7*, 70 (1987)
Potassium bromate	40, 207 (1986); *Suppl. 7*, 70 (1987); 73, 481 (1999)
Potassium chromate (*see* Chromium and chromium compounds)	
Potassium dichromate (*see* Chromium and chromium compounds)	
Prazepam	66, 143 (1996)

Prednimustine	*50*, 115 (1990)
Prednisone	*26*, 293 (1981); *Suppl. 7*, 326 (1987)
Printing processes and printing inks	*65*, 33 (1996)
Procarbazine hydrochloride	*26*, 311 (1981); *Suppl. 7*, 327 (1987)
Proflavine salts	*24*, 195 (1980); *Suppl. 7*, 70 (1987)
Progesterone (*see also* Progestins; Combined oral contraceptives)	*6*, 135 (1974); *21*, 491 (1979) (*corr. 42*, 259)
Progestins (*see* Progestogens)	
Progestogens	*Suppl. 7*, 289 (1987); *72*, 49, 339, 531 (1999)
Pronetalol hydrochloride	*13*, 227 (1977) (*corr. 42*, 256); *Suppl. 7*, 70 (1987)
1,3-Propane sultone	*4*, 253 (1974) (*corr. 42*, 253); *Suppl. 7*, 70 (1987); *71*, 1095 (1999)
Propham	*12*, 189 (1976); *Suppl. 7*, 70 (1987)
β-Propiolactone	*4*, 259 (1974) (*corr. 42*, 253); *Suppl. 7*, 70 (1987); *71*, 1103 (1999)
n-Propyl carbamate	*12*, 201 (1976); *Suppl. 7*, 70 (1987)
Propylene	*19*, 213 (1979); *Suppl. 7*, 71 (1987); *60*, 161 (1994)
Propyleneimine (*see* 2-Methylaziridine)	
Propylene oxide	*11*, 191 (1976); *36*, 227 (1985) (*corr. 42*, 263); *Suppl. 7*, 328 (1987); *60*, 181 (1994)
Propylthiouracil	*7*, 67 (1974); *Suppl. 7*, 329 (1987)
Ptaquiloside (*see also* Bracken fern)	*40*, 55 (1986); *Suppl. 7*, 71 (1987)
Pulp and paper manufacture	*25*, 157 (1981); *Suppl. 7*, 385 (1987)
Pyrene	*32*, 431 (1983); *Suppl. 7*, 71 (1987)
Pyrido[3,4-*c*]psoralen	*40*, 349 (1986); *Suppl. 7*, 71 (1987)
Pyrimethamine	*13*, 233 (1977); *Suppl. 7*, 71 (1987)
Pyrrolizidine alkaloids (*see* Hydroxysenkirkine; Isatidine; Jacobine; Lasiocarpine; Monocrotaline; Retrorsine; Riddelliine; Seneciphylline; Senkirkine)	

Q

Quartz (*see* Crystalline silica)	
Quercetin (*see also* Bracken fern)	*31*, 213 (1983); *Suppl. 7*, 71 (1987); *73*, 497 (1999)
para-Quinone	*15*, 255 (1977); *Suppl. 7*, 71 (1987); *71*, 1245 (1999)
Quintozene	*5*, 211 (1974); *Suppl. 7*, 71 (1987)

R

Radon	*43*, 173 (1988) (*corr. 45*, 283)

Reserpine	10, 217 (1976); 24, 211 (1980) (corr. 42, 260); Suppl. 7, 330 (1987)
Resorcinol	15, 155 (1977); Suppl. 7, 71 (1987); 71, 1119 (1990)
Retrorsine	10, 303 (1976); Suppl. 7, 71 (1987)
Rhodamine B	16, 221 (1978); Suppl. 7, 71 (1987)
Rhodamine 6G	16, 233 (1978); Suppl. 7, 71 (1987)
Riddelliine	10, 313 (1976); Suppl. 7, 71 (1987)
Rifampicin	24, 243 (1980); Suppl. 7, 71 (1987)
Ripazepam	66, 157 (1996)
Rockwool (see Man-made mineral fibres)	
Rubber industry	28 (1982) (corr. 42, 261); Suppl. 7, 332 (1987)
Rugulosin	40, 99 (1986); Suppl. 7, 71 (1987)

S

Saccharated iron oxide	2, 161 (1973); Suppl. 7, 71 (1987)
Saccharin and its salts	22, 111 (1980) (corr. 42, 259); Suppl. 7, 334 (1987); 73, 517 (1999)
Safrole	1, 169 (1972); 10, 231 (1976); Suppl. 7, 71 (1987)
Salted fish	56, 41 (1993)
Sawmill industry (including logging) (see Lumber and sawmill industry (including logging))	
Scarlet Red	8, 217 (1975); Suppl. 7, 71 (1987)
Schistosoma haematobium (infection with)	61, 45 (1994)
Schistosoma japonicum (infection with)	61, 45 (1994)
Schistosoma mansoni (infection with)	61, 45 (1994)
Selenium and selenium compounds	9, 245 (1975) (corr. 42, 255); Suppl. 7, 71 (1987)
Selenium dioxide (see Selenium and selenium compounds)	
Selenium oxide (see Selenium and selenium compounds)	
Semicarbazide hydrochloride	12, 209 (1976) (corr. 42, 256); Suppl. 7, 71 (1987)
Senecio jacobaea L. (see also Pyrrolizidine alkaloids)	10, 333 (1976)
Senecio longilobus (see also Pyrrolizidine alkaloids)	10, 334 (1976)
Seneciphylline	10, 319, 335 (1976); Suppl. 7, 71 (1987)
Senkirkine	10, 327 (1976); 31, 231 (1983); Suppl. 7, 71 (1987)
Sepiolite	42, 175 (1987); Suppl. 7, 71 (1987); 68, 267 (1997)
Sequential oral contraceptives (see also Oestrogens, progestins and combinations)	Suppl. 7, 296 (1987)
Shale-oils	35, 161 (1985); Suppl. 7, 339 (1987)
Shikimic acid (see also Bracken fern)	40, 55 (1986); Suppl. 7, 71 (1987)
Shoe manufacture and repair (see Boot and shoe manufacture and repair)	
Silica (see also Amorphous silica; Crystalline silica)	42, 39 (1987)
Silicone (see Implants, surgical)	

Simazine	53, 495 (1991); 73, 625 (1999)
Slagwool (see Man-made mineral fibres)	
Sodium arsenate (see Arsenic and arsenic compounds)	
Sodium arsenite (see Arsenic and arsenic compounds)	
Sodium cacodylate (see Arsenic and arsenic compounds)	
Sodium chlorite	52, 145 (1991)
Sodium chromate (see Chromium and chromium compounds)	
Sodium cyclamate (see Cyclamates)	
Sodium dichromate (see Chromium and chromium compounds)	
Sodium diethyldithiocarbamate	12, 217 (1976); Suppl. 7, 71 (1987)
Sodium equilin sulfate (see Conjugated oestrogens)	
Sodium fluoride (see Fluorides)	
Sodium monofluorophosphate (see Fluorides)	
Sodium oestrone sulfate (see Conjugated oestrogens)	
Sodium *ortho*-phenylphenate (see also *ortho*-Phenylphenol)	30, 329 (1983); Suppl. 7, 392 (1987); 73, 451 (1999)
Sodium saccharin (see Saccharin)	
Sodium selenate (see Selenium and selenium compounds)	
Sodium selenite (see Selenium and selenium compounds)	
Sodium silicofluoride (see Fluorides)	
Solar radiation	55 (1992)
Soots	3, 22 (1973); 35, 219 (1985); Suppl. 7, 343 (1987)
Spironolactone	24, 259 (1980); Suppl. 7, 344 (1987)
Stannous fluoride (see Fluorides)	
Steel founding (see Iron and steel founding)	
Steel, stainless (see Implants, surgical)	
Sterigmatocystin	1, 175 (1972); 10, 245 (1976); Suppl. 7, 72 (1987)
Steroidal oestrogens	Suppl. 7, 280 (1987)
Streptozotocin	4, 221 (1974); 17, 337 (1978); Suppl. 7, 72 (1987)
Strobane® (see Terpene polychlorinates)	
Strong-inorganic-acid mists containing sulfuric acid (see Mists and vapours from sulfuric acid and other strong inorganic acids)	
Strontium chromate (see Chromium and chromium compounds)	
Styrene	19, 231 (1979) (corr. 42, 258); Suppl. 7, 345 (1987); 60, 233 (1994) (corr. 65, 549)
Styrene-acrylonitrile-copolymers	19, 97 (1979); Suppl. 7, 72 (1987)
Styrene-butadiene copolymers	19, 252 (1979); Suppl. 7, 72 (1987)
Styrene-7,8-oxide	11, 201 (1976); 19, 275 (1979); 36, 245 (1985); Suppl. 7, 72 (1987); 60, 321 (1994)
Succinic anhydride	15, 265 (1977); Suppl. 7, 72 (1987)
Sudan I	8, 225 (1975); Suppl. 7, 72 (1987)
Sudan II	8, 233 (1975); Suppl. 7, 72 (1987)
Sudan III	8, 241 (1975); Suppl. 7, 72 (1987)
Sudan Brown RR	8, 249 (1975); Suppl. 7, 72 (1987)
Sudan Red 7B	8, 253 (1975); Suppl. 7, 72 (1987)
Sulfafurazole	24, 275 (1980); Suppl. 7, 347 (1987)
Sulfallate	30, 283 (1983); Suppl. 7, 72 (1987)

Sulfamethoxazole	*24*, 285 (1980); *Suppl. 7*, 348 (1987)
Sulfites (*see* Sulfur dioxide and some sulfites, bisulfites and metabisulfites)	
Sulfur dioxide and some sulfites, bisulfites and metabisulfites	*54*, 131 (1992)
Sulfur mustard (*see* Mustard gas)	
Sulfuric acid and other strong inorganic acids, occupational exposures to mists and vapours from	*54*, 41 (1992)
Sulfur trioxide	*54*, 121 (1992)
Sulphisoxazole (*see* Sulfafurazole)	
Sunset Yellow FCF	*8*, 257 (1975); *Suppl. 7*, 72 (1987)
Symphytine	*31*, 239 (1983); *Suppl. 7*, 72 (1987)

T

2,4,5-T (*see also* Chlorophenoxy herbicides; Chlorophenoxy herbicides, occupational exposures to)	*15*, 273 (1977)
Talc	*42*, 185 (1987); *Suppl. 7*, 349 (1987)
Tamoxifen	*66*, 253 (1996)
Tannic acid	*10*, 253 (1976) (*corr. 42*, 255); *Suppl. 7*, 72 (1987)
Tannins (*see also* Tannic acid)	*10*, 254 (1976); *Suppl. 7*, 72 (1987)
TCDD (*see* 2,3,7,8-Tetrachlorodibenzo-*para*-dioxin)	
TDE (*see* DDT)	
Tea	*51*, 207 (1991)
Temazepam	*66*, 161 (1996)
Terpene polychlorinates	*5*, 219 (1974); *Suppl. 7*, 72 (1987)
Testosterone (*see also* Androgenic (anabolic) steroids)	*6*, 209 (1974); *21*, 519 (1979)
Testosterone oenanthate (*see* Testosterone)	
Testosterone propionate (*see* Testosterone)	
2,2′,5,5′-Tetrachlorobenzidine	*27*, 141 (1982); *Suppl. 7*, 72 (1987)
2,3,7,8-Tetrachlorodibenzo-*para*-dioxin	*15*, 41 (1977); *Suppl. 7*, 350 (1987); *69*, 33 (1997)
1,1,1,2-Tetrachloroethane	*41*, 87 (1986); *Suppl. 7*, 72 (1987); *71*, 1133 (1999)
1,1,2,2-Tetrachloroethane	*20*, 477 (1979); *Suppl. 7*, 354 (1987); *71*, 817 (1999)
Tetrachloroethylene	*20*, 491 (1979); *Suppl. 7*, 355 (1987); *63*, 159 (1995) (*corr. 65*, 549)
2,3,4,6-Tetrachlorophenol (*see* Chlorophenols; Chlorophenols, occupational exposures to; Polychlorophenols and their sodium salts)	
Tetrachlorvinphos	*30*, 197 (1983); *Suppl. 7*, 72 (1987)
Tetraethyllead (*see* Lead and lead compounds)	
Tetrafluoroethylene	*19*, 285 (1979); *Suppl. 7*, 72 (1987); *71*, 1143 (1999)
Tetrakis(hydroxymethyl)phosphonium salts	*48*, 95 (1990); *71*, 1529 (1999)
Tetramethyllead (*see* Lead and lead compounds)	
Tetranitromethane	*65*, 437 (1996)
Textile manufacturing industry, exposures in	*48*, 215 (1990) (*corr. 51*, 483)
Theobromine	*51*, 421 (1991)
Theophylline	*51*, 391 (1991)
Thioacetamide	*7*, 77 (1974); *Suppl. 7*, 72 (1987)

4,4'-Thiodianiline	*16*, 343 (1978); *27*, 147 (1982); Suppl. *7*, 72 (1987)
Thiotepa	*9*, 85 (1975); Suppl. *7*, 368 (1987); *50*, 123 (1990)
Thiouracil	*7*, 85 (1974); Suppl. *7*, 72 (1987)
Thiourea	*7*, 95 (1974); Suppl. *7*, 72 (1987)
Thiram	*12*, 225 (1976); Suppl. *7*, 72 (1987); *53*, 403 (1991)
Titanium (*see* Implants, surgical)	
Titanium dioxide	*47*, 307 (1989)
Tobacco habits other than smoking (*see* Tobacco products, smokeless)	
Tobacco products, smokeless	*37* (1985) (*corr. 42*, 263; *52*, 513); Suppl. *7*, 357 (1987)
Tobacco smoke	*38* (1986) (*corr. 42*, 263); Suppl. *7*, 359 (1987)
Tobacco smoking (*see* Tobacco smoke)	
ortho-Tolidine (*see* 3,3'-Dimethylbenzidine)	
2,4-Toluene diisocyanate (*see also* Toluene diisocyanates)	*19*, 303 (1979); *39*, 287 (1986)
2,6-Toluene diisocyanate (*see also* Toluene diisocyanates)	*19*, 303 (1979); *39*, 289 (1986)
Toluene	*47*, 79 (1989); *71*, 829 (1999)
Toluene diisocyanates	*39*, 287 (1986) (*corr. 42*, 264); Suppl. *7*, 72 (1987); *71*, 865 (1999)
Toluenes, α-chlorinated (*see* α-Chlorinated toluenes and benzoyl chloride)	
ortho-Toluenesulfonamide (*see* Saccharin)	
ortho-Toluidine	*16*, 349 (1978); *27*, 155 (1982) (*corr. 68*, 477); Suppl. *7*, 362 (1987)
Toremifene	*66*, 367 (1996)
Toxaphene	*20*, 327 (1979); Suppl. *7*, 72 (1987)
T-2 Toxin (*see* Toxins derived from *Fusarium sporotrichioides*)	
Toxins derived from *Fusarium graminearum*, *F. culmorum* and *F. crookwellense*	*11*, 169 (1976); *31*, 153, 279 (1983); Suppl. *7*, 64, 74 (1987); *56*, 397 (1993)
Toxins derived from *Fusarium moniliforme*	*56*, 445 (1993)
Toxins derived from *Fusarium sporotrichioides*	*31*, 265 (1983); Suppl. *7*, 73 (1987); *56*, 467 (1993)
Tremolite (*see* Asbestos)	
Treosulfan	*26*, 341 (1981); Suppl. *7*, 363 (1987)
Triaziquone (*see* Tris(aziridinyl)-*para*-benzoquinone)	
Trichlorfon	*30*, 207 (1983); Suppl. *7*, 73 (1987)
Trichlormethine	*9*, 229 (1975); Suppl. *7*, 73 (1987); *50*, 143 (1990)
Trichloroacetic acid	*63*, 291 (1995) (*corr. 65*, 549)
Trichloroacetonitrile (*see also* Halogenated acetonitriles)	*71*, 1533 (1999)
1,1,1-Trichloroethane	*20*, 515 (1979); Suppl. *7*, 73 (1987); *71*, 881 (1999)
1,1,2-Trichloroethane	*20*, 533 (1979); Suppl. *7*, 73 (1987); *52*, 337 (1991); *71*, 1153 (1999)
Trichloroethylene	*11*, 263 (1976); *20*, 545 (1979); Suppl. *7*, 364 (1987); *63*, 75 (1995) (*corr. 65*, 549)

2,4,5-Trichlorophenol (*see also* Chlorophenols; Chlorophenols occupational exposures to; Polychlorophenols and their sodium salts)	*20*, 349 (1979)
2,4,6-Trichlorophenol (*see also* Chlorophenols; Chlorophenols, occupational exposures to; Polychlorophenols and their sodium salts)	*20*, 349 (1979)
(2,4,5-Trichlorophenoxy)acetic acid (*see* 2,4,5-T)	
1,2,3-Trichloropropane	*63*, 223 (1995)
Trichlorotriethylamine-hydrochloride (*see* Trichlormethine)	
T$_2$-Trichothecene (*see* Toxins derived from *Fusarium sporotrichioides*)	
Tridymite (*see* Crystalline silica)	
Triethylene glycol diglycidyl ether	*11*, 209 (1976); *Suppl. 7*, 73 (1987); *71*, 1539 (1999)
Trifluralin	*53*, 515 (1991)
4,4',6-Trimethylangelicin plus ultraviolet radiation (*see also* Angelicin and some synthetic derivatives)	*Suppl. 7*, 57 (1987)
2,4,5-Trimethylaniline	*27*, 177 (1982); *Suppl. 7*, 73 (1987)
2,4,6-Trimethylaniline	*27*, 178 (1982); *Suppl. 7*, 73 (1987)
4,5',8-Trimethylpsoralen	*40*, 357 (1986); *Suppl. 7*, 366 (1987)
Trimustine hydrochloride (*see* Trichlormethine)	
2,4,6-Trinitrotoluene	*65*, 449 (1996)
Triphenylene	*32*, 447 (1983); *Suppl. 7*, 73 (1987)
Tris(aziridinyl)-*para*-benzoquinone	*9*, 67 (1975); *Suppl. 7*, 367 (1987)
Tris(1-aziridinyl)phosphine-oxide	*9*, 75 (1975); *Suppl. 7*, 73 (1987)
Tris(1-aziridinyl)phosphine-sulphide (*see* Thiotepa)	
2,4,6-Tris(1-aziridinyl)-*s*-triazine	*9*, 95 (1975); *Suppl. 7*, 73 (1987)
Tris(2-chloroethyl) phosphate	*48*, 109 (1990); *71*, 1543 (1999)
1,2,3-Tris(chloromethoxy)propane	*15*, 301 (1977); *Suppl. 7*, 73 (1987); *71*, 1549 (1999)
Tris(2,3-dibromopropyl) phosphate	*20*, 575 (1979); *Suppl. 7*, 369 (1987); *71*, 905 (1999)
Tris(2-methyl-1-aziridinyl)phosphine-oxide	*9*, 107 (1975); *Suppl. 7*, 73 (1987)
Trp-P-1	*31*, 247 (1983); *Suppl. 7*, 73 (1987)
Trp-P-2	*31*, 255 (1983); *Suppl. 7*, 73 (1987)
Trypan blue	*8*, 267 (1975); *Suppl. 7*, 73 (1987)
Tussilago farfara L. (*see also* Pyrrolizidine alkaloids)	*10*, 334 (1976)

U

Ultraviolet radiation	*40*, 379 (1986); *55* (1992)
Underground haematite mining with exposure to radon	*1*, 29 (1972); *Suppl. 7*, 216 (1987)
Uracil mustard	*9*, 235 (1975); *Suppl. 7*, 370 (1987)
Uranium, depleted (*see* Implants, surgical)	
Urethane	*7*, 111 (1974); *Suppl. 7*, 73 (1987)

V

Vat Yellow 4	*48*, 161 (1990)
Vinblastine sulfate	*26*, 349 (1981) (*corr. 42*, 261); *Suppl. 7*, 371 (1987)
Vincristine sulfate	*26*, 365 (1981); *Suppl. 7*, 372 (1987)

Vinyl acetate	*19*, 341 (1979); *39*, 113 (1986); *Suppl. 7*, 73 (1987); *63*, 443 (1995)
Vinyl bromide	*19*, 367 (1979); *39*, 133 (1986); *Suppl. 7*, 73 (1987); *71*, 923 (1999)
Vinyl chloride	*7*, 291 (1974); *19*, 377 (1979) (*corr. 42*, 258); *Suppl. 7*, 373 (1987)
Vinyl chloride-vinyl acetate copolymers	*7*, 311 (1976); *19*, 412 (1979) (*corr. 42*, 258); *Suppl. 7*, 73 (1987)
4-Vinylcyclohexene	*11*, 277 (1976); *39*, 181 (1986) *Suppl. 7*, 73 (1987); *60*, 347 (1994)
4-Vinylcyclohexene diepoxide	*11*, 141 (1976); *Suppl. 7*, 63 (1987); *60*, 361 (1994)
Vinyl fluoride	*39*, 147 (1986); *Suppl. 7*, 73 (1987); *63*, 467 (1995)
Vinylidene chloride	*19*, 439 (1979); *39*, 195 (1986); *Suppl. 7*, 376 (1987); *71*, 1163 (1999)
Vinylidene chloride-vinyl chloride copolymers	*19*, 448 (1979) (*corr. 42*, 258); *Suppl. 7*, 73 (1987)
Vinylidene fluoride	*39*, 227 (1986); *Suppl. 7*, 73 (1987); *71*, 1551 (1999)
N-Vinyl-2-pyrrolidone	*19*, 461 (1979); *Suppl. 7*, 73 (1987); *71*, 1181 (1999)
Vinyl toluene	*60*, 373 (1994)

W

Welding	*49*, 447 (1990) (*corr. 52*, 513)
Wollastonite	*42*, 145 (1987); *Suppl. 7*, 377 (1987); *68*, 283 (1997)
Wood dust	*62*, 35 (1995)
Wood industries	*25* (1981); *Suppl. 7*, 378 (1987)

X

Xylenes	*47*, 125 (1989); *71*, 1189 (1999)
2,4-Xylidine	*16*, 367 (1978); *Suppl. 7*, 74 (1987)
2,5-Xylidine	*16*, 377 (1978); *Suppl. 7*, 74 (1987)
2,6-Xylidine (*see* 2,6-Dimethylaniline)	

Y

Yellow AB	*8*, 279 (1975); *Suppl. 7*, 74 (1987)
Yellow OB	*8*, 287 (1975); *Suppl. 7*, 74 (1987)

Z

Zearalenone (*see* Toxins derived from *Fusarium graminearum*, *F. culmorum* and *F. crookwellense*)

Zectran	*12*, 237 (1976); *Suppl. 7*, 74 (1987)
Zeolites other than erionite	*68*, 307 (1997)
Zinc beryllium silicate (*see* Beryllium and beryllium compounds)	
Zinc chromate (*see* Chromium and chromium compounds)	
Zinc chromate hydroxide (*see* Chromium and chromium compounds)	
Zinc potassium chromate (*see* Chromium and chromium compounds)	
Zinc yellow (*see* Chromium and chromium compounds)	
Zineb	*12*, 245 (1976); *Suppl. 7*, 74 (1987)
Ziram	*12*, 259 (1976); *Suppl. 7*, 74 (1987); *53, 423* (1991)

List of IARC Monographs on the Evaluation of Carcinogenic Risks to Humans*

Volume 1
Some Inorganic Substances, Chlorinated Hydrocarbons, Aromatic Amines, N-Nitroso Compounds, and Natural Products
1972; 184 pages (out-of-print)

Volume 2
Some Inorganic and Organometallic Compounds
1973; 181 pages (out-of-print)

Volume 3
Certain Polycyclic Aromatic Hydrocarbons and Heterocyclic Compounds
1973; 271 pages (out-of-print)

Volume 4
Some Aromatic Amines, Hydrazine and Related Substances, N-Nitroso Compounds and Miscellaneous Alkylating Agents
1974; 286 pages (out-of-print)

Volume 5
Some Organochlorine Pesticides
1974; 241 pages (out-of-print)

Volume 6
Sex Hormones
1974; 243 pages (out-of-print)

Volume 7
Some Anti-Thyroid and Related Substances, Nitrofurans and Industrial Chemicals
1974; 326 pages (out-of-print)

Volume 8
Some Aromatic Azo Compounds
1975; 357 pages

Volume 9
Some Aziridines, N-, S- and O-Mustards and Selenium
1975; 268 pages

Volume 10
Some Naturally Occurring Substances
1976; 353 pages (out-of-print)

Volume 11
Cadmium, Nickel, Some Epoxides, Miscellaneous Industrial Chemicals and General Considerations on Volatile Anaesthetics
1976; 306 pages (out-of-print)

Volume 12
Some Carbamates, Thiocarbamates and Carbazides
1976; 282 pages (out-of-print)

Volume 13
Some Miscellaneous Pharmaceutical Substances
1977; 255 pages

Volume 14
Asbestos
1977; 106 pages (out-of-print)

Volume 15
Some Fumigants, the Herbicides 2,4-D and 2,4,5-T, Chlorinated Dibenzodioxins and Miscellaneous Industrial Chemicals
1977; 354 pages (out-of-print)

Volume 16
Some Aromatic Amines and Related Nitro Compounds—Hair Dyes, Colouring Agents and Miscellaneous Industrial Chemicals
1978; 400 pages

Volume 17
Some N-Nitroso Compounds
1978; 365 pages

Volume 18
Polychlorinated Biphenyls and Polybrominated Biphenyls
1978; 140 pages (out-of-print)

Volume 19
Some Monomers, Plastics and Synthetic Elastomers, and Acrolein
1979; 513 pages (out-of-print)

Volume 20
Some Halogenated Hydrocarbons
1979; 609 pages (out-of-print)

Volume 21
Sex Hormones (II)
1979; 583 pages

Volume 22
Some Non-Nutritive Sweetening Agents
1980; 208 pages

Volume 23
Some Metals and Metallic Compounds
1980; 438 pages (out-of-print)

Volume 24
Some Pharmaceutical Drugs
1980; 337 pages

Volume 25
Wood, Leather and Some Associated Industries
1981; 412 pages

Volume 26
Some Antineoplastic and Immunosuppressive Agents
1981; 411 pages

Volume 27
Some Aromatic Amines, Anthraquinones and Nitroso Compounds, and Inorganic Fluorides Used in Drinking-water and Dental Preparations
1982; 341 pages

Volume 28
The Rubber Industry
1982; 486 pages

Volume 29
Some Industrial Chemicals and Dyestuffs
1982; 416 pages

Volume 30
Miscellaneous Pesticides
1983; 424 pages

---

*Certain older volumes, marked out-of-print, are still available directly from IARCPress. Further, high-quality photocopies of all out-of-print volumes may be purchased from University Microfilms International, 300 North Zeeb Road, Ann Arbor, MI 48106-1346, USA (Tel.: 313-761-4700, 800-521-0600).

Volume 31
Some Food Additives, Feed Additives and Naturally Occurring Substances
1983; 314 pages (out-of-print)

Volume 32
Polynuclear Aromatic Compounds, Part 1: Chemical, Environmental and Experimental Data
1983; 477 pages (out-of-print)

Volume 33
Polynuclear Aromatic Compounds, Part 2: Carbon Blacks, Mineral Oils and Some Nitroarenes
1984; 245 pages (out-of-print)

Volume 34
Polynuclear Aromatic Compounds, Part 3: Industrial Exposures in Aluminium Production, Coal Gasification, Coke Production, and Iron and Steel Founding
1984; 219 pages

Volume 35
Polynuclear Aromatic Compounds, Part 4: Bitumens, Coal-tars and Derived Products, Shale-oils and Soots
1985; 271 pages

Volume 36
Allyl Compounds, Aldehydes, Epoxides and Peroxides
1985; 369 pages

Volume 37
Tobacco Habits Other than Smoking; Betel-Quid and Areca-Nut Chewing; and Some Related Nitrosamines
1985; 291 pages

Volume 38
Tobacco Smoking
1986; 421 pages

Volume 39
Some Chemicals Used in Plastics and Elastomers
1986; 403 pages

Volume 40
Some Naturally Occurring and Synthetic Food Components, Furocoumarins and Ultraviolet Radiation
1986; 444 pages

Volume 41
Some Halogenated Hydrocarbons and Pesticide Exposures
1986; 434 pages

Volume 42
Silica and Some Silicates
1987; 289 pages

Volume 43
Man-Made Mineral Fibres and Radon
1988; 300 pages

Volume 44
Alcohol Drinking
1988; 416 pages

Volume 45
Occupational Exposures in Petroleum Refining; Crude Oil and Major Petroleum Fuels
1989; 322 pages

Volume 46
Diesel and Gasoline Engine Exhausts and Some Nitroarenes
1989; 458 pages

Volume 47
Some Organic Solvents, Resin Monomers and Related Compounds, Pigments and Occupational Exposures in Paint Manufacture and Painting
1989; 535 pages

Volume 48
Some Flame Retardants and Textile Chemicals, and Exposures in the Textile Manufacturing Industry
1990; 345 pages

Volume 49
Chromium, Nickel and Welding
1990; 677 pages

Volume 50
Pharmaceutical Drugs
1990; 415 pages

Volume 51
Coffee, Tea, Mate, Methyl-xanthines and Methylglyoxal
1991; 513 pages

Volume 52
Chlorinated Drinking-water; Chlorination By-products; Some Other Halogenated Compounds; Cobalt and Cobalt Compounds
1991; 544 pages

Volume 53
Occupational Exposures in Insecticide Application, and Some Pesticides
1991; 612 pages

Volume 54
Occupational Exposures to Mists and Vapours from Strong Inorganic Acids; and Other Industrial Chemicals
1992; 336 pages

Volume 55
Solar and Ultraviolet Radiation
1992; 316 pages

Volume 56
Some Naturally Occurring Substances: Food Items and Constituents, Heterocyclic Aromatic Amines and Mycotoxins
1993; 599 pages

Volume 57
Occupational Exposures of Hairdressers and Barbers and Personal Use of Hair Colourants; Some Hair Dyes, Cosmetic Colourants, Industrial Dyestuffs and Aromatic Amines
1993; 428 pages

Volume 58
Beryllium, Cadmium, Mercury, and Exposures in the Glass Manufacturing Industry
1993; 444 pages

Volume 59
Hepatitis Viruses
1994; 286 pages

Volume 60
Some Industrial Chemicals
1994; 560 pages

Volume 61
Schistosomes, Liver Flukes and *Helicobacter pylori*
1994; 270 pages

Volume 62
Wood Dust and Formaldehyde
1995; 405 pages

Volume 63
Dry Cleaning, Some Chlorinated Solvents and Other Industrial Chemicals
1995; 551 pages

Volume 64
Human Papillomaviruses
1995; 409 pages

Volume 65
Printing Processes and Printing Inks, Carbon Black and Some Nitro Compounds
1996; 578 pages

Volume 66
Some Pharmaceutical Drugs
1996; 514 pages

Volume 67
Human Immunodeficiency Viruses and Human T-Cell Lymphotropic Viruses
1996; 424 pages

Volume 68
Silica, Some Silicates, Coal Dust and *para*-Aramid Fibrils
1997; 506 pages

Volume 69
Polychlorinated Dibenzo-*para*-Dioxins and Polychlorinated Dibenzofurans
1997; 666 pages

Volume 70
Epstein-Barr Virus and Kaposi's Sarcoma Herpesvirus/Human Herpesvirus 8
1997; 524 pages

Volume 71
Re-evaluation of Some Organic Chemicals, Hydrazine and Hydrogen Peroxide
1999; 1586 pages

Volume 72
Hormonal Contraception and Post-menopausal Hormonal Therapy
1999; 660 pages

Volume 73
Some Chemicals that Cause Tumours of the Kidney or Urinary Bladder in Rodents and Some Other Substances
1999; 674 pages

Volume 74
Surgical Implants and Other Foreign Bodies
1999; 409 pages

Supplement No. 1
Chemicals and Industrial Processes Associated with Cancer in Humans (*IARC Monographs*, Volumes 1 to 20)
1979; 71 pages (out-of-print)

Supplement No. 2
Long-term and Short-term Screening Assays for Carcinogens: A Critical Appraisal
1980; 426 pages (out-of-print)

Supplement No. 3
Cross Index of Synonyms and Trade Names in Volumes 1 to 26 of the *IARC Monographs*
1982; 199 pages (out-of-print)

Supplement No. 4
Chemicals, Industrial Processes and Industries Associated with Cancer in Humans (*IARC Monographs*, Volumes 1 to 29)
1982; 292 pages (out-of-print)

Supplement No. 5
Cross Index of Synonyms and Trade Names in Volumes 1 to 36 of the *IARC Monographs*
1985; 259 pages (out-of-print)

Supplement No. 6
Genetic and Related Effects: An Updating of Selected *IARC Monographs* from Volumes 1 to 42
1987; 729 pages

Supplement No. 7
Overall Evaluations of Carcinogenicity: An Updating of *IARC Monographs* Volumes 1–42
1987; 440 pages

Supplement No. 8
Cross Index of Synonyms and Trade Names in Volumes 1 to 46 of the *IARC Monographs*
1990; 346 pages (out-of-print)

All IARC publications are available directly from
IARCPress, 150 Cours Albert Thomas, F-69372 Lyon cedex 08, France
(Fax: +33 4 72 73 83 02; E-mail: press@iarc.fr).

IARC Monographs and Technical Reports are also available from the
World Health Organization Distribution and Sales, CH-1211 Geneva 27
(Fax: +41 22 791 4857; E-mail: publications@who.int)
and from WHO Sales Agents worldwide.

IARC Scientific Publications, IARC Handbooks and IARC CancerBases are also available from
Oxford University Press, Walton Street, Oxford, UK OX2 6DP (Fax: +44 1865 267782).

www.ingramcontent.com/pod-product-compliance
Ingram Content Group UK Ltd.
Pitfield, Milton Keynes, MK11 3LW, UK
UKHW051258180426
11947UKWH00020B/1778